STEM CELLS IN HUMAN REPRODUCTION

STEM CELLS IN HUMAN REPRODUCTION

Basic Science and Therapeutic Potential

Editors

Carlos Simón MD PhD **and Antonio Pellicer** MD PhD

Instituto Valenciano de Infertilidad

Valencia University Centro de Investigación, Prince Felipe

Valencia, Spain

informa
healthcare

First published in the United Kingdom in 2007 by Informa Healthcare, 4 Park Square, Milton Park, Abingdon, Oxon OX14 4RN. Informa Healthcare is a trading division of Informa UK Ltd. Registered Office: 37/41 Mortimer Street, London W1T 3JH. Registered in England and Wales number 1072954.

Tel: +44 (0)20 7017 6000
Fax: +44 (0)20 7017 6699
Email: info.medicine@tandf.co.uk
Website: www.informahealthcare.com

A CIP record for this book is available from the British Library.
Library of Congress Cataloging-in-Publication Data

Data available on application

ISBN-10: 0 415 39777 4
ISBN-13: 978 0 415 39777 3

Distributed in North and South America by
Taylor & Francis
6000 Broken Sound Parkway, NW, (Suite 300)
Boca Raton, FL 33487, USA

Within Continental USA
Tel: 1 (800) 272 7737; Fax: 1 (800) 374 3401
Outside Continental USA
Tel: (561) 994 0555; Fax: (561) 361 6018
Email: orders@crcpress.com

Distributed in the rest of the world by
Thomson Publishing Services
Cheriton House
North Way
Andover, Hampshire SP10 5BE, UK
Tel: +44 (0)1264 332424
Email: tps.tandfsalesorder@thomson.com

Composition by Exeter Premedia Services Private Ltd., Chennai, India
Printed and bound in Great Britain by Antony Rowe Ltd., Chippenham, Wiltshire

Contents

Contributors

Begoña Aran PhD
Senior Embryologist
Servei de Medicina de la Reproducció
Institut Universitari Dexeus
Barcelona, Spain

Juan Carlos Izpisua Belmonte PhD
Professor
Gene Expression Laboratory
Salk Institute for Biological Studies
La Jolla, CA, USA
and
Centre de Medicina Regenerativa de Barcelona
Barcelona, Spain

Antonin Bukovsky MD PhD DSC
Professor of Obstetrics & Gynecology
Director, Laboratory of Development, Differentiation and Cancer
Department of Obstetrics & Gynecology
the University of Tennessee Graduate School of Medicine
Knoxville, TN, USA

Maria Vicenta Camarasa PhD
Banc de Linies Cel.lulars de Barcelona
Centre de Medicina Regenerativa de Barcelona
Barcelona, Spain

Keith HS Campbell Bsc DPhil
Professor of Animal Development
School of Biosciences
University of Nottingham
Sutton Bonington
Loughborough, Leics, UK

Hsu-Hsin Chen PhD
Harvard Stem Cell Institute
Massachusetts General Hospital – Center for Regenerative Medicine
Boston, MA, USA

Amparo Galán
Banco de Líneas Celulares
Centro de Investigación Príncipe Felipe (CIPF)
Valencia, Spain

Caroline E Gargett BAPPLSCI MAPPLSCI PhD
Senior Research Officer [NHMRC]
Senior Scientist
Centre for Women's Health Research
Monash Institute of Medical Research
Monash University Department of Obstetrics and Gynaecology
Monash Medical Centre
Clayton, Victoria
Australia

Niels Geijsen PhD
Assistant Professor of Medicine
Harvard Medical School
Harvard Stem Cell Institute
Massachusetts General Hospital – Center for Regenerative Medicine
Boston, MA, USA

Olga Genbacev PhD
Professor
Department of Cell and Tissue Biology
University of California San Francisco
San Francisco, CA, USA

Behzad Gerami-Naini
National Primate Research Center and Department of Obstetrics & Gynecology
University of Wisconsin School of Medicine and Public Health
University of Wisconsin-Madison
Madison, WI, USA

Thaddeus G Golos
National Primate Research Center and Department of Obstetrics & Gynecology
University of Wisconsin School of Medicine and Public Health
University of Wisconsin-Madison
Madison, WI, USA

Ellen Goossens PhD
Post-doctoral Researcher
Center for Reproductive Medicine
AZ-Vrije Universiteit Brussels
Brussels, Belgium

Vanessa Jane Hall PhD
Post-Doctoral Research Fellow
Neuronal Survival Unit
Department of Experimental Medical Science
Wallenberg Neuroscience Centre
Department of Physiological Sciences
Lund University
Lund, Sweden

Joshua Johnson PhD
Department of Obstetrics, Gynecology and Reproductive Sciences
Yale University School of Medicine
New Haven, CT, USA

Irina Klimanskaya PhD
Director of Stem Cell Biology
Advanced Cell Technology Inc.
Worcester, MA, USA

Ana Krtolica PhD
Chief Scientific Officer
StemLifeLine Inc
San Carlos, CA
and
Lawrence Berkeley National Laboratory
Berkeley, CA, USA

Emin Maltepe MD PhD
Departments of Cell and Tissue Biology and Pediatrics
University of California San Francisco
San Francisco, CA, USA

Queenie V Neri BSC
Research Associate
The Center for Reproductive Medicine and Infertility
Weill Medical College of Cornell University
New York, NY, USA

Gianpiero D Palermo MD PhD
Director of Andrology and Assisted Fertilization
The Center for Reproductive Medicine and Infertility
Weill Medical College of Cornell University
New York, NY, USA

Antonio Pellicer MD PhD
Dean of the School of Medicine
Valencia University Professor and Director
Instituto Valenciano de Infertilidad & Hospital Peset
Valencia, Spain

Ivan Araujo Penna MD MS
Postdoctoral Associate
Division of Reproductive Endocrinology and Infertility
Department of Obstetrics, Gynecology and Reproductive Sciences
Yale University School of Medicine
New Haven, CT, USA

Angel Raya MD PhD
ICREA Research Professor
Centre de Medicina Regenerativa de Barcelona
Barcelona, Spain

Paolo F Rinaudo MD PhD
Department of Obstetrics and Gynecology
University of California San Francisco
San Francisco, CA, USA

Mónica Romeu
Fundacion Instituto Valenciano de Infertilidad (IVI)
University of Valencia, Spain

Lisa Salvador PhD
Post-doctoral Fellow
Center for Research in Women's Health and Reproduction
University of Pennsylvania, Philadelphia, PA, USA

Emre Seli MD
Assistant Professor
Division of Reproductive Endocrinology and Infertility
Department of Obstetrics, Gynecology and Reproductive Sciences
Yale University School of Medicine
New Haven, CT, USA

Celso Silva MD
Senior Fellow
Division of Reproductive Endocrinology & Infertility
Department of Obstetrics & Gynecology,
University of Pennsylvania,
Philadelphia, PA and Center for Research in Women's Health and Reproduction
University of Pennsylvania, Philadelphia, PA, USA

Carlos Simón MD PhD
Associate Professor Valencia University
Scientific Director of IVI
Director of Stem Cell Bank CIPF
Valencia, Spain

Miodrag Stojkovic PhD
Deputy Director and Professor of Embryology and Stem Cell Biology
Cellular Reprogramming Principe Felipe
Centro de Investigación, Valencia, Spain

Jerome F Strauss III MD PhD
Dean & Executive Vice President for Medical Affairs
Virginia Commonwealth University School of Medicine and Health System
Richmond, VA, USA

Takumi Takeuchi MD PhD
Assistant Research Professor
The Center for Reproductive Medicine and Infertility
Weill Medical College of Cornell University
New York, NY, USA

Noriko Tanaka
The Center for Reproductive Medicine and Infertility
Weill Medical College of Cornell University
New York, NY, USA

Hugh S Taylor MD
Associate Professor and Associate Director of Reproductive Endocrinology and Infertility
Division of Reproductive Endocrinology and Infertility
Department of Obstetrics, Gynecology and Reproductive Sciences
Yale University School of Medicine
New Haven, CT, USA

Herman Tournaye MD PhD
Center for Reproductive Medicine
AZ-Vrije Universiteit Brussels
Brussels, Belgium

Anna Veiga PhD
Banc de Linies Cel.lulars de Barcelona
Centre de Medicina Regenerativa de Barcelona
Servei de Medicina de la Reproducció
USP Institut Universitari Dexeus
Barcelona, Spain

Irma Virant-Klun PhD
Assistant Professor
Directory of IVF Laboratory
Department of Obstetrics and Gynecology
University of Ljubljana Medical Center
Ljubljana
Slovenia

Danielle Vitiello MD PhD
Department of Obstetrics, Gynecology and Reproductive Sciences
Yale University School of Medicine
New Haven, CT, USA

Preface

The stem cell field owes much to developmental work by embryologists and researchers in reproductive medicine. This emerging field offers new avenues of understanding gametogenesis and early embryonic development to reproductive sciences. In mammals, primordial germ cells set aside during early embryonic development give rise to the production of male and female gametes. Once the sperm enters the egg, the two pronuclei become enveloped, fuse and begin the zygote's mitotic cycle. The earliest developmental events are regulated by maternally inherited mRNA, whereas genomic activation occurs at the 6- to 8-cell stage in humans. From the preimplantation embryo, at the morula or blastocyst stage or even from totipotent blastomeres, derivation of embryonic stem cells (ESCs) can be achieved. The possibility of accomplishing the differentiation of gametes from ESCs and/or from progenitor stem cells (PSCs) present in the gonads or other organs will complete this enigmatic 'circle of life'.

Stem Cells in Reproductive-Medicine, Basic Science and Therapeutic Potential is the first book to address the revolutionary advances in stem cell science that may potentially impact human reproductive medicine. Junior and senior leaders in the field have been invited to present their work. The first chapter covers the molecular biology of the gametes in an attempt to prepare the scientific framework that must be in place when differentiation of gametes is attempted. Section I covers the differentiation to the female gamete from ESCs of mouse and human origin, as well as insights into the progenitor stem cell (PSC) population in the rodent and human ovaries. Section II describes the differentiation of the male gamete from the mouse ESC and the search for the PSC population in the testis. In Section III, research on the differentiation of trophoblasts from human ESCs (hESCs) and the continuing search for the stem cell niche in other reproductive organs, such as the human endometrium, is presented. To understand these new achievements, it is important to pay attention to the new developments in hESC derivation and maintenance that are presented in Section IV. The selection of embryos for stem cell derivation, the use of embryo-friendly approaches that would offer a source of hESCs without causing the destruction of the human embryo, the culture in feeder-free, xeno-free conditions for their future therapeutic use, the role of polarization and the effect of oxygen on stem cell derivation and fate are carefully considered. Finally, Section V discusses the state-of-the-art of technologies such as reprogramming and nuclear transfer in relation to reproductive medicine. Although we are still a long way off for therapeutic applications, an attempt to hypothesize the potential clinical applications has been made by those authors.

We are fully aware that the novel and promising data presented in this book at the current state of the science will need more time and effort to be confirmed, sedimented and translated to the clinic. We hope that readers will find the contents of *Stem Cells in Reproductive Medicine, Basic Science and Therapeutic Potential* useful as a reference work, and we welcome opinions proposing additions or deletions to the next volume devoted to this avenue of knowledge.

Carlos Simon
Antonio Pellicer

CHAPTER 1

Molecular biology of the gamete

Danielle Vitiello and Emre Seli

INTRODUCTION

Nature operates in a conservative manner. The organism's existence is dependent upon tightly controlled metabolic pathways that capitalize on this evolutionary conservatism in an effort to maintain the species. Such established cellular pathways that allow the organism/species to thrive, and have been adapted through time, are the hallmark for the species' existence. The mechanisms that control and govern our most basic yet prized function, reproduction, are also tightly regulated, and share common features among evolutionarily distant species.

The large division of the animal kingdom that includes all multicellular animals whose cells become differentiated into tissues is called Metazoa. All sexually reproducing metazoans, regardless of their complexity, are the result of the union of two distinct gametes, an egg and a sperm. Their union forms the zygote, whose purpose is to develop into a functional organism that will propagate the species. Although the zygote represents an equal marriage of the two discrete germ cell lineages containing equal amount of genetic material, the precise cellular machinery that governs zygotic and early embryonic development is maternally regulated. This unequally distributed partition of function makes the biology of the gamete and early embryo quite distinct from that of the somatic cell. It is essential to characterize and to understand the mechanisms of these phases of embryonic–cellular regulation, as their implications in defining and predicting stem cell behaviors are paramount.

OOGENESIS AND EARLY EMBRYOGENESIS

Gametes originate from primordial germ cells (PGCs) that are set aside early in embryogenesis.[1] PGCs have an extragonadal origin in most metazoans, and migrate to reach the somatic gonad, where they proliferate by mitosis to form gametes.[1] In the female, PGCs differentiate into oocytes, which enter meiosis, and become arrested at the prophase of the first meiotic division (Figure 1.1).[2,3]

This first meiotic arrest may last as long as a few years in *Xenopus* (frog), and several decades in humans. Large quantities of dormant mRNA are synthesized and stored in the oocyte cytoplasm during this period.[4,5] When later translated, these maternal mRNAs regulate the oocytes' re-entry into meiosis[6–8] and control gene expression during the cleavage divisions of the early embryo.[9–11]

Release from the first meiotic arrest is hormonally mediated, and marks the onset of nuclear and cytoplasmic changes in the oocyte, termed oocyte maturation. In *Xenopus*, meiotic reactivation is mediated by progesterone,[12,13] while mouse and human oocytes respond to gonadotropins (see Figure 1.1).[14,15] In almost all vertebrates, oocyte maturation is completed by the metaphase of the second meiotic division, when oocytes become arrested for a second time and await fertilization.[3] A complex network of translational activation and repression of stored maternal mRNAs accompanies oocyte maturation,[6–8,10] while transcription is limited at best.

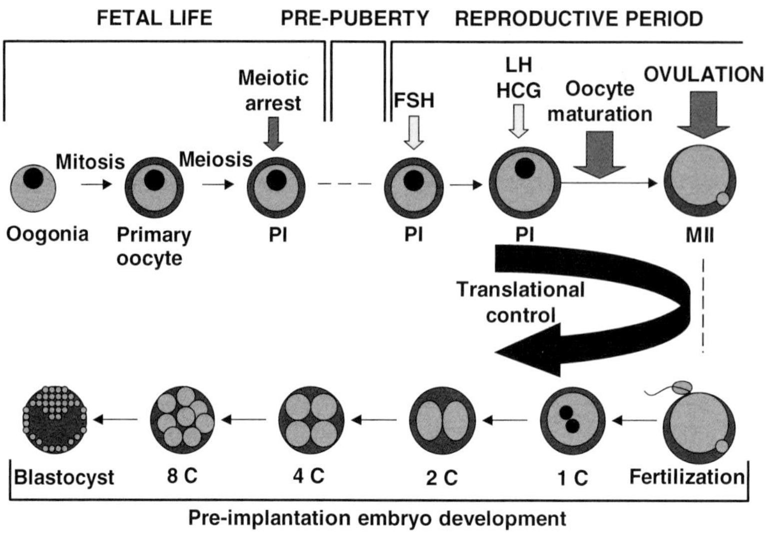

Figure 1.1 Regulation of gene expression during oocyte and pre-implantation embryo development. PGCs proliferate by mitosis and differentiate into oocytes. Primary oocytes enter meiosis, and become arrested at the prophase of the first meiotic division (PI). Release from the first meiotic arrest is hormonally mediated, and marks the onset of oocyte maturation. In *Xenopus*, meiotic reactivation is mediated by progesterone, while mouse and human oocytes respond to gonadotropins. In almost all vertebrates, oocyte maturation is completed by the metaphase of the second meiotic division (MII), when oocytes become arrested for a second time and await fertilization. Oocyte maturation is associated with suppression of transcription. Thereon, until the activation of transcription in the zygote (4- to 8-cell stage in human, and 2-cell stage in mouse), gene expression is regulated by activation and repression of stored maternal mRNAs. PI, prophase I oocyte with germinal vesicle and zona pellucida; MII, metaphase II oocyte (germinal vesicle breakdown has occurred) and the first polar body; 1C, 1-cell embryo; 2C, 2-cell embryo; 4C, 4-cell embryo; 8C, 8-cell embryo; FSH, follicle-stimulating hormone; LH, luteinizing hormone; HCG, human chorionic gonadotropin

The transcriptional silencing that begins with oocyte maturation persists during the initial mitotic divisions of the embryo. Activation of transcription in the zygote, also called zygotic genome activation (ZGA), occurs after 12 rapid synchronous cleavages in *Xenopus*, when the developing embryo is composed of approximately 4000 cells.[16,17] In mouse and human, ZGA occurs at the 2-cell, and 4- to 8-cell stages, respectively.[18–20] Despite the earlier occurrence of ZGA, activation of maternally inherited mRNAs in mammals seems to utilize mechanisms similar to those in other vertebrates, and to play a crucial role in early reproductive events.[10,21]

Nature demonstrates precision through molecular regulation and compartmentalization. This precision is essential for the function of gametes and somatic cells alike. In order to fully understand the unique nature of translational control of gene expression in gametes and early embryos, with its implications on stem cell biology, it is necessary to discuss the regulation of transcription and translation in somatic cells. From these parallels, we can begin to comprehend the exceptional role of embryonic translational control, the prime gatekeeper in metazoan reproductive life.

TRANSCRIPTION AND TRANSLATION IN SOMATIC CELLS

Transcription and processing of pre-mRNAs in somatic cells

From its inception within the nucleus, through its maturation and the following transport into the cytosolic compartment, nascent RNA does not exist as nucleic acid-only entities. Within the somatic cell, the formation and processing of pre-mRNA (Figure 1.2)

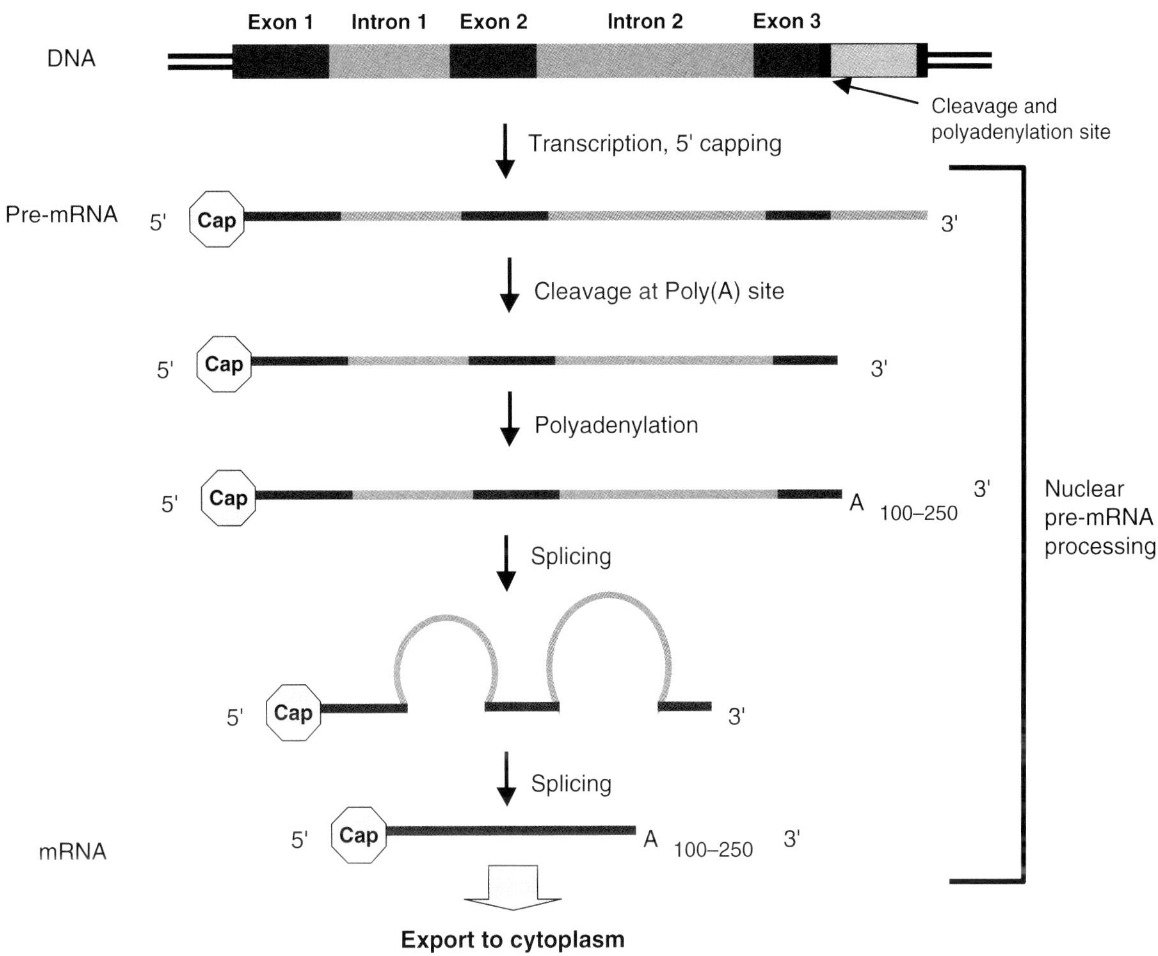

Figure 1.2 Pre-mRNA processing in eukaryotes. Soon after the initiation of transcription by RNA polymerase II, the 5′ end of the nascent RNA is capped with 7-methylguanylate. Next, the pre-mRNA transcript is cleaved at the poly(A) site, and adenosine (A) residues added. The poly(A) tail consists of approximately 250 A residues in mammals. Splicing may occur during transcription or following cleavage and polyadenylation

is mainly restricted to the nucleus. Within the nuclear confines, RNA polymerase II binds DNA and transcribes the first 25–30 nucleotides. This leader sequence is quickly bound by 7-methylguanosine (m^7Gppp) forming the 5′ cap (see Figure 1.2). The 5′ cap protects newly synthesized mRNA from enzymatic degradation.[22] In addition, the cap is also involved in splicing of introns, processing of the 3′ untranslated region (UTR), and export of mRNA into the cytoplasm.[23]

The now capped pre-mRNA transcript continues to be transcribed. The 3′ end of this newly formed pre-mRNA transcript is cleaved at a specific location and a series of approximately 250 adenosines (poly(A) tail) are added (see Figure 1.2). Recognition of the cleavage site at the 3′ UTR, and the addition of the poly(A) tail are well-coordinated events. A consensus sequence (the AAUAAA hexamer) that binds complementary multiprotein complex named cleavage and polyadenylation specificity factor (CPSF) guides this process,[24,25] while the addition of the poly(A) tail, called polyadenylation, is catalyzed by poly(A) polymerase (PAP).

A poly(A) binding protein – named poly(A) binding protein nuclear 1 (PABPN1) (previously termed poly(A) binding protein 2, PABII) – rapidly associates with the newly forming poly(A) tail and provides not only exonuclease protection but also accelerates the polyadenylation reaction. Once the mRNA is transported into the cytoplasm, PABPN1 will be replaced by poly(A) binding protein cytoplasmic 1 (PABPC1), which is significantly larger than its nuclear counterpart and protects the poly(A) tail from deadenylation. It is noteworthy that PABPC1 is ubiquitously expressed in all somatic cells, but not in oocytes or early embryos.

Only after these precisely ordered events (capping, cleavage and polyadenylation) occur can the mRNA be processed further in preparation for its directed exit out of the nucleus and into the cytosol for translation. The next and final process to occur is splicing where non-essential transcript sequences (introns) are removed (see Figure 1.2). Essentially, introns are spliced from existing pre-mRNAs through two sequential transesterification reactions.

The splicing reaction requires four essential elements determining the precise location of the intron to be removed. The first element is a transcript with a 5′ splice site that contains a conserved recognition consensus-sequence as well as a discrete 3′ splice site that delimits the exon–intron boundary. In between these two regions must exist a consensus branch point sequence to facilitate the transesterification and a variable-length polypyrimidine tract.[26,27] The splicesome, composed of 5 small nuclear ribonucleoproteins (snRNPs) that come together in a precise and deliberate sequence, orchestrates splicing. In addition, a larger number of proteins work in conjunction with the snRNPs to regulate this process and to complete transcription.

Central to splicing is its complexity, as interactions between regulatory factors and transcripts regulate processing and resultant expression. As a result, most immature pre-mRNAs undergo a process termed alternative splicing. Alternative pre-mRNA splicing affects approximately 70% of the human genes, is responsible for molecular diversity and contributes to morphologic complexity.[28] It involves the selection of alternate exon–intron combinations, the use of cell-specific promoters and alternate poly(A) sites employing different 3′ UTR regulatory sequences, which in concert, result in proteomic diversity. Tissue-specific factors can act to enhance alternative splicing in particular cells while repressing weaker splice sites in other cells.[29]

After the initial transcription and prior to splicing, select pre-mRNAs may also undergo RNA editing where the nucleotide sequence is altered, resulting in a nucleotide different than the one in its genomic DNA. RNA editing is a process that is common in protozoans, and rare in higher eukaryotes. It is the result of cytodine to uridine (C to U) deamination and currently is known to occur in two human genes, apolipoprotein B and neurofibromin.[29] Mechanistically, a guide RNA sequence attaches to imperfectly duplexed RNA containing the anchoring site. The select nucleotide is deaminated, and the guide RNA, with its associated deaminating enzyme, is undocked. This single deamination alters the incorporated amino acid and results in a functionally distinct protein.[30]

The result of this complex processing and transcript rearrangement is a mature mRNA destined to result in the synthesis of a functional protein. It is only after these modifications that the nuclear mRNA becomes associated within a ribonucleoprotein complex prior to its nuclear export. The 5′ cap that was placed at the transcript's inception guides the mRNA through the nuclear pore complex in conjunction with RNA transport proteins, delivering it to the cytosolic translational machinery.

Translation in somatic cells

The translation of mRNA into the protein product is mechanistically multifaceted. The cell is prudent in its expenditure of energy and only translates those messages inherent to its need at a particular time within the cell cycle.[9] Translational control mechanisms impact upon protein synthesis, and a familiarity with some key components is essential for understanding the regulation of translation.

The cap structure at the 5′ end of the mRNA, involved in 3′ UTR processing, splicing and mRNA transport into the cytoplasm, incurs yet another role in translation by binding the cap-binding protein complex (Figure 1.3). The cap-binding complex consists of the cap-binding protein eIF4E, the RNA helicase eIF4A and the modular scaffolding protein eIF4G (see Figure 1.3A). The protein eIF4G plays a pivotal role in translation initiation, not only by binding eIF4E and eIF4A but also by forming a bridge between the mRNA and the ribosome, and by binding the PABP to facilitate the translation of poly(A)-containing mRNAs (see Figure 1.3C).[31]

A translation pre-initiation complex (see Figure 1.3B) is formed when 40S ribosomal subunit–eIF3 complex

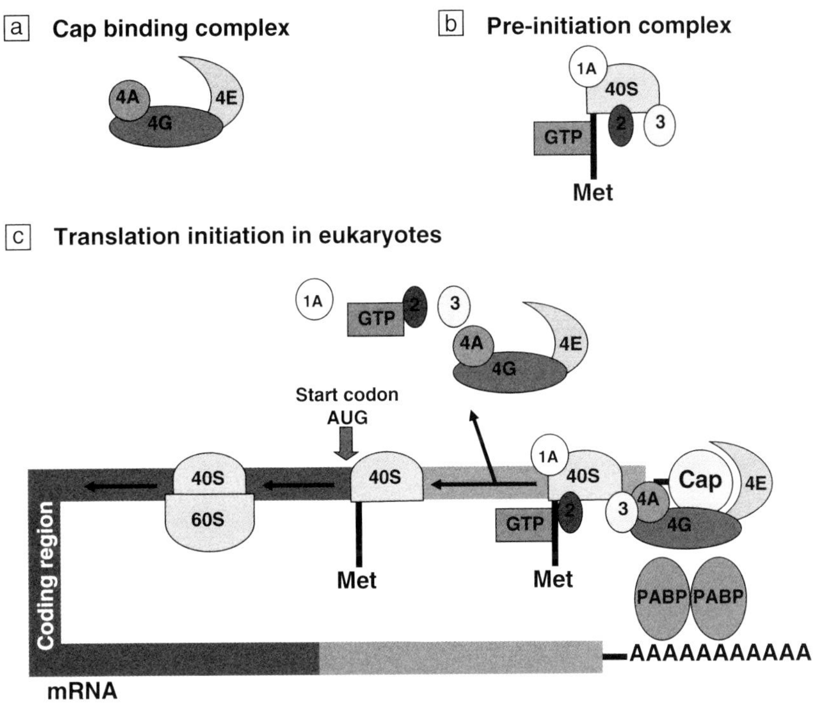

Figure 1.3 (a) The cap-binding complex consists of three eukaryotic initiation factors (eIF): the cap-binding protein eIF4E, the RNA helicase eIF4A and the modular scaffolding protein eIF4G. 4E, eIF4E; 4A, eIF4A; 4G, eIF4G. (b) The translation pre-initiation complex consists of a 40S ribosomal subunit–eIF3 complex bound by eIF1A and the ternary complex (Met-tRNA$_i$, eIF2 and GTP). 40S, 40S ribosomal subunit; 3, eIF3; Met, Met-tRNA$_i$; 2, eIF2. (c) When the translation pre-initiation complex becomes associated with the cap-binding complex and the mRNA, the 48S initiation complex is formed. Within the 48S initiation complex, eIF4G binds eIF4E and eIF4A, forms a bridge between the mRNA and the ribosome and also binds the PABP to facilitate the translation of poly(A)-containing mRNAs. Once bound to the cap structure, the 40S ribosomal subunit with associated proteins scans the mRNA toward the 3′ end until it reaches the initiation codon (AUG). At this point, initiation factors become released and the 60S ribosomal subunit is recruited, initiating translation. This model is simplified for clarity and not all the initiation factors are depicted

is bound by eIF1A and the ternary complex consisting of the transfer RNA charged with the initiation methionine (Met-tRNA$_i$), eIF2 and GTP. Cells can down-regulate protein synthesis by phosphorylating eIF2 and preventing the formation of the ternary complex.

When the translation pre-initiation complex becomes associated with the cap-binding complex and the mRNA, the 48S initiation complex is formed. Because mRNAs are usually produced in excess and compete with one another for the more limited translational machinery, the formation of the 48S initiation complex constitutes the rate-limiting step in translation.

Once bound to the cap structure, the 40S ribosomal subunit with associated proteins scans the mRNA toward the 3′ end until it reaches the initiation codon (AUG). At this point, initiation factors become released and the 60S ribosomal subunit is recruited, initiating translation.[31]

Although in a strict linear sense, the poly(A) tail is the last element reached by the translational machinery, it may be by far the most important factor in governing the translational fate of an mRNA. In addition to the complexes mentioned above, which bind and recruit the ribosomal complexes to the message, an interaction occurs between the 5′ and 3′ ends of mRNA and plays an important role in the initiation of translation. Indeed, the mRNA is circularized, intimating the essential components' of translational machinery (eIF4G-eIF4E at the 5′ end and poly(A) binding proteins at the 3′ end) and stimulating the translational initiation.[32]

Once translation is initiated, the polypeptide chain is elongated by the bound ribosomal complex. This complex pauses intermittently and may offer a means for translational control at this level. Translation is completed as the message is released upon reaching the poly(A) tail and its associated binding proteins.[33,34] The polypeptide undergoes post-translational modifications specific to its inherent function, resulting in a functional protein that is readied for its intended function.

TRANSLATIONAL CONTROL OF GENE EXPRESSION IN THE OOCYTE BY CYTOPLASMIC POLYADENYLATION

Although polyadenylation is a nuclear processing event that occurs on virtually every pre-mRNA,[35,36] it also takes place in the cytoplasm during oocyte maturation and early embryo development and plays a crucial role in the regulation of translation of many mRNAs.

Three key findings suggest that cytoplasmic polyadenylation regulates the translation of certain mRNAs in early development. First, in sea urchin eggs, poly(A) increases two-fold shortly after fertilization, a time when there is no de-novo transcription.[37,38] Secondly, this poly(A) increase is a cytoplasmic event because it can also occur in activated enucleated eggs.[38] Thirdly, these polyadenylated transcripts are preferentially polysomal.[37,38] Moreover, Northern analysis of specific mRNAs from surf clam, *Spisula*, demonstrate that poly(A) elongation is not an indiscriminate activity affecting all maternal mRNAs.[39,40] These observations and those in *Xenopus*[41–44] and mouse[6,10,45,46] establish a correlation between translation and polyadenylation and also demonstrate that the mechanism of control is likely to be mRNA-specific.

Not all maternal mRNAs are polyadenylated during oocyte maturation and early cleavage divisions. Some, such as those encoding ribosomal proteins[47,48] and actin,[49,50] are deadenylated at this time. In contrast to the effect of polyadenylation, deadenylation leads to the suppression of translation.[51]

Regulation of cytoplasmic polyadenylation

The molecular mechanisms regulating cytoplasmic polyadenylation have been studied primarily in mouse[45,46] and *Xenopus* oocytes[52–55] and appear to be highly conserved between the two.

In *Xenopus* oocytes, in addition to the nuclear cleavage and polyadenylation signal AAUAAA, a second sequence in the 3′ UTR, the cytoplasmic polyadenylation element (CPE), is necessary for cytoplasmic polyadenylation (Figure 1.4).[56] The CPE is located near the hexanucleotide (usually 20–30 nucleotides upstream) and has the consensus sequence $UUUUUA_{1-2}U$.[56] CPE is specific to mRNAs polyadenylated during meiotic maturation and binds CPE-binding protein (CPEB), a highly conserved zinc finger and RNA recognition motif (RRM) containing RNA binding protein.[57,58] Injection of antibody against CPEB into *Xenopus* oocytes inhibits polyadenylation and blocks progesterone-induced maturation.[8]

CPEB is also present in mammalian oocytes, where its function appears to be similar to that in *Xenopus*.[6,59] It is therefore noteworthy that the mRNA for synaptonemal complex protein 3 (SCP3), whose absence promotes female germ cell aneuploidy and embryo death in mice,[60] contains a CPE in its 3′ UTR and is probably subject to cytoplasmic polyadenylation during mammalian oogenesis and early development.

When *Xenopus* oocytes are stimulated by progesterone, the kinase aurora (Eg2) phosphorylates CPEB (see Figure 1.4),[7] helping CPEB stabilize CPSF on the AAUAAA.[61] However, simple extension of its poly(A) tail by a cytoplasmic form of PAP, which is recruited by CPSF binding to the AAUAAA sequence and stabilized by interactions with CPEB bound to CPE,[62,63] is not sufficient to explain maturation-induced translation of an oocyte mRNA. This is because there exists an inhibitory factor called maskin that interacts simultaneously with both CPEB and eIF4E[64] and inhibits the assembly of the eIF4G-mediated initiation complex on CPE-containing mRNAs (see Figure 1.4). Displacement of maskin, leading to initiation of translation, requires that a PABP become associated with the newly elongated poly(A) tail,[65] allowing the association of eIF4G with eIF4E (see Figure 1.4).

As previously described, the ubiquitous somatic cytoplasmic poly(A) binding protein, PABPC1, responsible for binding and stabilizing the poly(A) tail of mRNAs in the cytoplasm, is absent in oocytes and

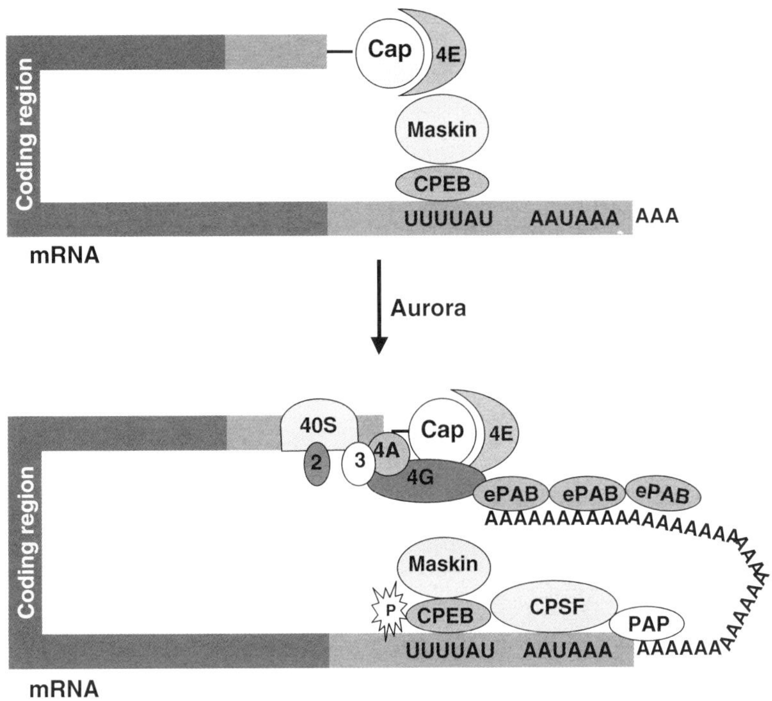

Figure 1.4 Model of polyadenylation-induced translation. (Adapted from Mendez and Richter.[31]) Dormant CPE-containing mRNAs (e.g. cyclin B1) in immature *Xenopus* oocytes are bound by CPEB, which in turn is bound to maskin, which in turn is bound to eIF4E, the cap-binding factor. The binding of maskin to eIF4E precludes the binding of eIF4G to eIF4E, thus inhibiting the formation of the translation initiation complex. Following stimulation, the kinase aurora is activated and phosphorylates CPEB, an event that causes CPEB to bind and recruit CPSF into an active cytoplasmic polyadenylation complex. CPSF recruits poly(A) polymerase (PAP) to the end of the mRNA, where it catalyzes poly(A) addition. The newly elongated poly(A) tail is then bound by a embryonic poly(A) binding protein (ePAB), which in turn associates with eIF4G. The protein eIF4G, when associated with ePAB, then displaces maskin from and binds to eIF4E, thereby initiating translation

early embryos. A cytoplasmic PABP present in significant amounts in vertebrate oocytes and embryos has recently been identified in *Xenopus*[66] and mouse.[67] This protein, called embryonic poly(A) binding protein (ePAB), is present only in oocytes, and early embryos prior to ZGA. ePAB binds maternal mRNAs and prevents their deadenylation. Moreover, it mediates the displacement of maskin, and initiation of translation in the oocytes and the early embryos.

TRANSLATION REGULATORY CASCADES IN THE OOCYTE

At a molecular level, meiotic reactivation depends on the timely translation of specific mRNAs stored in the oocyte cytoplasm. These include the rapid inducer of G2/M progression in oocytes/Speedy (RINGO/Spy), cyclin B1 and cyclin-dependent protein kinase 2 (Cdk2).[31,68–70]

Translation of the RINGO/Spy message is essential since the RINGO/Spy protein, a novel cell cycle regulator with unique kinase binding and activation domains, is required to activate Cdk2.[68,70–73] Cdk2 activates the protein kinase Aurora A/Eg2, which, in turn, promotes the polyadenylation and subsequent translation of CPE-containing messages, including mos serine/threonine kinase. Mos activates a mitogen-activated protein kinase (MAPK) cascade, resulting in progression through oocyte maturation.

Cytoplasmic polyadenylation appears to be the predominant translation regulator of the maternal mRNAs stored within the oocyte cytoplasm. However, in order to achieve timely expression of distinct genes necessary for specific steps of oocyte maturation and embryonic cleavage divisions, the presence of additional control mechanisms seems necessary.

Most recently, investigation of the activation of RINGO/Spy mRNA translation in *Xenopus* oocytes has revealed exciting information pertaining to the additional mechanisms that may play a role in regulating the translation of maternal mRNAs. In the oocyte cytoplasm, RINGO/Spy protein is absent, while RINGO/Spy mRNA is kept translationally silent. This is achieved by the binding of an RNA-binding protein, Pumilio-2, initially described as responsible for RNA silencing in lower organisms. Pumilio-2 binds to the consensus sequence called the pumilio-binding element (PBE) located in the 3′ UTR, and inhibits the translation of RINGO/Spy mRNA. Interestingly, in addition to Pumilio-2, 3′ UTR of RINGO/Spy mRNA is also bound by DAZL (deleted in azoospermia-like protein) and ePAB. It is postulated that Pumilio-2 recruits a repression complex to the RINGO/Spy mRNA and that DAZL and ePAB are co-repressors.[74]

Hormonal stimulation that causes meiotic reactivation (progesterone in *Xenopus*) results in the dissociation of the repressor protein (Pumilio-2) from the PBE and the DAZL/ePAB complex. This dissociation allows the DAZL/ePAB complex then to activate translation of the RINGO/Spy mRNA. Once translated, RINGO/Spy leads to the activation of a series of kinases described above. Finally, CPE-dependent polyadenylation and resultant translation of mos mRNA occurs and results in progression through oocyte maturation.

The recent findings pertaining to the regulation of RINGO/Spy mRNA translation have two important implications. First, they suggest the presence of additional mechanisms other than polyadenylation that regulate maternal mRNA translation in oocytes. Therefore, a translational control machinery that is activated in cascades, and uses specific binding sites in the 3′ UTR, seems to regulate the timely activation of maternal mRNAs.[75] Secondly, the identification of Pumilio-2, and DAZL, in addition to CPEB and ePAB, as regulators of maternal mRNA expression, suggests that an array of proteins with homologues in evolutionarily distant animals are involved in the regulation of maternal mRNA translation. Indeed, while CPEB, ePAB and Pumilio-2 were initially identified in model organisms, DAZL was first identified by its homology to DAZ (deleted in azoospermia), a gene on the long arm of the Y chromosome that is frequently deleted in infertile men with non-obstructive azoospermia. The presence of DAZL, as well as ePAB, CPEB and Pumilio-2, in numerous species, is suggestive that the mechanisms regulating maternal mRNA translation are evolutionarily conserved.

MOLECULAR ASPECTS OF SPERMATOGENESIS

Generation of the mature male gamete (spermatozoa) is termed spermatogenesis and occurs in three steps:

(1) Mitotic proliferation leads to the production of a large number of cells.

(2) Meiotic division halves the chromosome number and generates genetic diversity.

(3) Differentiation packages the chromosomes for effective delivery into the oocyte.

In mammals, spermatogenesis differs from oogenesis by the fact that it occurs continuously after puberty and results in the generation of millions of mature spermatozoa daily, compared with the limited number of oocytes ovulated in the lifetime of a female.

Early in the gestational life of a male embryo, PGCs are localized in the extraembryonic mesoderm. As these PGCs migrate toward the gonadal primordium, they proliferate, generating prospermatogonia that undergo cell cycle arrest at interphase. At puberty, under the influence of testosterone, and supported by both Sertoli and Leydig cells, prospermatogonia enter rounds of mitosis, generating spermatogonial stem cells. From within this reservoir of self-generating stem cells, groups of cells with a distinct morphology called A1 spermatogonia emerge at intervals, marking the beginning of spermatogenesis. Each of the A1 spermatogonia undergoes a predetermined and limited number of mitotic divisions, leading to the production of a clone of cells. The number of mitotic divisions that A1 spermatogonia undergo is specific for species (6 in mouse) and will determine the total number of cells in that clone, although cell death may reduce this number considerably. The morphology of the cells produced at each mitotic division can be distinguished from that of its parent, making it possible to subclassify spermatogonia. The end result of this series of mitotic divisions is the resting primary spermatocyte that will in turn enter meiotic division.

During the mitotic divisions of spermatogenesis, nuclear division is successfully completed at each step, while cytoplasmic division remains incomplete. Thus, all the primary spermatocytes derived from an A1 spermatogonium are linked together by thin cytoplasmic bridges, forming a large syncytium. This syncytial organization persists throughout the further meiotic divisions, and individual cells are only released during the last stages of spermatogenesis as mature spermatozoa.

Primary spermatocytes replicate their DNA and enter the prophase of meiosis I. The first meiotic division ends with separation of homologous chromosomes to opposite ends of the cell on the meiotic spindle, after which cytoplasmic division yields two secondary spermatocytes from each primary spermatocyte. Each secondary spermatocyte is haploid and contains a single set of chromosomes that consists of two chromatids joined at the centromere. The second meiotic division is characterized by the separation of sister chromatids, and generates two early round spermatids from each secondary spermatocyte. Therefore, in the case of the mouse, from a single A1 spermatogonium, a maximum of 64 primary spermatocytes and 256 early spermatids could result. However, the actual numbers are significantly less due to cell loss.

Meiosis is followed by cytoplasmic remodeling. The extensive differentiation that changes round spermatids into mature spermatozoa is called spermiogenesis. With the appearance of spermatozoa, the thin cytoplasmic bridges that make up the syncytium rupture, and cells are released into the lumen of the seminiferous tubules.[76]

It is noteworthy that the rate of progression through spermatogenesis is constant within a species. Therefore, type A1 spermatogonia within any male gonad of a given species advances through spermatogenesis at the same rate. Hormones or external agents do not seem to affect the rate of spermatogenesis, while they may influence whether or not the process occurs at all. In humans, spermatogenesis is completed in 64 days, while in rat it takes 48 days. The longest stage of the meiosis in the male is pachytene of the first meiotic prophase when crossing over of genetic material occurs. This is different from oogenesis, where the longest phase of meiotic division is the diplotene stage of prophase I characterized by the first meiotic arrest in oogenesis.

Transcriptional control in male germ cells

Germ cells utilize unique mechanisms of transcription initiation, including alternate forms of core promoter transcription factors, tissue-specific promoters, and somatic gene-expression silencing.[77] These common characteristics are seen not only in oogenesis but also in spermatogenesis.

Transcription factors are defined by their ability to bind promoter regions in the DNA upstream of the protein coding region, and regulate RNA transcription. Some transcription factors are ubiquitous and regulate many genes expressed in a multitude of tissues, while others are specific for certain tissues, and regulate tissue-specific gene expression. Transcription factors unique to spermatogenic cells have been identified (SPRM1, TAK-1, OCT-2, CREB, CREM).[78]

The best characterized male germ cell-specific transcription factors are the cAMP-responsive element binding protein (CREB) and the closely related cAMP-responsive element modulator (CREM) that are activated by cyclic AMP/protein kinase A signaling pathways.[79] CREM represents a regulatory element that itself is regulated during RNA processing.[80] During spermiogenesis, alternative splicing of the pre-mRNA renders the function of an isoform of the CREM protein from a transcriptional repressor to that of a potent activator. In addition, an alternate polyadenylation site is utilized, further up-regulating CREM expression.[81] These data support regulatory control of gamete-specific gene expression at the level of splicing and polyadenylation within the nucleus.

There are many transcripts specific to male germ cells. Often they are the result of alternate initiation of transcription within the coding sequence of the gene that is expressed in somatic cells. For example, transcription of the angiotensin-converting enzyme (ACE) gene begins within the 12th intron of the gene and produces a testes-specific protein that is both truncated from its somatic form and carries a novel string of N-terminal amino acids. Production of this altered gene product is the direct result of CREM activation.[82] Examples of other proteins expressed as a result of germ-cell-specific alterations to the transcriptional machinery include the proto-oncogenes *c-abl* and *c-mos*, proenkephalin, superoxide dismutase 1 and β-galactosyl transferase.[83]

Translational control in male germ cells

Translational repression during spermatogenesis

One of the most powerful modicums of translational regulation in both meiotic and haploid spermatogenic cells is translational repression.[84,85] In the mouse model, both spermatocytes and spermatids express lower levels of polysomal mRNA and increased concentrations of mRNA–protein complexes (mRNPs) when the cellular extracts are analyzed after gradient centrifugation.[86] This finding is opposite of what would be expected in an efficient, translationally active system. RNA-binding proteins that interact with the 3′ UTR of specific mRNAs seem to be important mediators of translational repression in male germ cells. One such protein is protamine 1 RNA-binding protein (PRBP), which binds to a 62 nucleotide region in the 3′ UTR of protamine 1 mRNA in spermatids, when the mRNA is repressed translationally.[87]

Translation repression/control also occurs secondary to specialization of the translational machinery. Interestingly, PABPC1 and eIF4E are over-expressed in spermatogenic cells;[88] however, greater concentrations of the rate-limiting proteins do not necessarily result in greater efficiency in translation. This phenomenon may be due to an increased nucleotide interval between bound ribosomes in spermatogenic cells (140 nt) when compared with somatic cell counterparts (100 nt).[76] In addition, the increased concentration of mRNPs may impede recruitment or sterically hinder interactions between the ribosome and mRNA.

Translational control of gene expression during spermatogenesis

Transcription terminates during spermiogenesis,[89] as the remodeled condensed chromatin structure of the late-stage spermatids is incompatible with transcription. Thereafter, the mechanisms that govern gene expression are post-transcriptional, and dependent upon dormant paternal mRNAs[90] for the production of functional spermatozoan proteins.

The pre-mRNAs destined to lie dormant are polyadenylated within the nucleus and exported into the cytosol where they await alteration to their poly(A) tails and subsequent activation.[91,92] Interestingly, unlike in the oocyte where the extension of the poly(A) tail results in translational activation, truncation of poly(A) tails in spermatids seems to trigger translation.[93] Indeed, the stored mRNAs in spermatids usually have poly(A) tails that are longer than 150 nucleotides, and are not associated with ribosomes. These appear to undergo shortening of the poly(A) tail to approximately 30 nucleotides coincident with their association with polysomes and translation.[94] However, the mechanisms regulating the shortening of poly(A) tail and translational activation in male germ cells are yet to be elucidated. It is also worthy of note that the translational activation of mRNAs associated with poly(A) tail truncation is exclusive to haploid cells, as dormant mRNAs expressed in meiotic male germ cells necessitate poly(A) lengthening for activation, akin to the mechanisms detailed in the oocyte.

Acknowledgments

Emre Seli is supported by National Institute of Health Grant K08 HD046581.

REFERENCES

1. Matova N, Cooley L. Comparative aspects of animal oogenesis. Dev Biol 2001; 231: 291–320.
2. Page AW, Orr-Weaver TL. Stopping and starting the meiotic cell cycle. Curr Opin Genet Dev 1997; 7: 23–31.
3. Sagata N. Meiotic metaphase arrest in animal oocytes: its mechanisms and biological significance. Trends Cell Biol 1996; 6: 22–8.
4. LaMarca MJ, Smith LD, Strobel MC. Quantitative and qualitative analysis of RNA synthesis in stage 6 and stage 4 oocytes of *Xenopus laevis*. Dev Biol 1973; 34: 106–18.
5. Rodman TC, Bachvarova R. RNA synthesis in preovulatory mouse oocytes. J Cell Biol 1976; 70: 251–7.
6. Gebauer F, Xu W, Cooper GM, Richter JD. Translational control by cytoplasmic polyadenylation of c-mos mRNA is necessary for oocyte maturation in the mouse. EMBO J 1994; 13: 5712.
7. Mendez R, Hake LE, Andresson T et al. Phosphorylation of CPE binding factor by Eg2 regulates translation of c-mos mRNA. Nature 2000; 404: 302–7.
8. Stebbins-Boaz B, Hake LE, Richter JD. CPEB controls the cytoplasmic polyadenylation of cyclin, Cdk2 and

c-mos mRNAs and is necessary for oocyte maturation in Xenopus. EMBO J 1996; 15: 2582–92.

9. Groisman I, Huang YS, Mendez R et al. CPEB, maskin, and cyclin B1 mRNA at the mitotic apparatus: implications for local translational control of cell division. Cell 2000; 103: 435–47.
10. Oh B, Hwang S, McLaughlin J, Solter D, Knowles BB. Timely translation during the mouse oocyte-to-embryo transition. Development 2000; 127: 3795–803.
11. Uto K, Sagata N. Nek2B, a novel maternal form of Nek2 kinase, is essential for the assembly or maintenance of centrosomes in early Xenopus embryos. EMBO J 2000; 19: 1816–26.
12. Bayaa M, Booth RA, Sheng Y et al. The classical progesterone receptor mediates Xenopus oocyte maturation through a nongenomic mechanism. Proc Natl Acad Sci USA 2000; 97: 12607–12.
13. Tian J, Kim S, Heilig E et al. Identification of XPR-1, a progesterone receptor required for Xenopus oocyte activation. Proc Natl Acad Sci USA 2000; 97: 14358–63.
14. Faiman C, Ryan RJ. Serum follicle-stimulating hormone and luteinizing hormone concentrations during the menstrual cycle as determined by radioimmunoassays. J Clin Endocrinol Metab 1967; 27: 1711–16.
15. Rao AJ, Moudgal NR, Raj HG, Lipner H, Greep RO. The role of FSH and LH in the initiation of ovulation in rats and hamsters: a study using rabbit antisera to ovine FSH and LH. J Reprod Fertil 1974; 37: 323–30.
16. Newport J, Kirschner M. A major developmental transition in early Xenopus embryos: II. Control of the onset of transcription. Cell 1982; 30: 687–96.
17. Newport J, Kirschner M. A major developmental transition in early Xenopus embryos: I. Characterization and timing of cellular changes at the midblastula stage. Cell 1982; 30: 675–86.
18. Clegg KB, Piko L. RNA synthesis and cytoplasmic polyadenylation in the one-cell mouse embryo. Nature 1982; 295: 343–4.
19. Flach G, Johnson MH, Braude PR et al. The transition from maternal to embryonic control in the 2-cell mouse embryo. EMBO J 1982; 1: 681–6.
20. Braude P, Bolton V, Moore S. Human gene expression first occurs between the four- and eight-cell stages of preimplantation development. Nature 1988; 332: 459–61.
21. Richter JD. Cytoplasmic polyadenylation in development and beyond. Microbiol Mol Biol Rev 1999; 63: 446–56.
22. Izaurralde E, Lewis J, McGuigan C et al. A nuclear cap binding protein complex involved in pre-mRNA splicing. Cell 1994; 78: 657–68.
23. Flaherty SM, Fortes P, Izaurralde E et al. Participation of the nuclear cap binding complex in pre-mRNA 3′ processing. Proc Natl Acad Sci USA 1997; 94: 11893–8.
24. Zhao J, Hyman L, Moore C. Formation of mRNA 3′ ends in eukaryotes: mechanism regulation and interrelationships with other steps in mRNA synthesis. Microbiol Mol Biol Rev 1999; 63: 405–45.
25. Proudfoot N. New perspectives on connecting messenger RNA 3′ end formation to transcription. Curr Opin Cell Biol 2004; 16: 272–8.
26. Staley J, Guthrie C. Mechanical devices of the splicesome: motors, clocks, springs and things. Cell 1998; 13: 302–9.
27. Jurica M, Moore M. Pre-mRNA splicing: awash in a sea of proteins. Mol Cell 2003; 12: 5–14.
28. Levine M, Tijan R. Transcription regulation and animal diversity. Nature 2003; 424: 147–51.
29. Soller M. Pre-messenger RNA processing and its regulation: a genomic perspective. Cell Mol Life Sci 2006; 63: 796–819.
30. Smith H, Gott J, Hanson M. A guide to RNA editing. RNA 1997; 3: 77–81.
31. Mendez R, Richter JD. Translational control by CPEB: a means to the end. Nature Rev Mol Cell Biol 2001; 2: 521–9.
32. Wells S, Hillner P, Vale R et al. Circularization of mRNA by eukaryotic translation initiation factors. Mol Cell 1998; 2: 135–40.
33. Mazumder B, Seshadri V, Fox PL. Translational control by the 3′-UTR: the ends specify the means. Trends Biochem Sci 2003; 28: 91–8.
34. Huang YS, Richter JD. Regulation of local mRNA translation. Curr Opin Cell Biol 2004; 16: 308–13.
35. Manley JL. A complex protein assembly catalyzes polyadenylation of mRNA precursors. Curr Opin Genet Dev 1995; 5: 222–8.
36. Wahle E. 3′-end cleavage and polyadenylation of mRNA precursors. Biochim Biophys Acta 1995; 1261: 183–94.
37. Slater DW, Slater I, Gillespie D. Post-fertilization synthesis of polyadenylic acid in sea urchin embryos. Nature 1972; 240: 333–7.
38. Wilt FH. Polyadenylation of maternal RNA of sea urchin eggs after fertilization. Proc Natl Acad Sci USA 1973; 70: 2345–9.
39. Rosenthal ET, Tansey TR, Ruderman JV. Sequence-specific adenylations and deadenylations accompany changes in the translation of maternal messenger RNA after fertilization of Spisula oocytes. J Mol Biol 1983; 166: 309–27.
40. Rosenthal ET, Ruderman JV. Widespread changes in the translation and adenylation of maternal messenger RNAs following fertilization of Spisula oocytes. Dev Biol 1987; 121: 237–46.

41. Dworkin MB, Dworkin-Rastl E. Changes in RNA titers and polyadenylation during oogenesis and oocyte maturation in *Xenopus laevis*. Dev Biol 1985; 112: 451–7.

42. Dworkin MB, Shrutkowski A, Dworkin-Rastl E. Mobilization of specific maternal RNA species into polysomes after fertilization in *Xenopus laevis*. Proc Natl Acad Sci USA 1985; 82: 7636–40.

43. McGrew LL, Dworkin-Rastl E, Dworkin MB, Richter JD. Poly(A) elongation during Xenopus oocyte maturation is required for translational recruitment and is mediated by a short sequence element. Genes Dev 1989; 3: 803–15.

44. Sheets MD, Wu M, Wickens M. Polyadenylation of c-mos mRNA as a control point in Xenopus meiotic maturation. Nature 1995; 374: 511–16.

45. Bachvarova R, De Leon V, Johnson A et al. Changes in total RNA, polyadenylated RNA, and actin mRNA during meiotic maturation of mouse oocytes. Dev Biol 1985; 108: 325–31.

46. Vassalli JD, Huarte J, Belin D et al. Regulated polyadenylation controls mRNA translation during meiotic maturation of mouse oocytes. Genes Dev 1989; 3: 2163–71.

47. Baum EZ, Hyman LE, Wormington WM. Post-translational control of ribosomal protein L1 accumulation in Xenopus oocytes. Dev Biol 1988; 126: 141–9.

48. Hyman LE, Wormington WM. Translational inactivation of ribosomal protein mRNAs during Xenopus oocyte maturation. Genes Dev 1988; 2: 598–605.

49. Bachvarova R, Cohen EM, De Leon V et al. Amounts and modulation of actin mRNAs in mouse oocytes and embryos. Development 1989; 106: 561–5.

50. Paynton BV, Bachvarova R. Polyadenylation and deadenylation of maternal mRNAs during oocyte growth and maturation in the mouse. Mol Reprod Dev 1994; 37: 172–80.

51. Varnum SM, Wormington WM. Deadenylation of maternal mRNAs during Xenopus oocyte maturation does not require specific cis-sequences: a default mechanism for translational control. Genes Dev 1990; 4: 2278–86.

52. McGrew LL, Richter JD. Xenopus oocyte poly(A) RNAs that hybridize to a cloned interspersed repeat sequence are not translatable. Dev Biol 1989; 134: 267–70.

53. McGrew LL, Richter JD. Translational control by cytoplasmic polyadenylation during Xenopus oocyte maturation: characterization of cis and trans elements and regulation by cyclin/MPF. EMBO J 1990; 9: 3743–51.

54. Paris J, Richter JD. Maturation-specific polyadenylation and translational control: diversity of cytoplasmic polyadenylation elements, influence of poly(A) tail size, and formation of stable polyadenylation complexes. Mol Cell Biol 1990; 10: 5634–45.

55. Paris J, Swenson K, Piwnica-Worms H et al. Maturation-specific polyadenylation: in vitro activation by p34cdc2 and phosphorylation of a 58-kD CPE-binding protein. Genes Dev 1991; 5: 1697–708.

56. Bilger A, Fox CA, Wahle E et al. Nuclear polyadenylation factors recognize cytoplasmic polyadenylation elements. Genes Dev 1994; 8: 1106–16.

57. Hake LE, Richter JD. CPEB is a specificity factor that mediates cytoplasmic polyadenylation during Xenopus oocyte maturation. Cell 1994; 79: 617–27.

58. Hake LE, Mendez R, Richter JD. Specificity of RNA binding by CPEB: requirement for RNA recognition motifs and a novel zinc finger. Mol Cell Biol 1998; 18: 685–93.

59. Stutz A, Conne B, Huarte J et al. Masking, unmasking, and regulated polyadenylation cooperate in the translational control of a dormant mRNA in mouse oocytes. Genes Dev 1998; 12: 2535–48.

60. Yuan L, Liu JG, Hoja MR et al. Female germ cell aneuploidy and embryo death in mice lacking the meiosis-specific protein SCP3. Science 2002; 296: 1115–18.

61. Mendez R, Murthy KG, Ryan K et al. Phosphorylation of CPEB by Eg2 mediates the recruitment of CPSF into an active cytoplasmic polyadenylation complex. Mol Cell 2000; 6: 1253–9.

62. Dickson KS, Bilger A, Ballantyne S et al. The cleavage and polyadenylation specificity factor in *Xenopus laevis* oocytes is a cytoplasmic factor involved in regulated polyadenylation. Mol Cell Biol 1999; 19: 5707–17.

63. Dickson KS, Thompson SR, Gray NK et al. Poly(A) polymerase and the regulation of cytoplasmic polyadenylation. J Biol Chem 2001; 276: 41810–16.

64. Stebbins-Boaz B, Cao Q, de Moor CH et al. Maskin is a CPEB-associated factor that transiently interacts with elF-4E. [Erratum in Mol Cell 2000; 5(4): following 766.] Mol Cell 1999; 4: 1017–27.

65. Cao Q, Richter JD. Dissolution of the maskin-eIF4E complex by cytoplasmic polyadenylation and poly(A)-binding protein controls cyclin B1 mRNA translation and oocyte maturation. EMBO J 2002; 21: 3852–62.

66. Voeltz GK, Ongkasuwan J, Standart N et al. A novel embryonic poly(A) binding protein, ePAB, regulates mRNA deadenylation in Xenopus egg extracts. Genes Dev 2001; 15: 774–88.

67. Seli E, Lalioti MD, Flaherty SM et al. An embryonic poly(A)-binding protein (ePAB) is expressed in mouse oocytes and early preimplantation embryos. Proc Natl Acad Sci USA 2005; 102: 367–72.

68. Ferby I, Blazquez M, Palmer A et al. A novel p34(cdc2)-binding and activating protein that is

necessary and sufficient to trigger G(2)/M progression in Xenopus oocytes. Genes Dev 1999; 13: 2177–89.

69. Eichenlaub-Ritter U, Peschke M. Expression in in-vivo and in-vitro growing and maturing oocytes: focus on regulation of expression at the translational level. Hum Reprod Update 2002; 8: 21–41.

70. Dekel N. Cellular, biochemical and molecular mechanisms regulating oocyte maturation. Mol Cell Endocrinol 2005; 234: 19–25.

71. Lenormand JL, Dellinger RW, Knudsen KE et al. Speedy: a novel cell cycle regulator of the G2/M transition. EMBO J 1999; 18: 1869–77.

72. Terret TE, Ferby I, Nebreda AR, Verlhac MH. RINGO efficiently triggers meiosis resumption in mouse oocytes and induces cell cycle arrest in embryos. Biol Cell 2001; 93: 89–97.

73. Cheng A, Xiong W, Ferrell JE Jr, Solomon MJ. Identification and comparative analysis of multiple mamalian Speedy/Ringo proteins. Cell Cycle 2005; 4: 155–65.

74. Padmanabhan K, Richter JD. Regulated Pumilio-2 binding controls RINGO/Spy mRNA translation and CPEB activation. Genes Dev 2006; 20: 199–209.

75. Vasudevan S, Seli E, Steitz JA. Metazoan oocyte and early embryo development program: a progression through translation regulatory cascades [comment]. Genes Dev 2006; 20: 138–46.

76. Kleene KC. Patterns, mechanisms, and functions of translation regulation in mammalian spermatogenic cells. Cytogenet Genome Res 2003; 103: 217–24.

77. DeJong J. Basic mechanisms for the control of germ cell gene expression. Genes 2006; 366: 39–50.

78. Eddy EM. Regulation of gene expression during spermatogenesis. Semin Cell Dev Biol 1998; 9: 451–7.

79. Sassone-Corsi P. Transcriptional checkpoints determining the fate of male germ cells. Cell 1997; 88: 163–6.

80. Foulkes NS, Mellstrom B, Benusiglio E et al. Developmental switch of CREM function during spermatogenesis: from antagonist to activator. Nature 1992; 355: 80–4.

81. Foulkes NS, Schlotter F, Pevet P et al. Pituitary hormone FSH directs the CREM functional switch during spermatogenesis. Nature 1993; 362: 264–7.

82. Zhou Y, Sun Z, Means AR et al. cAMP-response element modulator tau is a positive regulator of testis angiotensin converting enzyme transcription. Proc Natl Acad Sci USA 1996; 93: 12262–6.

83. Hecht NB. Molecular mechanisms of male germ cell differentiation. Bioessays 1998; 20: 555–61.

84. Kleene KC. Patterns of translational regulation in the mammalian testis. Mol Reprod Dev 1996; 43: 268–81.

85. Kleene KC. A possible meiotic function of the peculiar patterns of gene expression in mammalian spermatogenic cells. Mech Dev 2001; 106: 3–23.

86. Cataldo L, Mastrangelo MA, Kleene KC. A quantitative sucrose gradient analysis of the translational activity of 18 mRNA species in testes from adult mice. Mol Hum Reprod 1999; 5: 206–13.

87. Lee K, Fajardo MA, Braun R. A testis cytoplasmic RNA-binding protein that has the properties of a translational repressor. Mol Cell Biol 1996; 16: 3023–34.

88. Gu W, Kwon Y, Oko R et al. Poly (A) binding protein is bound to both stored and polysomal mRNAs in the mammalian testis. Mol Reprod Dev 1995; 40: 273–85.

89. Kierszenbaum AL, Tres LL. RNA transcription and chromatin structure during meiotic and postmeiotic stages of spermatogenesis. Fed Proc 1978; 37: 2512–16.

90. Hecht NB. The making of a spermatozoon: a molecular perspective. Dev Genet 1995; 16: 95–103.

91. Kashiwabara S, Noguchi J, Zhuang T et al. Regulation of spermatogenesis by testis-specific, cytoplasmic poly(A) polymerase TPAP. Science 1999; 298: 1999–2002.

92. Elliot D. Pathways of post-transcriptional gene regulation in mammalian germ cell development. Cytogenet Genome Res 2003; 103: 210–16.

93. Kleene KC. Poly(A) shortening accompanies the activation of translation of five mRNAs during spermiogenesis in the mouse. Development 1989; 106: 367–73.

94. Kleene KC, Distel RJ, Hecht NB. Translational regulation and deadenylation of a protamine mRNA during spermiogenesis in the mouse. Dev Biol 1984; 105: 71–9.

CHAPTER 2

Differentiation of germ cells from stem cells

Celso Silva, Lisa Salvador and Jerome F Strauss III

INTRODUCTION

Developments during the past 10 years have brought stem cells to a place of prominence because of the potential that they have to serve as an invaluable tool for research, offering unique insights into areas of mammalian developmental biology that are not readily accessible to experimentation, and because they offer significant promise for cell-based therapies for degenerative diseases. Although embryonic stem (ES) cells were first isolated more than 25 years ago,[1] it was only after the successful isolation of human ES cells from blastocyst embryos and embryonic germ (EG) cells,[2] and the inherent ethical and moral controversy surrounding this technique, that they were elevated to the medical headlines.

There are different types of stem cells, including ES cells, EG cells, fetal stem cells, adult stem cells and embryonal carcinoma stem cells. These stem cells are classified as totipotent, pluripotent or multipotent according to their capacity to differentiate into different cell lineages. Only the fertilized oocyte was considered to be totipotent because of its ability to differentiate not only into tissues derived from the three major germinative layers (ectoderm, endoderm and mesoderm) but also into the extraembryonic cell lineages (trophoectodermal tissue) and into germ cells.

ES cells, which are derived from the inner cell mass of blastocyst stage embryos,[1,2] by definition are capable of maintaining pluripotency during indefinite propagation in vitro, while maintaining a normal karyotype. In earlier in-vivo assays, ES cells have been shown to be able to differentiate into the three major germinative layers, germ cells and even into the trophoectodermal layer, but only when supported by the developmental capacity of a recipient embryo. This was accomplished by experiments in which ES cells were aggregated with early diploid and tetraploid embryos or injected into blastocyts,[3,4] demonstrating the in-vivo totipotent capacity of ES cells.

In vitro, ES cells can be induced to recapitulate several aspects of early embryonic development, and can give rise to cell types from all three germ cell layers, including neural, hematopoietic, vascular, pancreatic, muscular and cardiac lineages.[5] However, up until recently there were no reports demonstrating that ES cells could differentiate into the trophoectodermal layer or germ cells. This inability of ES cells to spontaneously differentiate into germ cells and trophoectoderm led to the conclusion that they were only pluripotent. However, recent studies have challenged this concept, and the in-vitro totipotency of mouse ES cells has been demonstrated, with formation of germ cells in vitro that were capable of developing into male and female gametes. Furthermore, these gametes were, in some cases, capable of undergoing meiosis and supporting fertilization, or undergoing parthenogenesis, resulting in the formation of blastocyst-like structures that contain cells expressing trophoectoderm markers.[6–8] Human ES cells cultured in vitro can also express markers characteristic of germ cells.[9]

This significant advance towards in-vitro systems capable of generating germ cells from ES cells can potentially revolutionize the field of reproductive development, since it may provide a new approach to test the totipotency of ES cells. Furthermore, if generation of oocytes from ES cells proves to be successful, this technique may provide new tools for the development of new therapies for different forms of female infertility. Moreover, if the ES cell-derived oocytes can be subjected to somatic cell nuclear transfer, the creation of patient-specific stem cell lines will be facilitated. Furthermore, in-vitro systems of germ cell generation present a wonderful opportunity to study early germ cell development, while allowing for the establishment of models for the study of early embryonic development and for epigenetic reprogramming. However, many questions remain to be answered regarding the feasibility and reproducibility of this technology:

- How can we control the differentiation process of ES cells into the germ cell lineage?
- How can we properly identify and purify the population of formed germ cells/gametes?
- Is it possible to increase the yield of germ cell/gametes?
- Are these gametes competent to support the development of healthy offspring?
- Can oocytes generated from ES cells be used successfully for somatic cell nuclear transfer?

Here we outline the steps involved in mammalian germ cell specification in vivo, and their subsequent development and differentiation, including the ultimate entry into oogenesis and spermatogenesis, highlighting the current knowledge about the molecular signaling pathways involved in these processes. We believe that knowledge about the molecular signaling pathways required for primordial germ cell (PGC) formation in vivo will be essential for the efforts of generating germ cells and gametes in vitro. It is important to ensure that the in-vivo process is being replicated adequately in vitro. We also critically assess the currently available information about this topic, and what questions remain to be answered about the process of ES cell differentiation into the germ line.

MOLECULAR ASPECTS OF PGCs' DEVELOPMENT IN VIVO

The events involved in specification of the germ line are not completely understood, and most of the current knowledge is derived from studies of lower species or from the murine model. Unlike in lower species where germ line specification is dictated and mediated by the germ plasm, a unique portion of the oocyte cytoplasm, established by a mechanism of cytoplasmic partitioning that happens before fertilization, and that induces germ cell fate,[10] mammals segregate PGCs from other somatic cells in early embryogenesis, during gastrulation. In the mouse, germ cell competence is induced in the proximal epiblast cells of the egg cylinder at 6.5 days postcoitum (dpc) in response to signals that include the bone morphogenetic factors Bmp4 and Bmp8b from the extraembryonic ectoderm.[11] Fate mapping studies have demonstrated that germ cells are derived from the proximal epiblast.[12] Interestingly, the distal epiblast, originally determined to generate the neural or ectoderm lineage, can be reprogrammed to form germ cells when placed adjacent to extraembryonic ectoderm. Conversely, when the proximal epiblast is transplanted to distal regions of the embryo, it will not give rise to PGCs, and instead will form ectoderm lineages.[13] Therefore, at this stage, these cells are not yet lineage specific, as they give rise to both primordial germ cells and somatic cells, including the extraembryonic mesoderm and allantois. The first clearly recognizable population of approximately 40–60 founder germ cells is visible around 7.5 dpc in the extraembryonic mesoderm, at the base of the allantois, where they can be identified by alkaline phosphatase staining (TNAP). From these studies, it is reasonable to assume that the specification of this initial population of founder germ cells is a phenomenon that is attributable to a very specific niche that has the capacity to determine PGC fate as opposed to somatic differentiation.

Bmp4 and Bmp8b play a fundamental role during the specification of PGCs. The role of transforming growth factor-β (TGF-β) superfamily members and of BMP signaling as determinants of germ cell fate is supported by several studies.[11,14–19] Bmp4 homozygous null embryos do not form PGCs, and heterozygous embryos have fewer PGCs than wild type, due to a reduction in size of the founder population.[14] Bmp4 and Bmp8 appear to act synergistically during PGC specification, since epiblast cultures with Bmp4 and Bmp8b revealed both homodimers alone cannot induce PGCs formation, whereas they can in combination.[15] However, the homozygous mice lacking Bmp4 or Bmp8b also lack the allantois, an extraembryonic mesoderm tissue also derived from the epiblast, supporting the idea that after the initial stimulus for PGC specification, these cells have not yet completely escaped a somatic fate.

The mechanisms that prevent the PGCs from assuming a somatic cell fate remain to be clarified. Two novel genes that are unique to differentiating germ cells, *Fragilis* and *Stella*, were recently identified using dissection of the early allantois containing allantoic mesoderm, PGCs and surrounding mesoderm cells, with subsequent single cell evaluation with reverse transcription polymerase chain reaction (RT-PCR) amplification, and differential cDNA expression analysis.[20]

Fragilis belongs to the interferon-inducible transmembrane family,[21,22] and its true function remains unknown, although it has been thought that it may be involved in the formation of a conglomerate of cells through homotypic adhesion, from which the founder PGCs are recruited, therefore isolating these cells from the remaining surrounding cells destined to become somatic cells.[20] *Fragilis* is initially detected in the proximal epiblast, under the influence of Bmp4, and then in the base of the allantois, where the expression of *Stella* is initiated. Once nascent PGCs are established, expression of *Fragilis* is diminished by 8.0 dpc, freeing the PGCs from homotypic adhesion, allowing for their migration into the genital ridge.[10,23] The induction of *Fragilis* in epiblast cells may not, by itself, be sufficient for the expression of *Stella*, but it is clear that only the cells with the highest expression of *Fragilis* subsequently express *Stella*, which is expressed exclusively in lineage-restricted germ cells. *Stella*, a nuclear protein of unknown function, has an unclear role in PGCs development. However, a critical event involved in the specification of PGCs is repression of the region-specific homeobox genes. Cells that are positive for *Stella* show repression of homeobox genes, which may explain their escape from a somatic cell fate.[20]

Recent studies have demonstrated that expression of the *Oct4* gene is required for the survival of early PGCs.[24] *Oct4* is a POU domain transcription factor that has a very specific pattern of expression during embryogenesis, and it has been shown that *Oct4* may have a role in maintaining the pluripotency and germline potential of pluripotent embryonic cells. Initial studies performed in *Oct4* null mice could not evaluate the function of this gene in germ cells, because this mutation leads to a phenotype of peri-implantation lethality. However, when *Oct4* is ablated exclusively in germ cells, PGCs' maintenance is disrupted, usually starting around 10.0 dpc, as a result of massive premature apoptosis. This is a very different function in germ cells as compared to the function of *Oct4* in inner cell mass cells, mainly the maintenance of pluripotency. Nonetheless, further studies are necessary to elucidate the role of *Oct4* in PGC specification and survival.

Another gene that is involved in germ cell specification is *Blimp1*.[25] As mentioned previously, escape from a somatic fate is a fundamental step in the specification of PGCs, and repression of homeobox (Hox) genes plays an important role in this process. *Blimp1* (B-lymphocyte-induced maturation protein-1) is a gene that encodes a transcriptional repressor with an SET domain and Kruppel-type zinc fingers. Classically, *Blimp1* drives the terminal differentiation of B cells into immunoglobulin-secreting plasma cells,[26] by repressing the mature B-cell gene expression program.[27] During very early embryogenesis, *Blimp1* shows specific expression in PGCs, but not in somatic cells. Its expression precedes that of *Stella*, and only cells that express *Blimp-1* progress to express *Stella*, demonstrating that expression of *Blimp1* is the first known determinant of PGCs' specification. Indeed, *Blimp1*-deficient embryos show marked reduction in the number of PGCs.[25] Wild-type *Blimp1* embryos have PGCs that are *Blimp1*- and *Stella*-positive, and these cells showed characteristic repression of Hox genes, both *Hoxa1* and *Hoxb1*. Somatic cells that were negative for *Blimp1* also showed expression of these Hox genes. Interestingly, in *Blimp1*-deficient mutant embryos, the few *Stella*-positive PGC-like cells encountered also fail to repress Hox genes, reinforcing the notion that repression of Hox genes is temporally related to the expression of *Stella* and is a fundamental event in the early specification of PGCs. The mechanisms underlying the initiation of *Blimp1* expression in epiblast cells in still unknown. However, it is possible that repression on Hox genes in ES cells, which are also derived from the epiblast, will drive the ES cells to differentiate into germ cells.

After initial specification, the Fgf/Frfr, LIF/gp130/Jak/Stat3 and Steel/c-Kit/AKT/mTOR/Bax transduction pathways are active in migratory PGCs, promoting their growth and survival.[28] From an anatomical standpoint, it is known that PGCs start to migrate through the allantois at 8 dpc to the hindgut. From the hindgut, they move towards the gonadal ridge, reaching this area around 9.5–11 dpc. In the genital ridge, the site of the future gonad, the patterns of proliferation of male and female PGCs differ significantly and sexual differentiation depends on the expression of the *Sry* gene present on the Y chromosome.[29] In the mouse, expression of *Sry* by Sertoli cells between 11.5 and 12.5 dpc triggers the formation of a male genital ridge, where the male germ cells stop proliferating and become mitotically arrested at the prospermatogonial stage by 13.5 dpc. These male germ cells, now called gonocytes, become irreversibly committed to a spermatogenic fate by 14.5 dpc,[30] and will remain within the testis in a quiescent state until after 2 days post-birth, when they resume the cell cycle and start meiotic division, producing haploid spermatogonia. The genetics of female sexual differentiation is still a mystery, but it is known that without the expression of *Sry*, PGCs develop into female germ cells, which, after reaching the gonads, initiate the first meiotic division and become arrested at prophase of meiosis I by birth. At this stage, they become surrounded by a single layer of granulosa cells, forming primordial follicles. At puberty, under hormonal stimulation, primordial follicles are stimulated to grow, with oocytes eventually resuming meiosis in response to the midcycle surge of luteinizing hormone (LH).

The specification, growth, survival, migration and subsequent differentiation of PGCs do not happen as a result of a single event or mechanism, and how all the pathways involved in these processes interact with each other remains to be elucidated. This is not an easy task, considering the limited number of PGC precursor cells, their short lifespan in vitro and in vivo, and the lack of an appropriate culture model. Therefore, the possibility of generating germ cells and gametes in-vitro from embryonic stem cells assumes fundamental importance, because it could contribute to the resolution of some of the issues discussed above.

IN-VITRO DEVELOPMENT OF GERM CELLS

Studies on animal stem cells

Female germ cells

Despite recent advances in the understanding of the specification of germ cells in vivo, the precise mechanisms by which specification occurs remains unclear, especially in humans, where similar studies are not feasible. Recent studies revealed that cells with germ cell characteristics could be obtained in-vitro from ES cells.[6–9] These in-vitro systems of germ cell generation, and the increasing number of specific PGC markers, could help to establish the mechanisms by which germ cells are specified.

Hubner et al, in 2003, were the first to demonstrate the generation of germ-like cells and oocyte-like cells from male and female mouse ES cells.[8] In this study, ES cells were engineered to express eGFP under the control of a modified *Oct4* promoter specific to germ cells. ES cells were differentiated in monolayers and, on day 8 of culture, approximately 40% of the cells were expressing this germ line specific signal. These cells also expressed other markers of germ cell development, such as *Vasa* and *c*-kit. Upon extended culture of these ES cells, around day 12, colonies of variable size had formed, with large colonies generally exhibiting reduced GFP expression but a high percentage of *Vasa*-positive cells. Subsequently, these cells detached from the bottom of the dish and formed aggregates in the culture media. These were collected and cultured in new plates where they formed well-organized follicle-like structures over a 2-week period. Most of these structures degenerated upon further cultivation but approximately 20% of them formed oocyte-like cells. Evidence of functional somatic cell activity in these follicle-like structures was demonstrated by the presence of estradiol in the culture medium as well as by the expression of genes involved in steroidogenesis. Around day 26 of culture, oocyte-like cells were released from the follicle-like structures and were found floating in the culture media. These oocyte-like cells were enveloped by a coat resembling the zona pellucida and showed molecular markers of meiosis. Subsequently, these oocyte-like cells appeared to undergo spontaneous parthenogenesis, leading to the formation of blastocyst-like structures.

Lacham-Kaplan et al[31] subsequently reported that when mouse ES cells were allowed to differentiate using the embryoid bodies (EBs) technique, a method that resembles the early embryo environment, with the EBs being subsequently cultured in the presence of conditioned media collected from testicular cell cultures prepared from the testes of newborn males, they developed into ovarian-like structures which contained oocyte-like cells. These oocyte-like cells were surrounded by one or two layers of flattened cells resembling granulosa cells, but were not enveloped by a visible zona pellucida. However, these putative oocytes did express zona pellucida-related genes such as *Fig1-α* and *Zp3*. The authors noted that when they attempted to replicate the differentiation process employed by Hubner et al[8] using fetal calf serum, they were unsuccessful, but when they used conditioned medium from testicular cell cultures, the putative oocytes were formed. Since the testis is rich in numerous growth factors such as Bmp4, stem cell factor (SCF), leukemia inhibitory factor (LIF), β-fibroblast growth factor (β-FGF), growth differentiation factor 9 (GDF9) and many others,[32] the authors suggested that these growth factors were responsible for the transformation of ES cells into gametes.

More recently, Dyce et al[33] reported the potential of adult stem cells to differentiate into the germ line, when they showed that porcine fetal skin stem cells were able to differentiate into cells with characteristics of oocytes.[33] In this study, 'floating spheres' of stem cells from fetal porcine skin were cultured in monolayers, and induced to form germ cells in medium supplemented with porcine follicular fluid. After initial differentiation, *Oct4* expression was turned off by day 4, resuming expression again by day 10 of differentiation. Differentiated cells also expressed markers of PGCs, such as *Dazl, Gdf9b* and *Vasa*. Colony structures started to form in culture from approximately day 20 of differentiation. At days 30–40, some of these colonies detached from the dish, and formed cell aggregates in suspension. With subsequent 10–15 days, some of these aggregates appear to contain a large cell, resembling the cumulus–oocyte complex inside a follicle. These structures were then transferred into oocyte-growth medium containing gonadotropins, and after 5–10 days of culture, 12–35% of the aggregates extruded large cells with an oocyte-like morphology. These oocyte-like cells expressed transcripts for *c-Mos, Zp3, Zp1* and *Scp3*, all markers for oocytes. Evidence that steroidogenesis was active in these follicle-like structures was obtained by the detection of estradiol and progesterone in the culture media. Furthermore, RT-PCR was used to detect *P450arom* and *FSH* receptor expression in these cells. As reported by Hubner et al,[8] some of these oocyte-like cells underwent spontaneous parthenogenesis and formed embryo-like structures.

Male germ cells

Toyooka et al reported the derivation of sperm-like cells from mouse ES cells.[7] ES cells were initially transfected with vectors in which the promoter of the mouse vasa homologue (*mvh*), a germ cell-specific gene, was driving the expression of GFP or *lac*Z to allow the tracking of PGCs. Subsequently, ES cells were cultured either in monolayers or allowed to form EBs in suspension, in either the presence or absence of LIF, which acts to keep the ES cells in the undifferentiated stage. When the cells were cultured as EBs and in the absence of LIF, GFP- or *lac*Z-positive cells were identified around day 3 of differentiation. GFP- or *lac*Z-positive cells were purified by flow cytometry from dissociated EBs and examined to confirm their germ cell characteristics, by immunocytochemical staining with anti-MVH, -germ cell nuclear antigen 1 (GCNA1) and -synaptonemal complex 3 (SYCP3) antibodies. Interestingly, when the transfected ES cells were co-cultured with BMP4-producing M15 cells, the number of PGC-like cells increased in culture. Purified cells were then co-cultured with gonadal cells and transplanted under a host testis and in 6–8 weeks the transplants had formed testicular tubules separate from the host tubules, and ES cell-derived *lac*Z-positive cells were detected inside these tubules. Finally, there were mature sperm in the lumen of these tubules.

Geijsen et al demonstrated PGC and gamete formation from mouse ES cells.[6] In this study, ES cells were also allowed to form EBs in suspension; after they had undergone differentiation for 7–10 days, the cells were sorted, based on the presence of the surface antigen SSEA1, a marker of pluripotent ES cells that is also expressed by germ cells. Culture of ES cells engineered with an *Oct4*-GFP plasmid in the presence of retinoic acid, which promotes differentiation of ES cells while stimulating proliferation of germ cells, helped to sort out if the SSEA1-positive cells derived from EBs were in fact PGCs. To further characterize these cells as germ cells, SSEA1-positive cells were isolated from EBs and cultured in the presence of retinoic acid for 7 days. Individual retinoic acid-resistant colonies were isolated and expanded in the presence of LIF, SCF and basic fibroblast growth factor (bFGF), factors shown to support the derivation of germ cells. The methylation status of the differentially methylated region 2 (DMR2) of the *Igf2r* gene was analyzed in these individual colonies and found to have imprint erasure, a specific characteristic of germ cell development. If the EBs were cultured for longer periods of time, round spermatid-like cells were identified and isolated using FE-J1 antibody, which specifically recognizes male meiotic germ cells in the late pachytene spermatocyte and round spermatid stages. This purified cell population was enriched for haploid cells, and when injected into metaphase II oocytes led to the formation of blastocysts.

Differentiation of human embryonic stem cells into germ cells

The first evidence that human ES cells could also differentiate into germ cell-like cells came from Clark et al in 2004.[9] They compared the transcriptional profile of three pluripotent human ES cell lines after differentiation into EBs. Initially, they examined the expression of ES cell genes and/or germ cell-specific genes in undifferentiated ES cells. It was observed that these three lines expressed *Gdf3, Nanog* and *Stella*. In addition, they observed the expression of early premeiotic germ cell-specific genes *Dazl, c-Kit, Nanos1, Pum1* and *Pum2* in these cells. Immunoblot analysis and immunohistochemistry studies confirmed the presence of PUM2, OCT4, NANOS1 and DAZL proteins in these undifferentiated ES cells. When the ES cells were allowed to differentiate into EBs they started to observe the expression of the genes *Vasa, Sycp1, Sycp3, Gdf9* and *Tkt1* that are specific to postmeiotic germ cells, suggesting the onset of more mature gonocytes in these cultures. Interestingly, markers of both male and female germ cells were found, regardless of the sex chromosome complement (XX or XY) of the cell lineages.

CURIOSITY OR BREAKTHROUGH?

The findings from all of these studies suggest the potential of ES cells to differentiate in vitro into germ cells, and subsequent manipulation of these putative germ cells has shown that they can undergo meiosis and form haploid gametes, opening new and exciting possibilities for the study of the development of this lineage.

The efficiency of ES cell differentiation into different cell lineages varies significantly, with neuroectoderm, hematopoietic, vascular and cardiac lineages being relatively easy to obtain, whereas hepatocytes and pancreatic cells are considerably more difficult.[5] These studies demonstrated that the development of oocytes and sperm was not very efficient and, at least in the case where oocytes were generated, the process was unpredictable and most of the oocytes formed either degenerated or underwent spontaneous parthenogenesis. If these oocytes are to be used for assisted reproductive techniques or somatic cell nuclear transfer, it is imperative to block these processes. Furthermore, it is still necessary to demonstrate that these oocyte-like cells can be fertilized and are able to develop into normal progeny. Equally, the fertilization potential of the ES cell-derived sperm that was reported by Toyooka et al was not evaluated. Although Geijsen et al did demonstrate that the spermatid-like cells that were obtained were able to provide a haploid DNA complement for oocytes by intracytoplasmic sperm injection and form blastocysts, it is unclear if these blastocysts were normal and could lead to normal progeny. Other important questions are related to the epigenetic status of these in-vitro-generated gametes. Do they undergo normal meiosis and do they carry the correct maternal or paternal imprinting pattern?

An interesting finding from these studies is that the germ cell-like cells were produced in vitro from ES cells in a much shorter period of time than they are generated in vivo. This observation could be explained by some currently available theories that have hypothesized that ES cells and embryonic germ cells are part of related families of pluripotent cell lines.[34] Therefore, it is possible that there is a group of founder cells, already committed to the germ cell lineage within the initial population of apparently ‘undifferentiated’ ES cells, and this could explain the shortened differentiation process. Alternatively, and perhaps much more intriguing, the requirements of the in-vitro process for germ cell/gametes formation may not be entirely the same as the ones required for in-vivo development.

Finally, such in-vitro differentiation would potentially be more effective if culture conditions were developed to direct the ES cells to differentiate into the germ line and necessary supporting somatic cell components alone. With applications in regenerative and transplantation medicine in mind, this would theoretically prevent the risk of transplanting impure cell populations that would still retain pluripotent potential that could lead to the formation of teratomas. For the most part, these studies did not attempt to direct differentiation into the germ line alone and it is reasonable to consider that other cell lineages were present in these cultures as well.

Consequently, much work still needs to be done to improve the efficiency of ES cell entry into a germ line fate in vitro and the subsequent formation of normal gametes.

FUTURE DIRECTIONS FOR THE IN-VITRO DERIVATION OF GERM CELLS

Directed embryonic stem cell differentiation and stem cell 'niches'

The ability to direct the differentiation of ES cells into the germ line may provide a better system to generate oocytes and sperm in vitro. It is reasonable to hypothesize that if we could replicate the in-vivo process that allows induction of PGCs, we could potentially direct the ES cells to differentiate into PGCs. Clearly, many growth factors have been identified that are critical for PGC specification, including BMP2, BMP4 and BMP8B, all members of the TGF-β family. These growth factors signal through activation of the intracellular SMAD proteins and modulate the transcriptional program of the cell.[35] For example, addition of BMP4 to primary cultures of epiblast cells before the onset of gastrulation augmented the subsequent formation of PGCs.[36] Therefore, addition of these growth factors to current culture systems could be used experimentally to test the hypothesis that they would augment the formation of ES cell-derived PGCs. While ES cell differentiation remains for the most part a spontaneous process, this and other approaches should be employed to direct the differentiation into germ cells.

There are three different mechanisms that could potentially explain the in-vitro derivation of PGCs seen in both monolayer and EBs cultures:

(1) ES cells may differentiate first into an intermediate epiblast-like state.

(2) ES cells could differentiate directly into PGCs.

(3) Undifferentiated ES cells may contain a subpopulation of cells that are already committed to the germ cell lineage.

Taking this into account, and considering that the in-vivo effects of BMP4 are mainly exerted over the proximal epiblast, it is possible that the in-vitro formation of germ cells from ES cells does depend on BMP4 stimulation, but this effect was only observed when the EB technique is employed, perhaps because EBs could produce the necessary environment for an initial differentiation of the ES cells into the intermediate epiblast-like state. It is possible that these requirements may be different for ES cell differentiation into male or female germ cells.

After specification, PGCs must associate with surrounding somatic cells, which are thought to provide the signals for their subsequent development. This brings to light the issue of an appropriate somatic cell niche for the proper PGC development. In female gonads, PGCs must associate with pre-granulosa cells to form primordial follicles. Normal sperm development requires supportive Sertoli cells. The processes of normal oogenesis and spermatogenesis follow an endocrine-regulated developmental program that features the transformation of undifferentiated diploid cells into highly differentiated haploid cells. In the female gonad, association of PGCs with pre-granulosa cells seems to be dependent on the activity of estradiol, which promotes the development of gap junctions between these two cell types.[37] Many factors appear to promote the transition of primordial to primary follicles, including LIF, GDF9, kit-ligand, bFGF and BMP7.[38,39] Finally, it is well documented that the gonadotropins follicle-stimulating hormone (FSH) and LH are critical for inducing growth and development of primary follicles into mature follicles containing oocytes that are competent for maturation and subsequent fertilization. In the male gonad, the differentiation of germ cells into spermatozoa occurs in the tubular seminiferous epithelium and depends on a complex paracrine crosstalk with Sertoli cells. Testosterone secreted by Leydig cells under the influence of LH and FSH, acting on Sertoli cells, stimulates gene transcription and the secretion of growth factors and peptides that promotes germ cell differentiation.[40] All of the factors mentioned above could theoretically be tested for their ability to optimize the development of fertilization-competent oocytes and sperm from ES cells. Potential approaches would be the addition of these factors directly to 'fortify' the culture media currently used in the differentiation experiments, or the development of new culture systems, for example using granulosa cells or Sertoli cells as feeder layers. It is also important to highlight that most experiments to date have serum-containing media. Besides problems related to batch-to-batch variability, serum contains a number of unspecified components, which creates an important confounding factor when one is testing the addition of specific factors in order to select potential inducing agents. Therefore, the use of serum-free media seems to be more appropriate to develop a system that would allow directed differentiation of ES cells.

Despite the concrete evidence that these factors are important for germ cell specification and development in-vivo, their use to direct ES cell differentiation into the germ cell lineage presents formidable challenges. BMP4, for example, has been shown to support self-renewal of ES cells by inhibiting the mitogen-activated protein (MAP) kinase pathway,[41] potentially hindering its use as an inducer of germ cell differentiation. Moreover, it has been observed that BMP4-producing feeder cells lack an addictive effect on primary cultures of epiblast tissue.[15] Interestingly, as reported by Toyoka et al, when EBs were allowed to form in mixed aggregates with BMP4-producing cells, the observed number of PGCs formed increased significantly as compared to EBs either cultured in suspension alone or in aggregation with trophoblast cells that do not produce BMP4.[7] In addition, no PGC formation was observed when BMP4 was added to a suspension culture or when the ES cells were cultured as a monolayer using BMP4-producing feeder cells. Therefore, it appears that the addition of specific inductive factors to change the conditions in which the ES cells are cultured will have to respect not only a temporal pattern in which the balance has shifted from self-renewal towards differentiation but also respect unique structural configurations, both allowing for the formation of intermediate cell types that are competent to respond to the inducing effects of these factors.

Nonetheless, our own laboratory has found some of these factors to be important during preferential XY ES cell differentiation towards the male germ line. For example, murine XY ES cells were allowed to form EBs in suspension and retinoic acid, testosterone and FSH were added alone or in combination to these cultures. Assessment of germ cell and/or gamete formation was done by using quantitative real-time RT-PCR (QPCR) to determine the relative expression levels of a panel of genes that are sequentially and preferentially expressed at different stages of germ cell development and spermatogenesis, including *Piwi2, Stra8, Dazl, Msy2, Tex14, Sycp1, Sycp2, Act, Prm1* and *Prm2*. We found that retinoic acid significantly increased the expression of these genes and that testosterone selectively modified this retinoic acid effect. Furthermore, retinoic acid and testosterone worked synergistically to increase the expression of *Act*, a postmeiotic, round spermatid-specific gene. We concluded that murine XY ES cells could be coaxed by retinoic acid and testosterone to differentiate into the male germ cell lineage.[42] Recently, retinoic acid has been implicated in the regulation of sex-specific timing of meiotic initiation in mice,[43] and it has been shown that signaling by retinoic acid is required for *Stra8* expression, a gene required for the transition into meiosis in both male and female germ cells. Thus, the retinoic acid effect observed in our studies may be explained by these mechanisms. Mizuno et al[44] revealed that the formation of germ cells from ES cells in culture was affected by the glucose concentration of the medium. In low-glucose medium, the appearance of ES-derived PGCs was markedly reduced. Furthermore, they identified higher expression of genes specific to developing gonads and adult testis during in-vitro differentiation in high-glucose medium than in low-glucose medium, and they speculate that high glucose concentration promotes the differentiation of ES cells into PGCs. The studies of Lacham-Kaplan et al[31] also support the notion that one can manipulate the culture conditions to directly drive ES cells to differentiate into the germ line.

PGCs require the appropriate support of somatic cells for proper development, which characterizes the concept of 'cell niche'. The fact that oocyte- and sperm-like cells were derived from ES cells suggests that such an environment was at least partially present in-vitro, but one could speculate that certain problems encountered in these experiments, such as the low efficacy and some of the alterations seen with these oocyte-like cells generated in-vitro (lack of zona pellucida, spontaneous parthenogenesis, no recruitment of granulosa cells, etc.) could be secondary to an abnormal 'niche'. It will be important to determine if the ES cells are concomitantly being able to differentiate into the appropriate somatic cell types that are critical for normal oocyte and sperm formation, such as granulosa/theca cells and Leydig/Sertoli cells, respectively. To date, no studies have directly investigated this issue. Hubner et al[8] did demonstrate the presence of estradiol in their cultures, an indirect evidence of somatic granulosa/theca cell activity. Zhao et al[45] reported that mouse ES cells can give rise to mature gonadotrope-like cells in EBs, suggesting that they may contain the necessary factors to support gamete production.

Another important aspect pertaining to the 'appropriate niche environment' relates to the spatial distribution of the cells once they start to differentiate. Cell–cell interactions are important throughout germ cell development. From the current literature, it appears that differentiation into male germ cells is intrinsically dependent on the three-dimensional structure of EBs, since monolayer cultures were not successful.[6,7] Conversely, female germ cell differentiation appears to occur using either technique[8,31] (Figure 2.1). EBs are spherical three-dimensional structures that ES cells form when they are allowed to differentiate in suspension. When one considers their morphology, EBs offer the potential of allowing intimate intercellular contact, therefore favoring cell–cell interactions, mimicking in-vivo developmental niches.[5] This technique of ES cell differentiation has been employed to differentiate mouse ES cells into PGCs and sperm-like cells[6,7] and oocyte-like cells.[31] Interestingly, when monolayer cultures were employed, there was no successful differentiation into sperm-like cells.[7] In Hubner et al's studies, oocyte-like cells were obtained after extended culture of mouse ES cells in monolayers.[8] Although the EBs offer the advantage of a three-dimensional environment, they also allow for the differentiation of many other cell types within the same structure, and it is not easy to dissect the interaction of all the signals and cell types produced. Two-dimensional co-culture with feeder layers that provide the necessary elements involved in germ cell specification and differentiation may also lead to the formation of other cell types, since these feeder layers can also produce other unspecified, undesired factors. Furthermore, the apparently important three-dimensional spatial distribution is lost with this system. An alternative approach would be to use synthetic three-dimensional models,[46–48] as an attempt to reduce the complexity of the EBs approach and the drawbacks of the co-culture systems. These models usually use inert and known substrates, minimizing the influence of undesired neighboring cells and supportive stromal cells, and, using such a system, one could attempt to identify the specific components and pathways involved in germ cell specification and differentiation, and hopefully direct the ES cells to differentiate only into PGCs and gametes by specifically controlling the factors that are important in this process.

The development of an appropriate niche for the differentiation of ES cells into germ cells assumes an even more important aspect when one considers the potential to form teratomas, a property that is inherent in ES cells. It is important to point out that ES cells are not usually found in adult mammalian organisms. They are encountered in several different tissues, such as bone marrow and testis, are already committed to a specific lineage, and the absence of undifferentiated cells in adult tissues could be part of a defense mechanism against abnormal cell differentiation and subsequent tumor formation. The microenvironment of developing germ cells is very tightly regulated and sensitive to hormones and paracrine factors, and the differentiation of germ cells into mature gametes spans prolonged periods of time, allowing for gradual down-regulation of genes that maintain pluripotency, and up-regulation of genes that have specific functions in germ cell and gamete biology. Disturbances in this microenvironment may change this balance, leading to the formation of germ cells and gametes that would still retain pluripotent potential. This could have fundamental implications for the possible application of ES cells in therapeutic tissue regeneration, as transplantation of ES-derived cells into an adult organism could potentially lead to cancer.[49]

Are adult stem cells, theoretically already committed to a specific cell lineage, able to 'trans-differentiate' or de-differentiate and form tissues belonging to different cell lineages? The studies performed by Dyce et al[33] shed light on this question. The authors describe three possible mechanisms by which the skin-derived stem cells are capable of differentiation into oocyte-like cells:

- PGCs could be lost during migration, and reside in skin tissue, where they would retain their germ cell potential;
- the fate of PGCs is not yet determined at the fetal developmental stage;
- somatic stem cells may still have the intrinsic machinery necessary to form germ cells.[33]

These are intriguing issues, and other reports have described the presence of germline stem cells in the postnatal mammalian ovary.[50] If somatic stem cells can in fact generate competent, normal oocytes in vitro, such techniques will have an enormous impact on the field, in particular if human somatic stem cells possess the same ability.

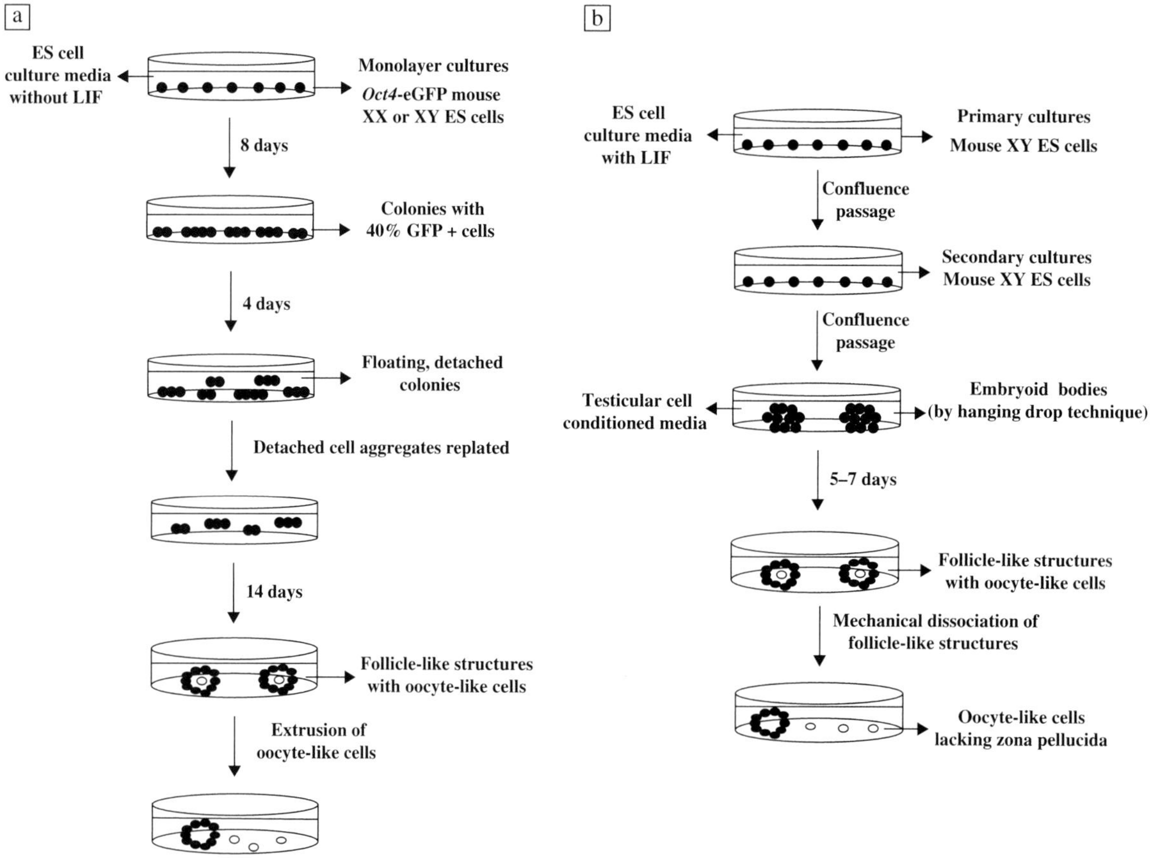

Figure 2.1 Overview of the different protocols used for the differentiation of germ cells from stem cells. (a) Hubner et al[8] employed ES cells engineered to express GFP under the control of *Oct4*. Cells were cultured in monolayers, and after a few days approximately 40% of the cells were expressing GFP. Aggregates formed and detached from the plates around day 12. These aggregates were collected, and replated. In 2 weeks, they observed the formation of follicle-like structures containing oocyte-like cells. (b) Lacham-Kaplan et al[31] used mouse male ES cells. When these cells were allowed to form embryoid bodies using the 'hanging drop' technique in testicular cell conditioned media, they observed the formation of follicle-like structures in 5–7 days. These structures were mechanically dissociated and released oocyte-like cells. (c) Dyce et al[33] employed porcine fetal skin cells. These cells were cultured in monolayers in media supplemented with porcine follicular fluid. In approximately 30–40 days, colonies detached from the plate, and in 2 weeks they formed follicle-like structures. These were replated, and cultured with oocyte growth medium containing gonadotropins. In 5–10 days, they observed extrusion of oocyte-like cells. (d) Tooyoka et al[7] were able to observe production of germ-like cells after they cultured mouse ES cells engineered to express GFP or lacZ under the control of *mvh* within embryoid bodies. After co-culture with gonadal cells, these *mvh*-GFP positive cells were transplanted and engrafted in host testis capsules. (e) Geijsen et al[6] differentiated mouse ES cells using the embryoid bodies technique, and were able to isolate potential germ-like cells by SSEA1 antibody sorting, and the addition of retinoic acid (RA) and growth factors to drive germ-like cells expansion. The were also able to isolate haploid, round spermatid-like cells by using the FE-J1 antibody. This purified haploid cell population was used to inject oocytes, and fertilization was accomplished with the generation of blastocysts

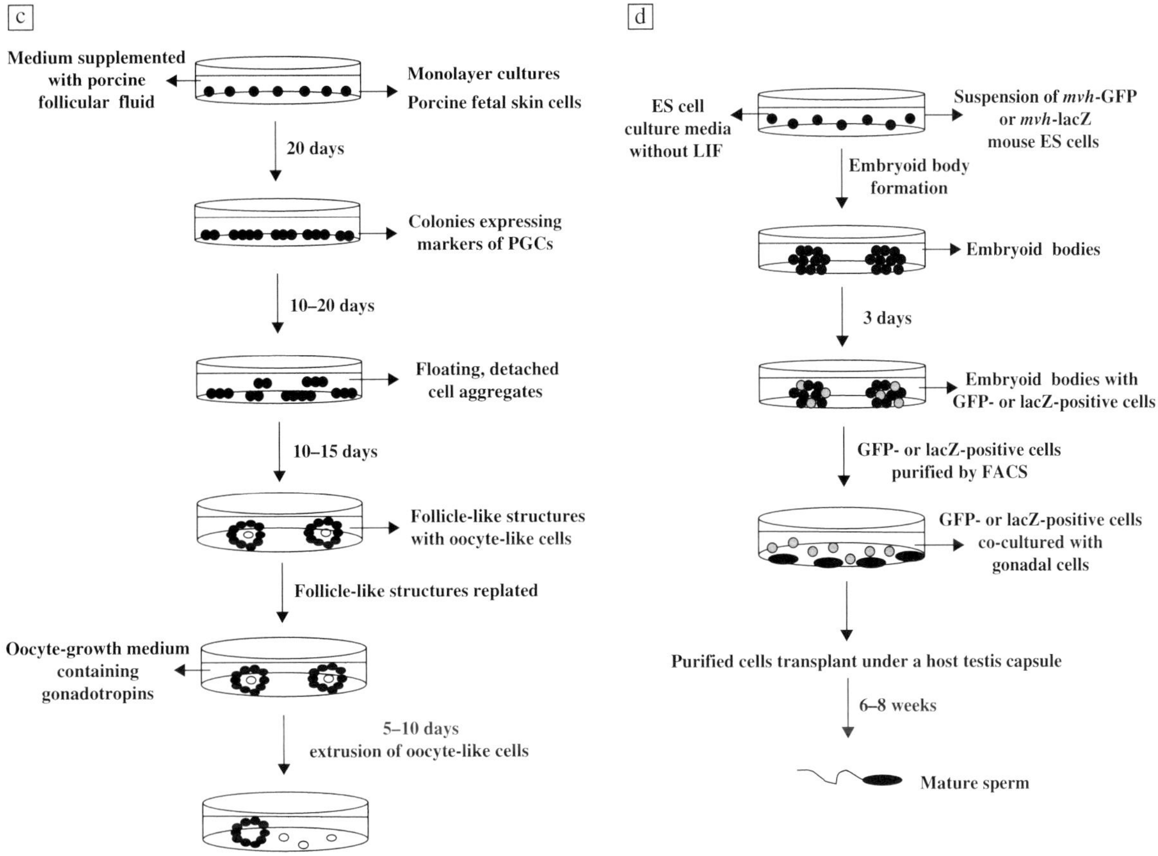

Figure 2.1 (*Continued*)

Identifying specific differentiated cell types: a major challenge

One of the most challenging aspects of the production of germ cells and gametes from ES cells has been the accurate identification of these cells once they have differentiated. Since ES cells and PGCs share the expression of many transcription factors and cell surface receptors, this task is difficult, and different approaches have been used in recent studies to overcome this problem. Early PGCs can be distinguished from ES cells and epiblast cells by their differential expression of *Oct4* transgenes containing germ cell-specific regulatory elements. This is possible because the expression of *Oct4* in ES cells, epiblast and PGCs relies on different promoter elements providing a means for identification of these different cell populations. Detection of postmigratory PGC markers such as *mvh* has also been used to demonstrate the presence of these cells and to isolate them from cultures of ES cells. In common, these methods targeted the identification of germ cells; subsequently, different culturing systems or transplantation methods were employed to assess further formation of gametes. Another approach that could be explored is the engineering of ES cells with transgenes that would express fluorescent reporters under the control of female or male germ cell-specific promoters. This system theoretically would allow the identification of mature gametes formed in culture and would facilitate their extraction from the cultures for further manipulation.

Our laboratory has been investigating the feasibility of two such systems. We generated an XY ES cell and an XX ES line that stably express promoter constructs driving the expression of fluorescent proteins that are male or female germ cell-specific, or which are expressed in associated somatic cells. These include *Acrosin*-GFP + *Pf20*-DsRed and *Gdf9*/GFP + *Sf-1*/DsRed,

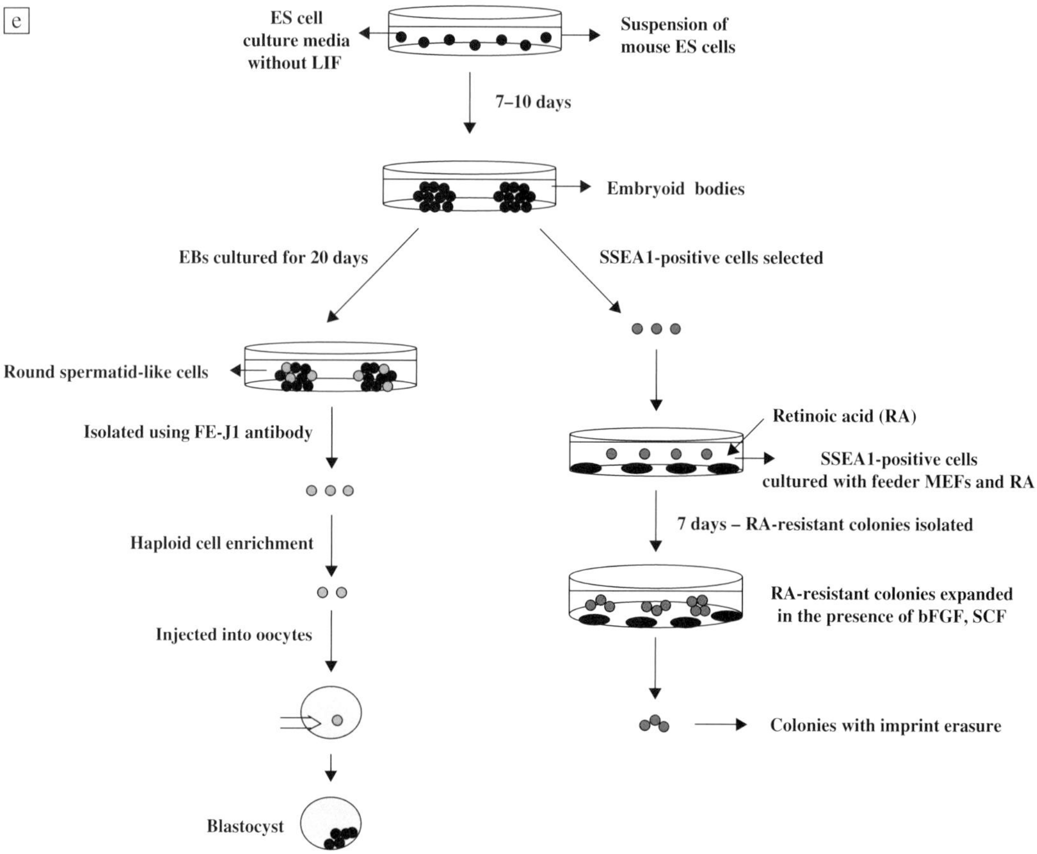

Figure 2.1 (*Continued*)

respectively. *Acrosin* and *Pf20* are sperm-specific markers expressed during the late stages of spermatogenesis,[51,52] *Gdf9* is an oocyte-specific marker expressed at the beginning of the primary follicle stage[53] and *Sf-1* is a marker normally expressed in steroidogenic cells of the ovaries (both theca and granulosa cells).[54] The promoter regions incorporated into these constructs induced appropriate cell-specific expression in transgenic animals (Figure 2.2).

When the ES cells are allowed to differentiate, these fluorescent reporter systems employing the *Acrosin*, *Pf20* and *Gdf9* promoters will serve as an in-vivo marker of the cells differentiating to become either a sperm or an oocyte, while the *Sf-1* construct serves as a marker for the somatic cells that usually surround the germ cells. In fact, when the XX ES cell line expressing GFP under the control of the *Gdf9* promoter was allowed to differentiate in monolayers in the presence of LIF, we observed the presence of GFP-positive cells with an oocyte-like morphology enclosed in a coat resembling the zona pellucida (Figure 2.3). QPCR was used to demonstrate that these cells expressed a number of germ cell- and oocyte-specific genes, including *Msy2, Gdf9, Fig1-α, Zp1, Zp2* and *Zp3.* Immunoblot analysis has confirmed expression of some of these proteins. Moreover, presumptive evidence of meiosis was obtained by demonstrating the expression of *Sycp1* and *Sycp3*.[55]

Once established successfully, these in-vitro models of generation of PGCs and gametes from ES cells create new opportunities to identify the biochemical factors that contribute to the unique niche needed to support germ cell specification and gametogenesis as well as the exploration of the function of germ cell-specific genes, an exercise which often requires the expensive and laborious creation of transgenic animals.

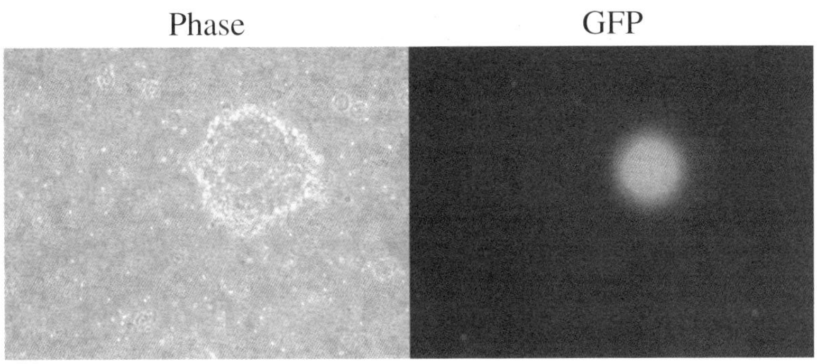

Figure 2.2 In-vivo expression of GFP in oocytes. Mouse ES cells transfected with a *Gdf9*/GFP plasmid were injected into blastocyst stage embryos, which were then subsequently transferred into host females. The mice that resulted were analyzed for agouti coat color and scored for percent of chimerism. Chimeric founders were then sacrificed and the oocyte–cumulus cell complexes were analyzed. This figure shows both GFP and phase-contrast images of such a complex. (See also color plate)

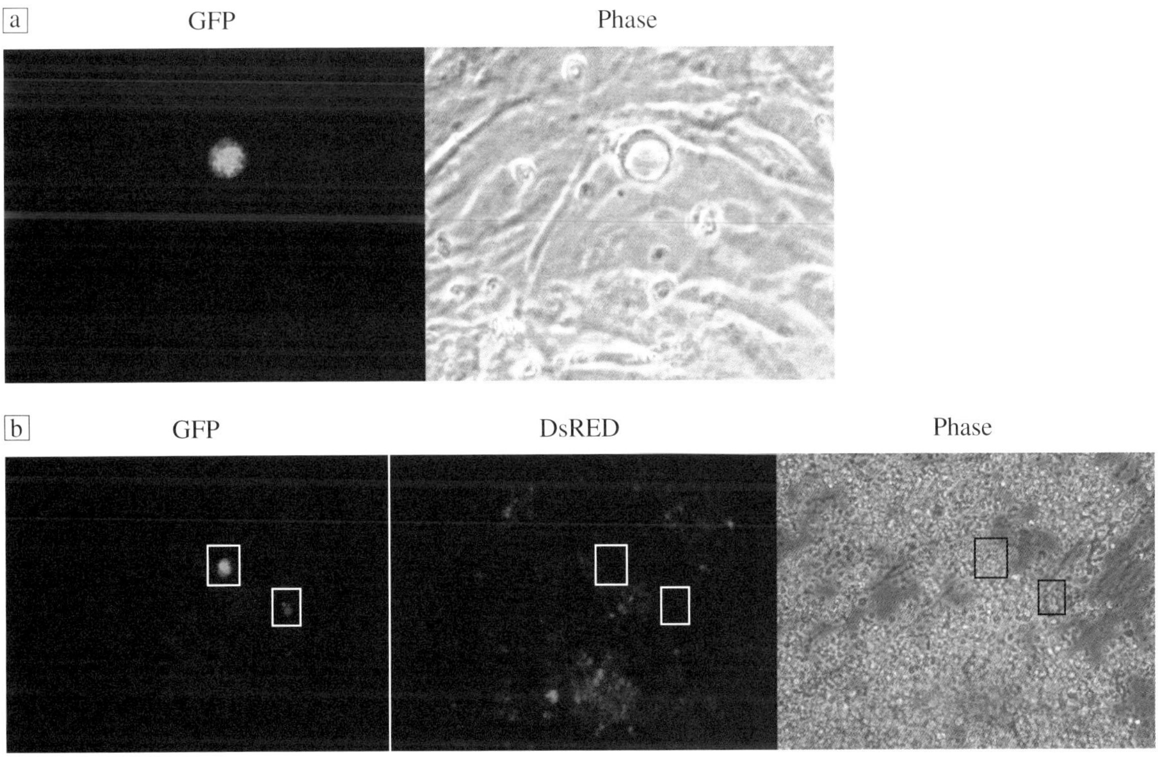

Figure 2.3 In-vitro expression of GFP and Ds-Red in transfected mouse ES cells. ES cells electroporated with *Gdf9*/GFP (M. Matzuk) and *Sf-1*/DsRed plasmids were selected for these constructs using G418 for 8 days. Screened clones were confirmed by PCR and Southern blot analysis. Positive ES cell clones were then cultured in the presence of LIF. Cells were examined for expression of GFP and DsRed by fluorescence microscopy (a) GFP and phase contrast images on day 2 of culture. (b) GFP, DsRed and phase contrast images on day 8 of culture. (See also color plate)

CONCLUSIONS

The fact that ES cells can contribute to the germ line in vivo supports the idea that they should also be able to differentiate into this lineage in vitro. Although still at an early stage, these studies can facilitate the understanding of reproductive development. Furthermore, the potential to generate an unlimited supply of gametes from ES cells provides a new approach for their use in assisted reproduction.

However, many obstacles must be overcome if we are to realize the potential of these studies. The development of culture conditions that would fully replicate the biochemical attributes of gametes is a very important topic, as it is the establishment of methods that would properly identify, enrich and purify the desired differentiated cell population. Furthermore, appropriate culture conditions could contribute to an increase in the method's efficiency.

It will be imperative to demonstrate the developmental capacity of these gametes and, to date, there is no published evidence for competency of in-vitro produced gametes from ES cells by documenting generation of viable offspring. Moreover, gametogenesis in vitro has only been observed in the murine system and the ability of human ES cells to form gametes in vitro remains to be demonstrated, an important point due to the inherent and fundamental differences between these two species. Moreover, it will be important to demonstrate that gametes developed in-vitro possess the correct imprinting characteristics, and undergo timely X-inactivation.

Finally, if we are going to continue with these lines of investigation, attention should be given to the ethical guidelines of this research. Generation of gametes in vitro will most certainly lead to the generation of embryos from these in-vitro formed gametes and such an accomplishment will for sure lead to moral debates.

Acknowledgments

The authors would like to acknowledge the contributions to this chapter made by Igor Kostetskii, Jennifer Wood, Glen Radice and Carmen Williams. In addition, the authors would like to thank their colleagues for generously providing the following materials: Gdf9/GFP construct (Martin Matzuk), *Sf-1*/DsRed construct (Keith Parker). This work was supported by grants from: NIH Grant T32 – HD 040135, NIH Grant T32 – HD 007305, NIH PO1 HD 06274 and the Pennsylvania Department of Health.

REFERENCES

1. Evans MJ, Kaufman MH. Establishment in culture of pluripotential cells from mouse embryos. Nature 1981; 292: 154–6.
2. Thomson JA, Itskovitz-Eldor J, Shapiro SS et al. Embryonic stem cell lines derived from human blastocysts. Science 1998; 282: 1145–7.
3. Nagy A, Gocza E, Diaz EM et al. Embryonic stem cells alone are able to support fetal development in the mouse. Development 1990; 110: 815–21.
4. Tam PP, Rossant J. Mouse embryonic chimeras: tools for studying mammalian development. Development 2003; 130: 6155–63.
5. Keller G. Embryonic stem cell differentiation: emergence of a new era in biology and medicine. Genes Dev 2005; 19: 1129–55.
6. Geijsen N, Horoschak M, Kim K et al. Derivation of embryonic germ cells and male gametes from embryonic stem cells. Nature 2004; 427: 148–54.
7. Toyooka Y, Tsunekawa N, Akasu R, Noce T. Embryonic stem cells can form germ cells in vitro. Proc Natl Acad Sci USA 2003; 100: 11457–62.
8. Hubner K, Fuhrmann G, Christenson LK et al. Derivation of oocytes from mouse embryonic stem cells. Science 2003; 300: 1251–6.
9. Clark AT, Bodnar MS, Fox M et al. Spontaneous differentiation of germ cells from human embryonic stem cells in vitro. Hum Mol Genet 2004; 13: 727–39.
10. Wylie C. Germ cells. Cell 1999; 96: 165–74.
11. Ying Y, Zhao GQ. Cooperation of endoderm-derived BMP2 and extraembryonic ectoderm-derived BMP4 in primordial germ cell generation in the mouse. Dev Biol 2001; 232: 484–92.
12. Lawson KA, Hage WJ. Clonal analysis of the origin of primordial germ cells in the mouse. Ciba Found Symp 1994; 182: 68–84, discussion 84–91.
13. Tam PP, Zhou SX. The allocation of epiblast cells to ectodermal and germ-line lineages is influenced by the position of the cells in the gastrulating mouse embryo. Dev Biol 1996; 178: 124–32.
14. Lawson KA, Dunn NR, Roelen BA et al. Bmp4 is required for the generation of primordial germ cells in the mouse embryo. Genes Dev 1999; 13: 424–36.
15. Ying Y, Qi X, Zhao GQ. Induction of primordial germ cells from murine epiblasts by synergistic action of BMP4 and BMP8B signaling pathways. Proc Natl Acad Sci USA 2001; 98: 7858–62.

16. Hayashi K, Kobayashi T, Umino T et al. SMAD1 signaling is critical for initial commitment of germ cell lineage from mouse epiblast. Mech Dev 2002; 118: 99–109.

17. Tremblay KD, Dunn NR, Robertson EJ. Mouse embryos lacking Smad1 signals display defects in extra-embryonic tissues and germ cell formation. Development 2001; 128: 3609–21.

18. Chang H, Matzuk MM. Smad5 is required for mouse primordial germ cell development. Mech Dev 2001; 104: 61–7.

19. Chu GC, Dunn NR, Anderson DC, Oxburgh L, Robertson EJ. Differential requirements for Smad4 in TGFbeta-dependent patterning of the early mouse embryo. Development 2004; 131: 3501–12.

20. Saitou M, Barton SC, Surani MA. A molecular programme for the specification of germ cell fate in mice. Nature 2002; 418: 293–300.

21. Tanaka SS, Matsui Y. Developmentally regulated expression of mil-1 and mil-2, mouse interferon-induced transmembrane protein like genes, during formation and differentiation of primordial germ cells. Mech Dev 2002; 119(Suppl 1): S261–7.

22. Lange UC, Saitou M, Western PS, Barton SC, Surani MA. The fragilis interferon-inducible gene family of transmembrane proteins is associated with germ cell specification in mice. BMC Dev Biol 2003; 3: 1.

23. Gomperts M, Garcia-Castro M, Wylie C, Heasman J. Interactions between primordial germ cells play a role in their migration in mouse embryos. Development 1994; 120: 135–41.

24. Kehler J, Tolkunova E, Koschorz B et al. Oct4 is required for primordial germ cell survival. EMBO Rep 2004; 5: 1078–83.

25. Ohinata Y, Payer B, O'Carroll D et al. Blimp1 is a critical determinant of the germ cell lineage in mice. Nature 2005; 436: 207–13.

26. Turner CA, Jr, Mack DH, Davis MM. Blimp-1, a novel zinc finger-containing protein that can drive the maturation of B lymphocytes into immunoglobulin-secreting cells. Cell 1994; 77: 297–306.

27. Shaffer AL, Lin KI, Kuo TC et al. Blimp-1 orchestrates plasma cell differentiation by extinguishing the mature B cell gene expression program. Immunity 2002; 17: 51–62.

28. McLaren A. Germ and somatic cell lineages in the developing gonad. Mol Cell Endocrinol 2000; 163: 3–9.

29. Albrecht KH, Eicher EM. Evidence that Sry is expressed in pre-Sertoli cells and Sertoli and granulosa cells have a common precursor. Dev Biol 2001; 240: 92–107.

30. Ohta H, Wakayama T, Nishimune Y. Commitment of fetal male germ cells to spermatogonial stem cells during mouse embryonic development. Biol Reprod 2004; 70: 1286–91.

31. Lacham-Kaplan O, Chy H, Trounson A. Testicular cell conditioned medium supports differentiation of embryonic stem cells into ovarian structures containing oocytes. Stem Cells 2006; 24(2): 266–73.

32. Huleihel M, Lunenfeld E. Regulation of spermatogenesis by paracrine/autocrine testicular factors. Asian J Androl 2004; 6: 259–68.

33. Dyce PW, Wen L, Li J. In vitro germline potential of stem cells derived from fetal porcine skin. Nat Cell Biol 2006; 8(4): 384–90.

34. Zwaka TP, Thomson JA. A germ cell origin of embry onic stem cells? Development 2005; 132: 227–33.

35. Chang H, Brown CW, Matzuk MM. Genetic analysis of the mammalian transforming growth factor-beta superfamily. Endocr Rev 2002; 23: 787–823.

36. Pesce M, Gioia Klinger F, De Felici M. Derivation in culture of primordial germ cells from cells of the mouse epiblast: phenotypic induction and growth control by Bmp4 signalling. Mech Dev 2002; 112: 15–24.

37. Zachos NC, Billiar RB, Albrecht ED, Pepe GJ. Developmental regulation of baboon fetal ovarian maturation by estrogen. Biol Reprod 2002; 67: 1148–56.

38. Nilsson EE, Kezele P, Skinner MK. Leukemia inhibitory factor (LIF) promotes the primordial to primary follicle transition in rat ovaries. Mol Cell Endocrinol 2002; 188: 65–73.

39. Nilsson EE, Skinner MK. Growth and differentiation factor-9 stimulates progression of early primary but not primordial rat ovarian follicle development. Biol Reprod 2002; 67: 1018–24.

40. Griswold MD. The central role of Sertoli cells in spermatogenesis. Semin Cell Dev Biol 1998; 9: 411–16.

41. Qi X, Li TG, Hao J et al. BMP4 supports self-renewal of embryonic stem cells by inhibiting mitogen-activated protein kinase pathways. Proc Natl Acad Sci USA 2004; 101: 6027–32.

42. Silva CK, Horowitz E, Leite R, Clement HO, Strauss JF. Retinoic acid-driven differentiation of mouse embryonic stem cells into male germ cells. J Soc Gynecol Investig 2005; 12(Suppl 2): 301A.

43. Koubova J, Menke DB, Zhou Q et al. Retinoic acid regulates sex-specific timing of meiotic initiation in mice. Proc Natl Acad Sci USA 2006; 103(8): 2474–9.

44. Mizuno K, Tokumasu A, Nakamura A et al. Genes associated with the formation of germ cells from embryonic stem cells in cultures containing different glucose concentrations. Mol Reprod Dev 2006; 73: 437–45.

45. Zhao X, Teng R, Asanuma K et al. Differentiation of mouse embryonic stem cells into gonadotrope-like cells in vitro. J Soc Gynecol Investig 2005; 12: 257–62.

46. Yim EK, Leong KW. Proliferation and differentiation of human embryonic germ cell derivatives in bioactive polymeric fibrous scaffold. J Biomater Sci Polym Ed 2005; 16: 1193–217.

47. Kreeger PK, Deck JW, Woodruff TK, Shea LD. The in vitro regulation of ovarian follicle development using alginate-extracellular matrix gels. Biomaterials 2006; 27: 714–23.

48. Pangas SA, Saudye H, Shea LD, Woodruff TK. Novel approach for the three-dimensional culture of granulosa cell–oocyte complexes. Tissue Eng 2003; 9: 1013–21.

49. Almstrup K, Sonne SB, Hoei-Hansen CE et al. From embryonic stem cells to testicular germ cell cancer – should we be concerned? Int J Androl 2006; 29: 211–18.

50. Johnson J, Canning J, Kaneko T, Pru JK, Tilly JL. Germline stem cells and follicular renewal in the postnatal mammalian ovary. Nature 2004; 428: 145–50.

51. Kremling H, Keime S, Wilhelm K et al. Mouse proacrosin gene: nucleotide sequence, diploid expression, and chromosomal localization. Genomics 1991; 11: 828–34.

52. Zhang Z, Kostetskii I, Moss SB et al. Haploinsufficiency for the murine orthologue of Chlamydomonas PF20 disrupts spermatogenesis. Proc Natl Acad Sci USA 2004; 101: 12946–51.

53. Dong J, Albertini DF, Nishimori K et al. Growth differentiation factor-9 is required during early ovarian folliculogenesis. Nature 1996; 383: 531–5.

54. Park SY, Meeks JJ, Raverot G et al. Nuclear receptors Sf1 and Dax1 function cooperatively to mediate somatic cell differentiation during testis development. Development 2005; 132: 2415–23.

55. Silva CS, Kostetskii I, Wood J, Strauss JF. Differentiation of mouse embryonic stem cells into oocyte like-cells in vitro. Fertil Steril 2005; 84(Suppl 1): S28.

CHAPTER 3

Stem cell support of ovary function and fertility

Joshua Johnson

INTRODUCTION

Understanding the mechanisms behind adult stem cell support of tissue function is of extreme importance when considering next-generation methods to treat damaged or diseased organs in humans. Two general translational approaches have been taken with adult stem cells in order to speed their introduction into the clinic. First, the understanding of the basal function(s) of endogenous adult stem cells has led to strategies to stimulate these cells into improved tissue support and repair. Protecting these cells from damage caused by disease – or damage caused by the treatment of disease – is a critical consideration. Secondly, adult stem cells are being coaxed to behave differently than their endogenous roles in the body. Such strategies seek to use non-essential biopsied cells to produce or protect the cells of their source organ or even completely unrelated tissues. A general paradigm for these two modes of use of stem cells may be seen in the cases of bone marrow-resident stem cells, hematopoietic stem cells (HSCs) and mesenchymal stem cells (MSCs). HSCs are routinely extracted from donors or patients themselves within bone marrow biopsies or mobilized stem cell blood products, and redelivered for therapy. More recently, attempts are being made to stimulate these cells via drug or biomolecule treatment to modulate the production of blood and other hematopoietic lineages within the clinic. Advances in the handling of both HSCs and MSCs have allowed for the directed differentiation of these cell types into cells that may contribute to peripheral organs (e.g. endothelial cells from HSCs and various stromal support cells from MSCs) (See References 1–3 for reviews.)

As evidenced by this book, stem cells are now viewed as potential therapeutic tools for the treatment of reproductive tract disease and/or infertility. This chapter considers the special case of ovarian failure in females, due to the natural loss or destruction of the pool of oocytes within the ovary. If, indeed, new oocytes are produced by stem cells during adult life by circulating progenitor cells,[4] the ovary may be a uniquely tractable model for the study of stem cell support of other organs. After all, oocytes in mammalian ovaries generally number in the few thousands in rodents and the tens of thousands in young humans, and that number only declines with advancing age. And it is relatively easy, if time consuming, to accurately measure the actual number of oocytes in the ovary at any given time or after experimental treatments.[5,6] Thus, the exact numerical contribution of a pool of stem cells to a tractable pool of differentiated cells (e.g. oocytes) can be measured. Perhaps more general mechanisms of stem cell support of other tissues will be uncovered by the study of these processes affecting oocyte number and thereby ovary function.

It has long been accepted that in mammals, all female germ cells commit to meiosis entrance and oocyte development at or soon after birth,[7,8] or are deleted via apoptosis – atresia (see Reference 9 for a review). This 'endowment' is thus a fixed pool of oocytes within follicles that are capable of maturation into fertilization-competent eggs. If women are endowed with all of their oocytes around birth, the loss of oocytes due to atresia or ovulation will inevitably and irreversibly result in ovarian failure. Ovarian failure that occurs within the fourth or fifth decade of life is considered natural menopause. Whether 'premature' or menopausal, ovarian failure has essentially been considered an untreatable condition due to the accepted notion of a fixed oocyte pool.

The question of whether stem cell technologies may be brought to bear for the generation of new human oocytes to treat ovarian failure and female infertility is for now an open one. However, some recent advances using mammalian model systems, and even analyses of human ovaries and stem cells, threaten to change the rules of how oocytes are produced both in vivo and in vitro from stem cells. First, I will introduce highlights from the historical literature supporting the dogma of a total oocyte endowment at birth. Next, I will attempt to resolve those data with conflicting modern reports that show that oocytes are or are not generated de novo after birth. Special emphasis has been placed on experimental results that address the question of whether or not oocytes are produced from extragonadal sources, e.g. the bone marrow and peripheral blood.[4,10] Last, an exciting group of contemporary manuscripts show that oocyte-like cells and sperm-like cells may be generated using embryonic and, separately, adult stem cells. There is hope that 'untreatable' ovarian failure may be addressed by the production of new functional, fertilizable, and perhaps most importantly, patient-matched oocytes at some time in the future.

OOCYTE ENDOWMENT AT BIRTH: GONADAL GERM CELL DEVELOPMENT

As mentioned, germ cell endowment in the context of the mammalian female germ line refers to a total commitment of germ cells to meiosis entrance and oocyte development at or soon after birth.[7,8] In the early mammalian embryo, the germ line starts with primordial germ cell (PGC) development.[11,12] PGCs are first detectable at e7.5 and arise via inductive origins in the proximal epiblast near the base of the allantois; signals from the extraembryonic ectoderm, including Bmp4 and Bmp8b,[11,13] are required for PGC specification. Cells in the proximal epiblast respond to those inductive signals and an increasingly restricted expression pattern of the genes *Fragilis*, and then *Stella*, result and reveal the committed PGCs.[11,13] During gastrulation, PGCs migrate through the posterior embryo, into the hindgut, and finally arrive at the developing gonad between e9.0 and e9.5 (see Reference 12 for a review). In females, gonadal arrival of germ cells results in a transition from PGCs into a proliferative stage, termed 'oogonia.' As an important aside here, it may be noted that in developing avian embryos during these same stages, PGCs are known to enter the peripheral circulation, and are found in the bloodstream prior to, during and after the colonization of the fetal gonad by PGCs.[14,15] Circulating chicken PGCs have directly been shown to give rise to functional gametes in adults.[14] In mammals,[16–18] it has been assumed, but not definitively proven, that all primordial germ cells that do not engraft within the gonad are fated for death via apoptosis.

Beginning at day 13.5, germ cells that have entered the ovary undergo a regulated entrance into meiosis that involves interconnected nests of oogonia (Reference 19; see Reference 20 for a review) interacting with ovarian somatic cells. The nests eventually break down, leaving so-called primordial follicles consisting of an oocyte and its surrounding pregranulosa somatic cells.[21] Meiosis entrance and follicle formation proceed as a 'major wave' across the ovary that begins at day 13.5 postcoitum (dpc) and is completed just after birth as all gonadal germ cells have entered prophase-I arrest.[22] While little is known about the control of the timing of this wave, meiosis entrance and follicle formation define an irreversible transition of mitotic oogonia into oocytes that are committed to the completion of meiosis. As we will see below, it is meiosis entrance that is the key determinant for the detection of the production of new oocytes. The early stages of meiosis are easily recognized in histological preparations, and the rarity of ovarian germ cells in these stages in most postnatal mammals made it difficult to understand how new oocytes could be formed after birth.[23,24]

Overlaid onto these developmental stages is the apoptotic loss of oogonia and oocytes, known as atresia, initiated around 15 dpc and continuing throughout life both at baseline levels and in response to environmental insults.[9] Also, as mentioned, the loss of oocytes beneath a threshold level results in menopause or, if during reproductive years, premature ovarian failure.[9] Those few oocytes that survive to ovulate have completed an elaborate program of oocyte and somatic cell maturation and growth that results in the production of fertilization-competent eggs.

THE DOGMA OF A TOTAL ENDOWMENT OF OOCYTES AT BIRTH: OOGONIA AND MEIOTIC ENTRY

Sir Solomon Zuckerman's book *The Ovary*[24,25] is still the gold standard for information on the comparative function of the female gonad across the animal kingdom, and especially within mammals. *The Ovary* bound together several key investigations into the nature and timing of oogenesis, instigated by the question: 'Is oogenesis on a par with spermatogenesis as a process continuing throughout reproductive life?'[24] Zuckerman and colleagues highlight the anatomist Wilhelm Waldeyer's 1870 monograph *Eierstock und Ei* (*Ovary and Egg*)[23] and its support of a total endowment of oocytes at birth in both adult mammals and birds. The stages and histological features of oogenesis within the ovary were quite well described by Waldeyer's time, and it was known that female gonadal germ cells pass through a mitotic 'oogonial' phase prior to a coordinated entrance into the characteristic stages that we call meiosis. Waldeyer felt keenly that neo-oogenesis could only occur if oogonia persisted in the adult ovary. To Waldeyer, the absence of oogonia and the succeeding stages of meiosis in adult ovaries meant that oocyte production had ceased around birth.

As recently as 1962, Sir Solomon Zuckerman had presented both sides of the debate, conceding that neo-oogenesis in adult life was 'the majority view of [that] day.'[25] Zuckerman cited an influential study performed by the American Edgar Allen in which histological evidence was interpreted to show that new oocytes are formed in the cortex of the ovary in waves that correspond to the estrous cycle.[26] Allen concluded that 400–500 new oocytes are produced in adult females during each estrous cycle, with the highest number of immature oocytes seen in metestrus/diestrus, and the lowest numbers observed during estrus. Similar findings, showing fluctuating numbers of oocytes within rodent estrous cycles, were reported by others.[27,28] However, Zuckerman surveyed these studies and others and concluded that in each case, the sample size was either too small or other experimental design flaws rendered the data uninterpretable.[24,25] Even so, modern histomorphometric measurements of the number of immature follicles across the estrous cycle[4] closely correspond to those generated in Allen's study. But what of a scenario where new follicle production occurs at a rate that is slightly less than that of follicle death and clearance? The follicle pool would then appear to be either static or slowly declining, and would deceptively fit the model of total endowment at birth. Figure 3.1 is a cartoon showing oocyte number as depicted by 'drips' of liquid exiting and, in the case of oocyte replenishment, entering buckets that contain the oocyte reserve. Note that the net loss of oocyte 'drips' are equivalent, regardless of the responsible mechanism.

Allen's work was performed at a time when the developmental source of oocytes was controversial, and he and others[27,28] postulated that oocytes arise via a 'transformative mechanism.'[25] This mechanism was thought to consist of the direct transformation of cells in the ovary that are not oocytes (i.e. cells of

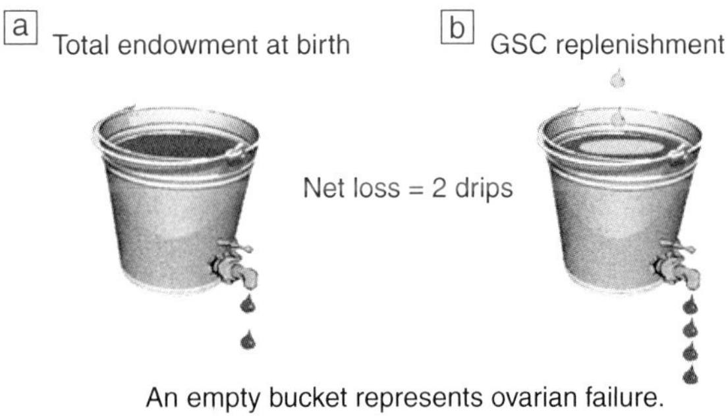

Figure 3.1 Simple cartoon representation of diminishing oocyte number over postnatal life in mammals. Here, oocyte number is represented by the level of water inside buckets. Drips of liquid from the bottom of the buckets represent oocyte loss via growth activation, ovulation, or atresia. (a) The dogma of a total endowment of oocytes at birth is represented; 2 drips have been lost. No input of new oocytes (input drips) exists. (b) A more rapid loss of oocytes (4 drips) is offset by the input of new drips. Here, input drips offset and slow the more rapid loss of liquid. Critically, the net loss of drips/oocytes is equal in both cases. Static histomorphometric analyses of oocytes within histological preparations over postnatal life (e.g. measuring the water level) would show the same trend of oocyte loss in either situation. (See also color plate)

the unfortunately named[25] germinal epithelium) into new oocytes. For obvious reasons, holding that a transformative mechanism exists required that 'an unequivocal demonstration of a consecutive series of intermediate cellular stages' be shown.[24] The Birmingham group rightfully demanded direct, stepwise evidence that the squamous/cuboidal somatic cells of the ovarian surface epithelium transform into oocytes. Interestingly, a modern proposal for a transformative mechanism of oocyte development in the human ovary was published by Bukovsky et al in 2004[29] and 2005.[30] Using histological and immunohistochemical approaches, that group proposed that bipotential progenitor cells (e.g. may produce both somatic cells of the ovary and new oocytes) exist near the surface of the human ovary in the tunica albuginea and are responsible for the production of new oocytes.[29] Also, tissue culture of cells isolated from the surface epithelium/tunica albuginea of human ovaries resulted in the apparent production of oocyte-like cells from putative progenitors.[30] Time will tell whether the models offered by Bukovsky et al are to be regarded as the start of 'unequivocal' evidence for human neo-oogenesis that has been lacking for more than 100 years.

A detailed histological study of pre- and postnatal mouse ovaries by Brambell in 1927 is featured prominently in the historical literature.[31] By that time, it was at least known that, early in development, germ cells could be found in extraembryonic tissues, especially within the yolk sac, and that these PGCs were probably migrating to the embryonic gonads. Brambell created one of the first comprehensive germ lineage tracing studies to show the direct development of migratory PGCs into ovary-resident oogonia, then oocytes. Brambell first sought to contrast his findings with earlier interpretations that germ cells arise solely in the so-called germinal epithelium. A model consisting of a combination of oocyte production by migratory PGCs and a separate, 'secondary' set of germinal epithelium-resident germ cells postulated by earlier workers[23,32] was also considered and rejected. Brambell concluded that (1) those PGCs that migrate to the gonad represent the sole source of germ cells, and (2) a total commitment to meiosis begins soon after arrival at the genital ridge and ends soon after birth. In fact, Brambell's ability to trace female germ cells from their origins to their entry into meiosis seemed to close the case upon this matter entirely. The manuscript did note that germ cells reside in the germinal epithelium of the ovary throughout life, but held that after postnatal day 4 all of these cells were dictyate oocytes.[31]

In 1961, Kirstine Borum[33] confirmed Brambell's results tracing meiotic entry by both extending previous histological analyses and by carefully categorizing the stages of meiosis in all germ cells between prenatal days 10–19 and postnatal days 1–5. Squash preparations were prepared of ovaries from these stages to score the meiotic stages. Soon afterwards, the Peters group[34] showed that those same stages of meiotic entry, as revealed by tritiated thymidine incorporation, are detectable in new oocytes of the prenatal mouse. The Peters[35] and Borum[36] groups also provided further key information in studies designed to determine the approximate length of the stages of oocyte meiotic entry during late fetal development. Meiotic oocytes were assessed in histological preparations and the timing of the stages of meiosis were reported as follows: premeiotic S phase, 10.5–12 hours; premeiotic S + G2 phase, 14 hours (in which the G2 phase is very short and may be <0.5 hours); leptotene, 3–6 hours; zygotene, 12–40 hours; and the pachytene stage lasting a minimum of 60 hours prior to the diplotene arrest. These measurements demonstrate clearly that if oocyte development is occurring postnatally, it is not occurring under the same time constraints as seen during fetal development.

JHM Pinkerton and others in 1961[37] provided what is now a common citation for a total endowment of oocytes at birth in humans. This study made use of histochemical and histological preparations of human fetal and prepubertal ovaries. The authors' conclusions regarding oocyte development and endowment were based on the apparent end of germ cell mitoses at the time of birth and the onset of atresia in developing follicles. As meiotic synapsis was never detected in the germ cells of postnatal human ovaries, those authors held that the total endowment of oocytes at birth was conserved in humans as well as lower mammals.

In the end, Zuckerman and the Birmingham group laid down a set of common 'rules' of mammalian oogenesis:

> 'In [mammals] the number of germ cells increases to a peak (usually before birth) as a result of the mitotic division of oogonia. The number then declines with increasing age due

> to cessation of mitotic divisions and to 'waves' of degeneration affecting germ cells at all stages of their development.'[38]

The Birmingham group contended that only direct histological detection of mitotic germ cells and germ cells displaying the hallmarks of the early stages of meiosis in the adult ovary would support the existence of postnatal neo-oogenesis.

POSTNATAL OOCYTE PRODUCTION IN THE MOUSE

In contrast to the concept of a total germ cell endowment at birth in mammalian females, it has been demonstrated that juvenile and adult mouse ovaries are supported by mitotically active germ cells that, based on rates of oocyte degeneration and clearance, are needed to continuously replenish the follicle pool.[39] The initial data that called a total endowment of oocytes at birth into question consisted of histomorphometric measurements of the number of healthy oocytes that exist in the ovary at different time points after birth. Strikingly, the number of total immature oocytes did not significantly decrease between postnatal days 4 and 40. Even when the number of primordial oocytes was considered separately on those days, there was no significant difference between days 4 and 40.

If a fixed pool of oocytes exists at day 4, the only possible explanation for unchanged numbers of healthy oocytes at day 40 is a lack of loss of oocytes to growth activation or atresia. We also counted the number of atretic follicles during the same time points and found that high levels of atretic follicles are seen after day 30 of life. The morphological measurement of atretic follicles is more subjective that the measurement of health follicles and our attempts to do so have been met with strong criticism from the field.[40–42] Even if the data describing follicular atresia are disregarded, the stability of healthy follicle numbers remains. As will be mentioned below, the data of Kerr et al[6] essentially replicate these findings while extending them via their impressively broad postnatal time course and their 'unbiased' assessment of healthy follicle numbers.

Further evidence for the production of new oocytes in adult life came from ovarian graft experiments. It was hypothesized that if new follicles were forming in adult life, they could be identified as mosaic follicles within grafts. Here, ovary 'halves' from wild-type adult mice were grafted to intact half-ovaries in transgenic mice that ubiquitously express green fluorescent protein. Two months after graft establishment, 'hybrid' follicles were seen in the wild-type grafts. These hybrid follicles contained green-fluorescent oocytes and endothelial cells, but wild-type granulosa and theca cells. Importantly, the reciprocal grafting experiments performed as controls resulted in the reciprocal result: wild-type oocytes within green fluorescent follicles. We interpreted those cases as representing new host-derived oocytes that formed new follicles via interaction with the somatic cells of the graft(s).

Proliferative germ cells, identifiable by their expression of the cardinal germ cell marker mouse vasa homolog (*MVH*)[43–49] concurrent with bromodeoxyuridine (BrdU) incorporation, were detected in the surface epithelium of the ovary. These cells were the original candidate sources of new oocyte production.[39] Initial measurements of the number of these cells at different times in juvenile/young adult life were compatible with the production of tens to hundreds of new oocytes per day. And it was the relatively low number of these cells in young adult mice (63 ± 8; $n = 4$ animals) that suggested that a small pool of proliferative cells were functioning as a germ stem cell population. In contrast, if the proliferative germ cells functioned as symmetrically dividing oogonia, maintenance of the oocyte pool would require hundreds, if not thousands of these cells. However, by day 40 of life, the number of germ cells found in the surface epithelium drops to 6 ± 3, $n = 5$.[4] Therefore, stem cell support of the oocyte pool by cells that reside outside of the ovary was considered as a viable hypothesis.

Highlights of the primary data and conclusions from work investigating the source of 'new' oocytes follow here. First, when approximately 80% of immature oocytes are killed by the chemotherapeutic agent doxorubicin (DOX), those dead oocytes are cleared within 24 hours of treatment. Strikingly, a significant number of new oocytes (approximately 30% of the original number of oocytes) regenerate de novo by 30 hours' post-treatment.[4] In a set of separate experiments, it was shown that application of the histone deacetylase inhibitor trichostatin A (TSA) resulted in an approximately 50% increase in the number of primordial oocytes (Reference 4, supplemental data). It is important to emphasize that if no new oocytes may be generated after birth, neither regeneration as seen in the case of DOX treatment, nor the production of new oocytes above the baseline number are possible. An intriguing possible alternative explanation has been offered in which oocytes under certain experimental treatments might alter their appearance such that they are unrecognizable as oocytes; then, after a recovery period, the characteristic appearance of oocytes is regained. Therefore, histomorphometric measurements might underestimate the actual number of oocytes under certain conditions, within a certain time frame (M Skinner, pers comm). However, this explanation does not address the outcome after TSA treatment (above) in which the number of oocytes increases above baseline.

Direct evidence of oocyte production, including evidence of meiotic entry in a large group of cells within the ovary, was lacking during these experiments. Also, the appearance of new oocytes occurred more rapidly than expected, expecially considering the timing of the fetal stages of meiotic entrance determined by Borum (above).[33] In total, these data supported the consideration of an extragonadal source of new oocytes. The results from several experiments show that the bone marrow (BM) and peripheral blood (PB) compartments contain cells capable of engrafting as oocytes in adult female mice. Transplantation studies were performed to test whether transplanted marked BM could contribute to oocyte production. Wild-type and ataxia-telangiectasia mutated gene deficient (AtmKO)[50–52] recipient female mice were treated with one of the following chemical sterilization regimens: 12 mg/kg body weight (b.w.) busulfan and 120 mg/kg b.w. Cytoxan (BuCy); or, 10 mg/kg b.w. DOX. Transplantation of BM from wild-type and transgenic (germline-specific green fluorescent protein [GFP] expressing pOct4-GFP [OG2]) donors followed. Critically, it must be noted that treatment with 10 mg/kg busulfan alone resulted in the complete loss of the primordial pool of oocytes after 20 days.[39] Delivery of wild-type BM to wild-type BuCy-treated recipients resulted in significant de novo primordial oocyte production, while control animals contained zero primordial oocytes (Reference 4, Figure 4A). AtmKO recipients, which otherwise harbor zero oocytes in their ovaries,[50–52] contained rare primordial and growing follicle-enclosed oocytes that both appeared histologically normal (Reference 4, Figure 5C–G) and expressed the oocyte-specific gene *MVH*. Wild-type and AtmKO recipients of OG2+ perpheral blood mononuclear cells (PBMNCs), after DOX conditioning, contained GFP-positive follicle-enclosed oocytes as soon as 24 hours post-transplant (Reference 4, Figure 6). In several cases, dual fluorescence-immunolabeling showed that GFP-positive oocytes within follicles also specifically co-stained for germ cell markers. And in what amounted to confirmatory gene expression analyses, every gene reported to be 'germ cell-specific' is also expressed within bone marrow, albeit at low levels as detected by reverse transcription polymerase chain reaction (RT-PCR). These data support the existence of putative mammalian female germline cells that exist outside of the ovary, within hematopoietic compartments, and validate their ability to contribute to postnatal oocyte production in the mouse.

These studies have resulted in the following surprising, but experimentally supported, model: putative GSCs capable of long-term support of oogenesis reside in an extragonadal location, in adult BM, and germ progenitor cells are released from BM into circulating PB. Once circulating, germ cells may then engraft in the adult ovary and participate in follicle formation.[4] This is in accordance with that seen for HSCs and MSCs, their respective progenitors, and the potential for their contribution to adult tissues.[1–3] Figure 3.2a shows cartoon representations of the two proposed models of neo-oogenesis. A mechanism making use of extragonadal production of new oocytes via bone marrow-derived stem cells in adult life is shown in Figure 3.2a; compare with Figure 3.2b, which depicts the transformative mechanism mentioned above.[26,29,30]

Recently, an independent confirmation that the production of new oocytes in postnatal life may, and indeed must, occur came from Kerr et al, a collaborative group from Australia and the United Kingdom.[6] That group used a variety of histological and immunohistochemical approaches to carefully assess the location, mitotic status and meiotic status of the postnatal oocyte pool in the C57Bl/6 mouse. In keeping with Johnson et al's[39] demonstration of BrdU incorporation within postnatal germ cells, PCNA (proliferating cell nuclear antigen) staining revealed that proliferating germ cells do exist postnatally, but only rarely as late as postnatal day 25, and never afterwards. It was also found that GCNA (germ cell nuclear antigen), a marker of oocyte development that

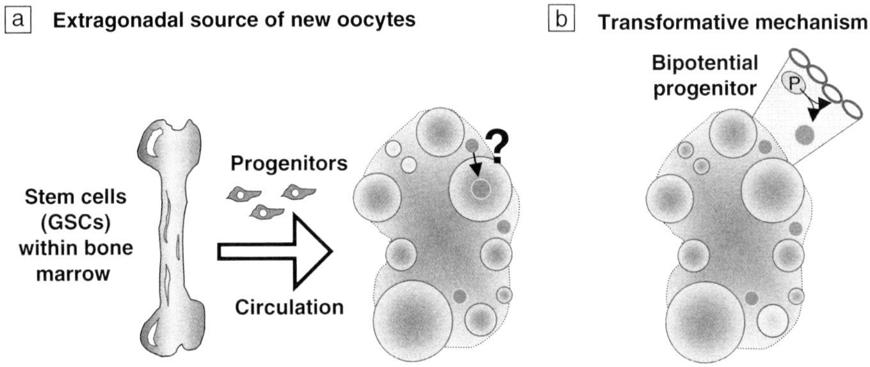

Figure 3.2 Two proposed mechanisms for the generation of new oocytes in postnatal mammals. (a) New oocytes are produced via germ stem cells that reside in an extragonadal location, the bone marrow.[4] Germ progenitor cells are released to the peripheral circulation, and these progenitors home to the ovary, where they may engraft as new oocytes (depicted in green) within new follicles. The question of the developmental potential of labeled oocytes after bone marrow transplantation remains unclear.[10] (b) New oocytes (green) are produced by a transformative mechanism. Bipotential progenitor cells (depicted in blue) produce both new oocytes and somatic cells within the ovary.[26,29,30] (See also color plate)

comes on only after the diplotene stage of meiotic arrest, and then only for a period of hours to days, also labels oocytes as late as postnatal day 25.

Additionally, using a sophisticated histomorphometric protocol deemed an 'unbiased stereological (method),' those authors measured the number of healthy oocytes in C57Bl/6 mouse ovaries between postnatal days 1 and 200. Remarkably, Kerr et al's estimate of oocyte number on day 1 of postnatal life only differs from that of Johnson et al[39] by 5%, suggesting that the techniques used by the two groups are at least comparable. Thereafter, Kerr et al's oocyte numbers are consistently lower for primordial oocytes, but different criteria for follicle categorization, including location, are used. In the end, in keeping with several other groups' findings, Kerr et al show that the pool of primordial oocytes is stable even beyond postnatal day 40 of life, as late as day 100. At day 200 of life, the number of primordial oocytes significantly decreases, suggesting that important events in the control of oocyte number occur between those two times.

OPPOSITES ATTRACT: CAN WE RESOLVE DIAMETRICALLY OPPOSED DATA?

Unsurprisingly, a number of experts in the field have produced commentaries upon and criticisms of the data that support neo-oogenesis during postnatal life.[40,41,53–55] In general, the tone of these commentaries has been critical and cautious. The caution called for by these experts has been well warranted, especially as regards any theoretical prospects for postnatal oocyte production in women. Independent experimental evidence for or against neo-oogenesis has been slightly slower in coming. As described above, an independent analysis of the number of healthy follicles during a broad postnatal time course supported new oocyte production[6] although that group only speculated as to the origins of said new oocytes.

Reports that contradict postnatal oocyte production are beginning to be published. Byskov et al in Copenhagen[42] provide one such report. Their conclusions strongly disagreed with the initial report of neo-oogenesis in mice,[39] especially as regards the quantification of follicular atresia (above). They found that the amount of immature follicle atresia only represented a fraction of the amount that was estimated in the Johnson et al study.[39] If the histomorphometric analysis of atresia is so subjective as to render comparisons between laboratory results meaningless, these data may be impossible to resolve. Whether this problem has been successfully overcome by Kerr et al's technique of unbiased estimates of healthy follicle numbers over time,[6] mentioned above, remains to be seen.

In a clever turn, Byskov et al went on to take advantage of BrdU labeling in an attempt to measure the rate of clearance of dying large follicles. By detecting BrdU incorporation in surviving cells 8 days after a series of closely spaced pulses of BrdU, it was shown that non-dividing cells within follicular remnants remain stained (e.g. were interpreted to be remnants of follicles that were growing 8 days previously), while very few BrdU-positive cells could be found elsewhere in the ovary. As this experiment was performed using otherwise-untreated animals, this is a well-designed technique to estimate the rate of clearance of large growing follicles. Follicular remnants that are present and positive for BrdU labeling must have been growing (e.g. healthy) during the pulse(s) of BrdU. Unfortunately, just how large those growing follicles were between their labeling and eventual fixation is unknown. Whether this technique applies to smaller follicles is also unclear, as it is likely that smaller atretic follicles are cleared from the ovary more quickly. Perhaps this strategy can be modified to address the problem of the morphological assessment of atresia? The remainder of Byskov et al's publication was essentially commentary upon published work that has been rebutted elsewhere.[56] Suffice it to say that a significant amount of data exist that calls into question Byskov et al's final statement that '[there does not exist] any evidence for neo-folliculogenesis in the adult mammalian ovary.'

More impressive has been the demonstration that ovulated eggs always match the genotype of a host animal when bloodborne cells are introduced. Eggan et al[10] show that in the case of reciprocal transplantation of BM between wild-type animals and those that express GFP ubiquitously, ovulated eggs match the host/recipient in all cases. This experiment was performed in accordance with the protocol used by the Tilly group,[4] including the type and dosage of chemotherapeutic conditioning. The major contrasting point between the two studies was the endpoint analyzed. Eggan et al assessed the contribution of BM or PB cells to the pool of ovulated eggs, whereas the Tilly laboratory assessed contributions to the immature oocyte pool. In an elegant series of studies, parabiosis, or, the surgical fusing of the circulation of two animals, was used to detect any peripheral transfer of cells from one 'parabiont' to the other. Here, parabiosis was created between a wild-type female mouse and one expressing GFP ubiquitously. Animals were 'superovulated,' or hormonally primed to ovulate a maximal number of mature oocytes either 2 weeks or 2 months later. In some cases, the wild-type parabiont was treated with ovotoxic chemotherapy prior to parabiosis to test whether any extraovarian contribution to the mature egg pool was dependent on ovarian damage. In all experiments presented, ovulated oocytes always matched the genotype of their host animal and bloodborne cells derived from the opposite parabiont did not contribute to the generation of a single mature ovulated egg.

These data in total offer 665 out of 665 host-matched ovulated eggs, strong evidence in the authors' view that the production of ovulated eggs by circulating or transplanted cells is very unlikely to occur, if ever. And 665 eggs would appear to be a sufficiently large total sample size amongst the different experiments; however, careful analysis of the experimental design forces some caution in interpretation. It is very important to note that although mature, ovulated eggs arise from the pool of immature oocytes within the ovary, they must be considered separately in order to compare these data. Indeed, in the critical experiment in which long-term (2 months) effects of chemotherapy and parabiosis or BM transplantation were measured, only 11 total eggs (parabiosis, 7; marrow transplant, 4) were retrieved – and all were shown to be host-matched. Given that, in Eggan et al's hands, some of the mature, growing pool of oocytes survives chemotherapy when no parabiosis or transplant is performed, the maintenance of host-matched oocytes within large follicles is no surprise. A believable alternative outcome is that immature oocytes derived from the transplanted cells or parabiont exist within the ovaries of the recipients and the efficiency of their survival to ovulation is low. The assessment of 11 oocytes does not allow for this particular question to be addressed. One thing is certain: if donor-derived oocytes do exist, they exist alongside the recipient's surviving oocytes. One hopes that a complete assessment of the identity of all oocytes, from primordial oocytes through ovulated eggs, is performed under such experimental conditions soon. Indeed, extraordinary conclusions require extraordinary proofs. It remains to be tested whether producing ovulated, fertilization-competent oocytes in vivo from transplanted cells or parabiosis is a strict impossibility, or just a very inefficient process requiring greater sample size(s).

IN-VITRO PRODUCTION OF GAMETE-LIKE CELLS FROM EMBRYONIC STEM CELLS AND ADULT STEM CELLS

Along with the reports assessing postnatal oocyte production in rodents have come exciting reports of the production of oocyte-like[57–59] and sperm-like[60,61] cells in vitro from embryonic stem cells (ES cells). ES cells are the totipotent cells derived from the inner cell mass of the blastocyst stage of embryo development (see References 62 and 63 for reviews). Certainly more surprising, given the source of the cells, is the recent example of oocyte-like cell production from cells within porcine skin using similar techniques.[64] In these cases, the development of cells with many inarguable hallmarks of oocytes, including size and general morphology, the presence of zona pellucidae, and interaction with (specification of?) steroidogenic[57–59] somatic cells, raises the tantalizing possibility of an unlimited supply of these precious cells. However, the continued description of these cells as 'oocyte-like or sperm-like' is fair and perhaps generous, as no demonstration that these cells are capable of leading to normal embryos or offspring has been offered yet.

Nayernia et al[65] recently provided another link between the germline and adult stem cells, here BM resident cells. Marrow cells were used from a transgenic mouse line in which GFP is placed downstream of the control elements of the germ cell-specific gene *Stra8*.[22,66] Classically, when whole BM is placed into culture, the hematopoietic fraction of cells remains non-adherent while mesenchymal cells, including stem cells, adhere to culture plastic.[2,3] A small fraction of *Stra8*:GFP bone marrow adherent cells became positive for GFP in culture. This cell fraction was shown to express molecular markers of the primordial germ cells, including *Fragilis, Mvh, Oct4, Rnf17* and *Stella/Dppa3*. Further, these cells expressed Rbm, c-Kit, Tex18, Stra8, Piwil2, Dazl, Hsp90a, and the β_1- and α_6-integrins, all known markers of spermatogonial stem cells and spermatogonia. Quite impressively, the authors show that colonies that develop from GFP+ cells show an organization reminiscent of the organization of the testis tubule in vivo as evidenced by spatial gene expression in cell colonies. When the cells were delivered into chemotherapy-ablated testis tubules, they participated in spermatogenesis, forming cells reminiscent of round spermatids. However, their colonization of testis tubules did not result in their development into functional or even elongating spermatids. These data are strongly reminiscent of results after the delivery of ES cells to testis tubules.[60]

A very recent manuscript from the Höög laboratory[58] offers a potential simple explanation as to the lack of offspring produced by oocyte-like cells derived from ES cells. Their data may also relate to functionality of the sperm-like cells produced from BM-resident stem cells by Nayernia et al.[65] Here, Novak et al convincingly show that oocyte-like cells that develop from ES cells do not enter meiosis. In fact, other than the expression of a single protein component of the synaptonemal complex required for meiotic entry, SYCP3, these clearly oocyte-like cells demonstrate almost no evidence of participation in meiosis at all. These data suggest that meiotic entry may not be required for oocyte and follicle development at all – and, if true for all of the previous studies that generated these cells,[57–59] it may be that many markers of the germline are maintained in gamete-like cells whether meiosis entry occurs or not. However, meiosis entry seems to be required for the development of fertilization-competent eggs. Several remarkable paths lie ahead for these studies and we may be on the cusp of solving the key technical problems that have prevented the generation of stem cell-derived fertilization-competent oocytes. Novak et al rightly point out that since meiotic entry is apparently a default condition of fetal female germ cells,[58] it may be that simple adjustment of culture conditions will lead to proper meiotic entry of ES cell-derived oocytes or oocytes generated from adult stem cells harvested from other tissues.

MECHANISM(S) OF ACTION OF CANCER THERAPIES UPON FEMALE FERTILITY: CONSIDERATION OF PUTATIVE GERM STEM CELLS

It is well-known that therapeutic intervention, especially radio- and chemotherapy, often compromises fertility by destroying oocytes and damaging the ovary. Many strategies have been used to protect gonadal function during these treatments, with varying levels of success (see Reference 67 for a comprehensive review). Strategies for oocyte and/or embryo retrieval followed by cryopreservation or vitrification are entering the mainstream for the preservation of fertility in cancer survivors. However, any additional damage to the reproductive tract due to treatment that compromises fertility may only be helped by understanding how to protect these sites.

For women and girls, total body irradiation (TBI) often results in permanent ovarian failure.[67,68] The use of physical radioprotective shielding of the ovaries during TBI has been shown to protect some patients against therapy-induced ovarian failure.[69] Another approach uses the delivery of an antiapoptotic molecule directly to the ovary during radio- and/or chemotherapy. In mice, the application of sphingosine-1-phosphate (S1P)[70] prevents the vast damage to the oocyte pool caused by treatments. Whether the delivery of S1P or other molecules may protect the human ovary via the reduction of ovarian apoptosis remains to be determined. Either physical or molecular protection of the ovary may also be protecting any ability of the mammalian ovary to regenerate follicles. If this is true, damage to either extragonadal (e.g. bone marrow sites of GSCs) or gonadal stem cells may prevent the recovery of ovarian function after treatment.

Chemotherapeutic treatment regimens have become sufficiently sophisticated and reliable such that fertility preservation may be a consideration. However, one chemotherapeutic agent in particular is associated strongly with permanent ovarian failure – and by extension, may relate to the existence of female GSCs in mice. Busulfan is known to be cytotoxic to stem and progenitor cells, notably host HSCs during preparation for BM transplants[71] and dividing male germ stem cells and spermatogonia within the testis.[72–75] It was hypothesized that busulfan would act in female mice in an analogous fashion to males, at the level of dividing germ stem or progenitor cells. Postpartum day 25 female mice were injected with vehicle or busulfan (20 mg/kg b.w.): 20 days post-injection, busulfan treatment resulted in 95% fewer healthy primordial follicles than in vehicle-treated females, with only a minimal induction of primordial oocyte death in the first 10 days post-treatment.[39] Although there was no precedent in the literature for busulfan inducing the growth activation of primordial follicles, the number of (growth-activated) primary follicles during the time course were used to calculate the average ratio of primordial follicles to primary follicles over the time course. No significant change in the ratio of primordial to primary follicles was seen between busulfan and vehicle treatment, indicating that busulfan treatment did not decrease the primordial pool by increasing follicle growth activation (J Tilly, pers comm). These data supported the interpretation that busulfan interferes with the production of new oocytes, resulting in a gradual loss of the primordial follicle pool by halting oocyte and follicle renewal.

Chemotherapeutic treatments of human females that included busulfan resulted in a near-total incidence of premature ovarian failure (POF), regardless of other drugs used in combination therapy. Data combined from two studies of ovarian function in childhood showed that 15 of 15 (mean age = 12.6 years old) girls treated with chemotherapeutic regimens containing busulfan experienced POF, whereas comparable treatments that lacked busulfan resulted in POF for 22 of 37 girls (mean age = 8.7 years old).[75,76] In another study, busulfan treatment in women between the ages of 16 and 40 years old (mean age = 28.2 years old; raw ages used to calculate mean age provided by A Grigg, pers comm) caused POF in 19 of 19 cases.[77] Last, in a study where combined busulfan and cyclophosphamide therapy was compared with cyclophosphamide alone, 72 of 73 patients treated with both agents underwent POF (ages 14–57 years old, median = 38 years old), whereas cyclophosphamide alone resulted in POF in 47 of 103 patients [Sanders et al[71] (ages 13–58 years old, median = 28 years old; raw ages, J Sanders, pers comm)].

All told, busulfan inclusion resulted in POF in 106 of 107 patients, whereas other treatments lacking busulfan were associated with POF in 69 of 140 cases. Although busulfan treatment may induce death in human oocytes, such a result may also indicate an irreversible destruction of human female GSCs by busulfan in similar fashion, as was reported for the mouse.[39] Treatments (lacking busulfan) are known to target and kill oocytes, and it is possible that GSCs capable of repopulating the ovary with new oocytes are spared in these situations, allowing the continuation of ovarian function post-therapy. The interpretation of data from ongoing and retrospective analyses of ovarian failure after various treatments may be profoundly different when possible effects on a regenerative pool of oocytes are considered.

It is important to remember that in the case of fertility-compromising therapies, the ovaries are not the only potential targets. Proven and potential damaging effects upon the rest of the female reproductive tract should be considered with care. Finding less-damaging treatments or stem cell therapies that are capable of ensuring the proper function of the uterus or fallopian tube(s) is a more than worthy goal.

THE PRODUCTION OF NEW, FERTILIZATION-COMPETENT EGGS: CAN WE REVERSE THE 'IRREVERSIBLE'?

Stem cell-based therapies that successfully treat POF may only be in the distant future, if ever. The critical issue in this chapter is the determination of whether new fertilizable eggs capable of offspring production may be generated, whether in vivo or in vitro, from tissues derived from postnatal women. To date, there is no evidence that oocyte-like cells may participate in offspring production, regardless of the method or source cell type of their 'stem cell' derivation. As mentioned, the lack of meiotic entry of both oocyte-like cells produced from ES cells[58] and sperm-like cells generated from BM[65] is one possible explanation for the difficulty in producing offspring from the oocyte-like cells derived in vitro from ES cells[57–59] and cells found in porcine skin.[64] Whether oocytes generated from BM-resident or other stem cells are capable of development into fertilization-competent eggs and offspring production remains an open and exciting question. A fascinating race is afoot to see if 'the impossible' can be performed: the reversal of ovarian failure and perhaps the recovery of fertility in the oocyte-barren patient.

SUMMARY

For more than 50 years it has been generally accepted that most if not all mammalian females are endowed with their entire complement of oocytes at birth. If this is true, the loss of oocytes below a threshold number will result in irreversible ovarian failure. Recently, the question of whether new oocyte cells may be produced in adult life ('neo-oogenesis') has been re-addressed. Several lines of evidence supported neo-oogenesis in adult mice. It was initially shown that the level of dying, or atretic oocytes, was far higher during adult life than expected if compared to the number of healthy oocytes across the same time span. These data were in accordance with independent studies assessing oocyte dynamics in both rodent and primate ovaries. The stability of the primordial oocyte pool in rodents in the face of significant losses early in life has now been confirmed by multiple groups. It was hypothesized that neo-oogenesis must take place to offset the amount of oocyte death if the normal fertile life span of mice is to be achieved. Pharmacological treatments were shown to significantly increase the number of primordial oocytes above baseline and, separately, reveal primordial oocyte regeneration after destruction. Quite surprisingly, bone marrow, and by extension, the peripheral circulation, were evaluated and were supported as locations harboring extraovarian cells that can develop into immature oocytes within transplant recipients. A model was then proposed in which the bone marrow is one location of putative GSCs that support oocyte numbers in adult mice. It remains to be confirmed whether these extragonadal cells differentiate under normal physiological conditions into oocyte-like cells or whether pluripotent cells trans-differentiate under certain experimental conditions. In conflict with these data, a recent high-profile manuscript was published in which zero donor-derived ovulated oocytes were found after bone marrow transplantation. This work did not address the issue of the origins of immature oocytes within host ovaries. There are no data to date that show that stem cells of any kind may develop into fertilization-competent oocytes. However, the detection of donor-derived immature oocytes raises the possibility that this process is inefficient but not impossible. Last, if GSCs exist in human females, there will be important implications for the preservation of fertility given choices between treatment agents and methodologies. It is crucial to emphasize that the utility of oocytes and oocyte-like cells from adult stem cells and, separately, embryonic stem cells, will only be proven when fertilization-competent eggs are produced. In the end, significant advances in oocyte production using stem cells shows that regeneration of the oocyte pool in patients is a goal worth fighting towards, instead of a strict biological impossibility.

REFERENCES

1. Weissman IL. Stem cells: units of development, units of regeneration, and units in evolution. Cell 2000; 100: 157–68.
2. Orkin SH. Hematopoietic stem cells: molecular diversification and developmental interrelationships.

In: Marshak DR, Gardner RL, Gottlieb D, eds. Stem Cell Biology. Cold Spring Harbor, NY: CSHL Press, 2001: 289–327.

3. Pittenger MF, Marshak DR. Mesenchymal stem cells of human adult bone marrow. In: Marshak DR, Gardner RL, Gottlieb D, eds. Stem Cell Biology. Cold Spring Harbor, NY: CSHL Press 2001: 349–73.
4. Johnson J, Bagley J, Skaznik-Wikiel M et al. Oocyte generation in adult mammalian ovaries by putative germ cells in bone marrow and peripheral blood. Cell 2005; 122: 303–15.
5. Tilly JL. Ovarian follicle counts – not as simple as 1, 2, 3. Reprod Biol Endocrinol 2003; 1: 11.
6. Kerr JB, Duckett R, Myers M et al. Quantification of healthy follicles in the neonatal and adult mouse ovary: evidence for maintenance of primordial follicle supply. Reproduction 2006; 132: 95–109.
7. Zuckerman S. The number of oocytes in the mature ovary. Rec Prog Horm Res 1951; 6: 63.
8. Saffman EE, Lasko P. Germline development in vertebrates and invertebrates. Cell Mol Life Sci 1999; 55: 1141–63.
9. Tilly JL. Commuting the death sentence: how oocytes strive to survive. Nat Rev Mol Cell Biol 2001; 2: 838–48.
10. Eggan K, Jurga S, Gosden R, Min IM, Wagers A. Ovulated oocytes in adult mice derive from non-circulating germ cells. Nature 2006; 441: 1109–14.
11. Saitou M, Payer B, Lange UC et al. Specification of germ cell fate in mice. Philos Trans R Soc Lond B Biol Sci 2003; 358: 1363–70.
12. Molyneaux K, Wylie C. Primordial germ cell migration. Int J Dev Biol 2004; 48: 537–44.
13. Lange UC, Saitou M, Western PS, Barton SC, Surani MA. The fragilis interferon-inducible gene family of transmembrane proteins is associated with germ cell specification in mice. BMC Dev Biol 2003; 3: 1.
14. Naito M, Matsubara Y, Harumi T et al. Differentiation of donor primordial germ cells into functional gametes in the gonads of mixed-sex germline chimaeric chickens produced by transfer of primordial germ cells isolated from embryonic blood. J Reprod Fertil 1999; 117: 291–8.
15. Mozdziak PE, Angerman-Stewart J, Rushton B, Pardue SL, Petitte JN. Isolation of chicken primordial germ cells using fluorescence-activated cell sorting. Poult Sci 2005; 84: 594–600.
16. McLaren A. Development of primordial germ cells in the mouse. Andrologia 1992; 24: 243–7.
17. Stallock J, Molyneaux K, Schaible K, Knudson CM, Wylie C. The pro-apoptotic gene Bax is required for the death of ectopic primordial germ cells during their migration in the mouse embryo. Development 2003; 130: 6589–97.
18. McLaren A. Primordial germ cells in the mouse. Dev Biol 2003; 262: 1–15.
19. Pepling ME, Spradling AC. Female mouse germ cells form synchronously dividing cysts. Development 1998; 125: 3323–8.
20. Pepling ME, de Cuevas M, Spradling AC. Germline cysts: a conserved phase of germ cell development? Trends Cell Biol 1999; 9: 257–62.
21. Pepling ME, Spradling AC. Mouse ovarian germ cell cysts undergo programmed breakdown to form primordial follicles. Dev Biol 2001; 234: 339–51.
22. Menke DB, Koubova J, Page DC. Sexual differentiation of germ cells in XX mouse gonads occurs in an anterior-to-posterior wave. Dev Biol 2003; 262: 303–12.
23. Waldeyer W. Eierstock und Ei. Leipzig: Engelmann, 1870.
24. Zuckerman S, Baker TG. In: Zuckerman S, Weir BJ, eds. The Ovary, 2nd edn. New York: Academic Press 1977.
25. Franchi LL, Mandl AM, Zuckerman S. In: Zuckerman S, ed. The Ovary, 1st edn. New York: Academic Press. 1962.
26. Allen E. Ovogenesis during sexual maturity. Am J Anat 1923; 31: 439.
27. Swezy O. The ovarian chromosome cycle in a mixed rat strain. J Morphol 1929; 48, 445.
28. Evans HM, Swezy O. Ovogenesis and the normal follicular cycle in adult mammalia. Mem Univ Calif 1931; 9: 119–224.
29. Bukovsky A, Caudle MR, Svetlikova M, Upadhyaya NB. Origin of germ cells and formation of new primary follicles in adult human ovaries. Reprod Biol Endocrinol 2004; 2: 20.
30. Bukovsky A, Svetlikova M, Caudle MR. Oogenesis in cultures derived from adult human ovaries. Reprod Biol Endocrinol 2005; 3: 17.
31. Brambell FWR. The development and morphology of the gonads of the mouse. Part I. The morphogenesis of the indifferent gonad and of the ovary. Proc Roy Soc Lond 1927; 101: 391.
32. Rubaschkin W. The germ cell cycle of the guinea pig. 1909; 39: 605. [in German]
33. Borum K. Oogenesis in the mouse: a study of the meiotic prophase. Exp Cell Res 1961; 24: 495–507.
34. Peters H. Migration of gonocytes into the mammalian gonad and their differentiation. Phil Trans Roy Soc Lond Biol Sci 1970; 259: 91–101.
35. Crone M, Levy E, Peters H. The duration of the premeiotic DNA synthesis in mouse oocytes. Exp Cell Res 1965; 39: 678–88.
36. Borum K. Oogenesis in the mouse. A study of the origin of the mature ova. Exp Cell Res 1966; 45: 39.

37. Pinkerton JHM, McKay DG, Adams EC, Hertig AT. Development of the human ovary – a study using histochemical techniques. Obstet Gynecol 1961; 18: 152–81.

38. Baker TG. In: Balin H, Glasser SR, eds. Reproductive Biology, Amsterdam: Excerpta Medica Foundation, 1972; 398–437.

39. Johnson J, Canning J, Kaneko T, Pru JK, Tilly JL. Germline stem cells and follicular repopulation in the postnatal mammalian ovary. Nature 2004; 428: 145–50.

40. Albertini DF. Micromanagement of the ovarian follicle reserve – do stem cells play into the ledger? Reproduction 2004; 127: 513.

41. Telfer EE. Germline stem cells in the postnatal mammalian ovary: a phenomenon of prosimian primates and mice? Reprod Biol Endocrinol 2004; 2: 24.

42. Byskov AG, Faddy MJ, Lemmen JG, Andersen CY. Eggs forever? Differentiation 2005; 73: 438–46.

43. Roussell DL, Bennett KL. glh-1, a germ-line putative RNA helicase from Caenorhabditis, has four zinc fingers. Proc Natl Acad Sci USA 1993; 90: 9300–4.

44. Komiya T, Itoh K, Ikenishi K, Furusawa M. Isolation and characterization of a novel gene of the DEAD box protein family which is specifically expressed in germ cells of *Xenopus laevis*. Dev Biol 1994; 162: 354–63.

45. Rongo C, Broihier HT, Moore L et al. Germ plasm assembly and germ cell migration in Drosophila. Cold Spring Harb Symp Quant Biol 1997; 62: 1–11.

46. Braat AK, Zandbergen T, van de Water S, Goos HJ, Zivkovic D. Characterization of zebrafish primordial germ cells: morphology and early distribution of vasa RNA. Dev Dyn 1999; 216: 153–67.

47. Castrillon DH, Quade BJ, Wang TY, Quigley C, Crum CP. The human VASA gene is specifically expressed in the germ cell lineage. Proc Natl Acad Sci USA 2000; 97: 9585–90.

48. Fabioux C, Pouvreau S, Le Roux F, Huvet A. The oyster vasa-like gene: a specific marker of the germline in *Crassostrea gigas*. Biochem Biophys Res Commun 2004; 315: 897–904.

49. Fujiwara Y, Komiya T, Kawabata H et al. Isolation of a DEAD-family protein gene that encodes a murine homolog of *Drosophila vasa* and its specific expression in germ cell lineage. Proc Natl Acad Sci USA 2004; 91: 12258–62.

50. Xu Y, Ashley T, Brainerd EE et al. Targeted disruption of ATM leads to growth retardation, chromosomal fragmentation during meiosis, immune defects, and thymic lymphoma. Genes Dev 1996; 10: 2411–22.

51. Barlow C, Liyanage M, Moens PB et al. Atm deficiency results in severe meiotic disruption as early as leptonema of prophase I. Development 1998; 125: 4007–17.

52. Di Giacomo M, Barchi M, Baudat F et al. Distinct DNA-damage-dependent and -independent responses drive the loss of oocytes in recombination-defective mouse mutants. Proc Natl Acad Sci USA 2005; 102: 737–42.

53. Greenfeld C, Flaws JA. Renewed debate over postnatal oogenesis in the mammalian ovary. Bioessays 2004; 26: 829–32.

54. Telfer EE, Gosden RG, Byskov AG et al. On regenerating the ovary and generating controversy. Cell 2005; 12: 821–2.

55. Kayisli UA, Seli E. Stem cells and fertility: what does the future hold? Curr Opin Obstet Gynecol 2006; 18: 338–43.

56. Johnson J, Skaznik-Wikiel M, Lee HJ et al. Setting the record straight on data supporting postnatal oogenesis in female mammals. Cell Cycle 2005; 4: 1471–7.

57. Hubner K, Fuhrmann G, Christenson LK et al. Derivation of oocytes from mouse embryonic stem cells. Science 2003; 300: 1251–6.

58. Novak I, Lightfoot DA, Wang H et al. Mouse embryonic stem cells from follicle-like ovarian structures but do not progress through meiosis. Stem Cells 2006; Apr 27 [Epub ahead of print].

59. Silva C, Strauss JF III. Differentiation of germ cells from stem cells, Vol. I, 2006; 15–30.

60. Toyooka Y, Tsunekawa N, Akasu R, Noce T. Embryonic stem cells can form germ cells in vitro. Proc Natl Acad Sci USA 2003; 100: 11457–62.

61. Geijsen N, Horoschak M, Kim K et al. Derivation of embryonic germ cells and male gametes from embryonic stem cells. Nature 2004; 427: 148–54.

62. Semb H. Human embryonic stem cells: origin, properties and applications. APMIS 2005; 113: 743–50.

63. Tutter AV, Baltus GA, Kadam S. Embryonic stem cells: a great hope for a new era of medicine. Curr Opin Drug Discov Devel 2006; 9: 169–75.

64. Dyce PW, Wen L, Li J. In vitro germline potential of stem cells derived from fetal porcine skin. Nat Cell Biol 2006; 8: 384.

65. Nayernia K, Lee JH, Drusenheimer N et al. Derivation of male germ cells from bone marrow stem cells. Lab Invest 2006; 86: 654–63.

66. Nayernia K, Li M, Jaroszynski L et al. Stem cell based therapeutical approach of male infertility by teratocarcinoma derived germ cells. Hum Mol Genet 2004; 1: 1451–60.

67. Lobo RA. Potential options for preservation of fertility in women. N Engl J Med 2005; 353: 64–73.

68. Greskovich JF Jr, Macklis RM. Radiation therapy in pregnancy: risk calculation and risk minimization. Semin Oncol 2000; 27: 633–45.

69. Nakagawa K, Kanda Y, Yamashita H et al. Preservation of ovarian function by ovarian shielding when undergoing total body irradiation for hematopoietic stem cell transplantation: a report of two successful cases. Bone Marrow Transplant 2006; 37: 583–7.

70. Morita Y, Perez GI, Paris F et al. Oocyte apoptosis is suppressed by disruption of the acid sphingomyelinase gene or by sphingosine-1-phosphate therapy. Nat Med 2000; 6: 1109–14.

71. Sanders JE, Hawley J, Levy W et al. Pregnancies following high-dose cyclophosphamide with or without high-dose busulfan or total-body irradiation and bone marrow transplantation. Blood 1996; 87: 3045–52.

72. Bucci LR, Meistrich ML. Effects of busulfan on murine spermatogenesis: cytotoxicity, sterility, sperm abnormalities, and dominant lethal mutations. Mutat Res 1987; 176: 259–68.

73. Brinster CJ, Ryu BY, Avarbock MR et al. Restoration of fertility by germ cell transplantation requires effective recipient preparation. Biol Reprod 2003; 69: 412–20.

74. Brinster RL, Zimmermann JW. Spermatogenesis following male germ-cell transplantation. Proc Natl Acad Sci USA 1994; 91: 11298–302.

75. Thibaud E, Rodriguez-Macias K, Trivin C et al. Ovarian function after bone marrow transplantation during childhood. Bone Marrow Transplant 1998; 21: 287–90.

76. Teinturier C, Hartmann O, Valteau-Couanet D, Benhamou E, Bougneres PF. Ovarian function after autologous bone marrow transplantation in childhood: high-dose busulfan is a major cause of ovarian failure. Bone Marrow Transplant 1998; 22: 989–94.

77. Grigg AP, McLachlan R, Zaja J, Szer J. Reproductive status in long-term bone marrow transplant survivors receiving busulfan-cyclophosphamide (120 mg/kg). Bone Marrow Transplant 2000; 26: 1089–95.

CHAPTER 4

Adult stem cells in the human ovary: hope or fiction?

Mónica Romeu, Carlos Simon and Antonio Pellicer

INTRODUCTION

For more than half a century, reproductive biologists have upheld the theory that, in most mammalian species, oocytes are formed before or shortly after birth, but never in adulthood. This doctrine was established[1] and germline stem cells have not been recorded in juvenile or adult ovaries, apart from a few isolated exceptions in certain species. In fact, although spermatogenesis is maintained throughout adult life, oocyte production in mammalian females is considered to cease before birth. This cornerstone of reproductive science has stood strong despite the rapid development of new technology and knowledge, remaining virtually unchallenged until the publication of two reports.[2,3]

It is a dogma within reproductive biology that females are born with a finite and non-renewable number of germinal cells, all of which are arrested in the first phase of meiosis and surrounded by somatic cells in structures known as follicles.[1] The number of follicles decreases during postnatal life[4] through mechanisms involving apoptosis. Three waves of this dramatic apoptosis have been described. The first wave, and most important, takes place in the prophase of the first meiotic division. From a maximum of 6–7 million around week 20 of gestation, the total follicle number drops to approximately 1 million in the female newborn. The second wave occurs just before puberty, and sees the ovarian reserve drop to around 400 000 primordial follicles during puberty. The third wave is gradual and cyclic, and takes place in response to the monthly deprivation of follicle-stimulating hormone (FSH), leading to the total depletion of germ cells in the ovaries in what represents the menopause, which occurs around the fifth decade of life.[4]

Although this dogma has only recently been challenged, it is a debate that was first raised in the 1920s. At that time, the consensus was that the oocyte supply was fixed,[5] until challenged in 1923 by Allen,[6] who claimed he had evidence that oocytes continued to be formed throughout reproductive life. It was proposed that cyclical proliferation of the germinal epithelium gave rise to oocytes.[6,7] This was a widely held view until the 1950s, when Zuckerman[1] demonstrated, through extensive studies based on differential counting of follicles, that oocytes were not produced throughout the life span in most mammals. Further evidence using tritiated thymidine labeling of oocyte nuclei suggested that juvenile and adult ovaries are direct descendants of the fetal germ cells, and that germ cells do not increase in number throughout life. However, exceptions to this rule had previously been demonstrated in mammals; in some species of prosimian primates (*Loris tardigradus lydekkerianus* and *Nycticebus coucang*), the most ancient of primate families, mitotically active germ cells had been found in adult ovaries.[8,9] These studies found that germ cells, clustered in nests within the ovarian cortex, incorporated tritiated thymidine. However, it was not clarified whether any of these proliferating germ cells undergo a process of follicular growth and ovulation, which is a question that remains unanswered.

THE DOGMA CHALLENGED

Of all the tenets of mammalian female reproductive biology, the concept that a non-renewing oocyte reserve is present in the ovaries at birth is probably the most long-standing and widely held. Tilly and his co-workers were studying ovarian failure in cancer patients in order to compare it with normal ovarian aging. To establish a benchmark, they harvested ovaries from mice at different stages of life and counted the healthy follicles and the number of dying egg cells in the same animals. When, unexpectedly, data from their studies of oocyte apoptosis began to challenge the aforementioned theory, they embarked on an investigation, unbiased by any preconceived dogmas, to determine whether or not oocyte production continued in adult female mice.[2]

In a first report, they showed that mouse germline stem cells replaced ovarian follicles that had been rapidly lost through follicle death. As in previous studies, they found that about a third of the number of follicles present at peak levels were lost during development into young adults. However, the total number of follicles only gradually declined over time. If the rate of atresia continued at the aforementioned rate, ovarian function would not extend for as long as it did.

Employing immunohistochemistry, the group found cells that expressed a conserved germ cell protein called vasa MVH (mouse vasa homologue), a gene that is only expressed in the germ cells of vertebrates and invertebrates.[10] It is a reliable marker of germ cells in any state, and allows their numbers to be estimated. Moreover, the cells were found to divide and, importantly, to express the meiotic entry protein synaptonemal complex protein 3 (SCP3).[2]

These researchers confirmed that the germ stem cells did indeed develop into mature follicles by grafting parts of wild-type ovaries into a transgenic mouse that expressed green-fluorescent protein in all its cells. The wild-type piece of ovary was infiltrated with fluorescent germ cells that went on to form follicles.[2]

Other investigators have observed follicular death and clearance of resulting cellular detritus, and have thus concluded that follicle generation in the adult mammalian ovary is possible.[11–17] That said, follicles do atresiate at a slightly higher rate than that at which they are generated from stem germ cells, which explains the slight decrease of the follicular reserve.

The cells found on the superficial epithelium of the ovary were germ stem cell candidates, but their numbers decreased dramatically from 63 ± 8 on postpartum day 30 to 6 ± 3 on postpartum day 40. This scarce population is not capable of completely restocking the ovaries following damage. A second report showed how the adult mouse ovary can produce hundreds of new oocytes.[3]

With the intention of investigating a possible extraovarian niche, the group analyzed the bone marrow provided that:

- germ and hematopoietic stem cells originate in the same region
- both stem cell types initiate their migration to the genital ridge and the liver, respectively, at the same developmental moment
- the hematopoietic system is maintained by stem cells that reside in the bone marrow
- the abundant evidence demonstrating the multilineage potential of bone marrow-derived cells.[18–20]

Mice were treated with a toxic cocktail and then transplanted with compatible, untreated mouse bone marrow. Two months later, their ovaries were analyzed under the microscope and were found to contain very few, if any, immature oocytes or follicles. When bone marrow transplantation was performed 1 or 7 days after chemotherapy, ovarian histology showed several hundreds of follicles at different stages of development, including the primordial stage. The same results were obtained with ataxia-telangiectasia mutated (Atm) mice, which are unable to produce mature germ cells and whose ovaries lack follicles and were found to contain normal follicles and oocytes thereafter.[3] Moreover, the results were identical to those obtained after peripheral blood transfusion, which is how bone marrow cells reach the different organs. Experiments carried out with Atm null female chemoablated mice provided the same satisfactory results. The number of oocytes observed depended on the stage of the cycle at which blood had been collected.

Given the magnitude of its implications, the work of Johnson et al[2,3] has been critically dissected by many scientists. The methodology employed to count follicles,[21–25] the effects of the gonadotoxic substances employed,[26] the nature of the stem cells described,[25,27] and the grafting experiments with transgenic animals[28,29] have all been criticized. Similarly, the short time interval necessary for oocytes generated in the bone marrow to reach full development has also been questioned.

Although the concept requires further backing up, there is a slowly increasing acceptance that adult mammalian females are capable of producing new oocytes. The aforementioned findings raise many important questions. Determining the exact number and location of these functional germline stem cells requires tagging germ cells and demonstrating that their descendants form follicles and, ultimately, mature oocytes. Such lineage-tracing experiments will also address whether the progeny of mouse germline stem cells differentiate directly into oocytes or whether they first increase their numbers by forming interconnected 'germ-cell cysts'. There is still a lack of direct evidence of the existence of germ stem cells or their capacity to rescue and sustain oocyte production.

In the future, it will need to be demonstrated that the cells that travel from the bone marrow to the ovaries can trigger ovulation and give rise to normal offspring, but Johnson et al's experiments have certainly led the scientific community to readdress a reproductive biology creed. There is presently a healthy skepticism in this field of ovarian biology, which should bear fruit in new lines of investigation.

Another quest is to compare the destiny of follicles that originate while the fetus is in the uterus to those generated during adult life by adult stem cells. Do the follicles produced before birth expire before reproductive maturity, so that female fertility depends on the presence of young follicles recently produced from germline stem cells? And does the loss of these stem cells soon lead to follicle aging and depletion, and reproductive decline?[30]

EVIDENCE IN HUMANS

Few studies have been performed in humans with respect to the presence of adult stem cells in the ovaries. Bukovsky and co-workers have recently published two reports[31,32] in which they hypothesize a mesenchymal–epithelial transition to explain how mesenchymal cells in the tunica albuginea are bipotent progenitors for both granulosa and germ cells. They analyzed the ovaries of 12 adult women through single-, double-, and triple-color immunohistochemistry, and showed that these mesenchymal cells differentiated into surface epithelium cells through a mesenchymal–epithelial transition. Segments of the surface epithelium directly associated with the ovarian cortex were described as overgrown with tunica albuginea, which formed solid epithelial cords that fragmented into small epithelial nests descending into the lower ovarian cortex, before assembling with zona pellucida + oocytes. The authors described how germ cells originated via asymmetric division from superficial epithelium cells covering the tunica albuginea. The germ cells subsequently divided symmetrically and entered the adjacent cortical vessels. During vascular transport, these putative germ cells increased to oocyte size, and were picked up by epithelial nests associated with the vessels. During follicle formation, extensions of granulosa cells entered the oocyte cytoplasm, forming a single paranuclear Balbiani body that supplied all the oocyte's mitochondria. This follicular turnover represented an adaptable mechanism that eliminated the spontaneous and environmentally induced genetic alterations in oocytes arrested in meiosis.[31]

In a subsequent report, Bukovsky et al[32] investigated the possible differentiation of oocytes and granulosa cells in cultures derived from adult human ovaries. They scraped cells from the surface of ovaries and cultured them for 5–6 days in the presence or absence of estrogenic stimuli (phenol red). The cells cultured in the medium without phenol red differentiated into small cells of a granulosa phenotype, and epithelial-, neural- and mesenchymal-type cells. In contrast, the cells cultured with phenol red differentiated directly into large cells of the oocyte phenotype. Such cells exhibited germinal vesicle breakdown, expulsion of the polar body and surface expression of zona pellucida proteins. The luteal phase seemed to be the most adequate period for both cell types to form follicles.

Bukovsky et al[31,32] employed simple methodology, such as immunohistochemistry and cell culture, in these pioneering studies. It must be said that their findings would need to be reconfirmed employing appropriate updated methodology. Although their publications are rather difficult to follow, they certainly deserve the merit of being the first reports to challenge the previously mentioned consensus concerning human beings.

In addition to the presence of adult stem cells in the human ovary, the origin of these precursors should be considered. With respect to this, allogenic transplantation is a biological experiment that needs to be explored in detail. Although transplanted women are not expected to experience a restoration of ovarian function and tend to show a poor response to multifollicular development treatments or develop low-quality follicles that are incapable of leading to full-term pregnancies, results in mice[3] could explain a number of surprising reports of cancer patients and other individuals who were expected to be infertile but who gave birth to children after receiving bone marrow transplants. For example, one patient with Fanconi's anemia had a single menstrual period and then entered the menopause at 12 years old. After receiving a bone marrow transplant from a sibling, her periods resumed and she later gave birth to two children.[33]

It remains to be seen whether or not autologous transfusions are beneficial in any way. It seems that recolonization of adult human ovaries with new primary follicles requires the presence of nests of primitive granulosa cells, which makes them receptive to be repopulated. Could the said cells also be present in peripheral blood? According to the report by Johnson et al,[3] germ cell markers were found in the bone marrow of human female donors between 24 and 36 years old. Similarly, germ cell markers were detected in the peripheral blood of human females between 23 and 33 years old. Unfortunately, their report provided no data to confirm this.

ADULT STEM CELLS AS A POSSIBLE SOLUTION TO INFERTILITY PROBLEMS

The claim that these adult stem cells generate new oocytes to replace those perishing in atretic follicles is of great interest. If true, a complete revision of the underlying mechanisms of the menopause and oocyte aging will be fundamental. Moreover, it might herald breathtaking advances in reproductive technology. The new paradigm is as revolutionary for ovarian biology as the breakthrough in nuclear transfer was for reproductive cloning some years ago.

The finding opens up avenues for delaying the menopause and preserving fertility in female chemotherapy patients. The number of adults with a history of childhood cancer is increasing due to rising rates of the disease among young people and advances in its treatment.[34,35] Survival rates among young people with malignancies have reached 90–95%, but most cancer therapies have the unfortunate shortcoming of producing non-reversible consequences for the reproductive system that are age- and dose-dependent.[36,37]

Several strategies have been explored to overcome this unfortunate secondary effect (Figure 4.1). Ovarian stimulation and preservation of oocytes or

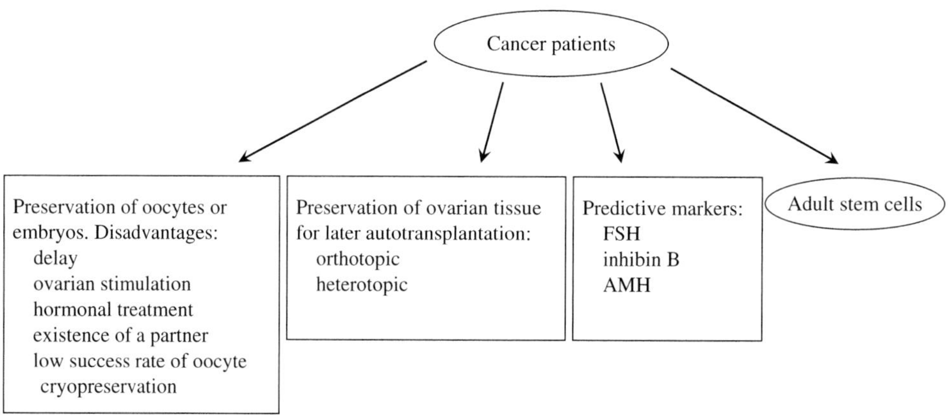

Figure 4.1 Strategies for solving infertility problems in cancer patients. FSH, follicle-stimulating hormone; AMH, antimüllerian hormone

embryos is an option that carries the disadvantage that relatively few oocytes/embryos can be preserved. Further drawbacks are the delay caused to the initiation of cancer treatment while ovarian stimulation is carried out in order to retrieve oocytes, and the potential contraindication and detrimental effect of hormonal treatment for some cancers. In addition, cryopreservation of embryos implies the existence of a partner, and the current success rate of oocyte cryopreservation is low.[38]

A second strategy for preserving fertility in cancer patients is cryopreservation of ovarian tissue for later auto-transplantation, which can be performed at a heterotopic or orthotopic site. Orthotopic transplantation is preferable in that it permits natural fertility using fresh[39] or frozen and thawed ovarian cortex.[40] When natural conception fails, in-vitro fertilization (IVF) remains an option.[41] The report of the first three full-term pregnancies achieved with ovarian orthotopic transplantation has promoted its application. Nevertheless, it must be said that the long-term accumulated experience of ovarian grafting is as yet limited.

The aim from now is to identify those women who could benefit from ovarian cortex cryopreservation. We know that as many as 42% of cancer-treated patients will never recover ovarian function,[42] and only 5% of bone marrow transplanted women will conceive.[43] Several markers of ovarian reserve, such as serum FSH, antimüllerian hormone and inhibin B, have been employed[44–46] to predict ovarian function, but only to a certain extent. The question posed here is whether the presence of a high or low population of adult stem cells in the ovaries and/or bone marrow of these patients is a more accurate marker of ovarian function after cancer therapy. This is an issue to be investigated in future trials.

Women are fertile when relatively young; after 30 years old they produce an increasing fraction of defective oocytes, which leads to an increased rate of aneuploidies in human embryos.[47] Women aged $\geq$37 years old have a reduced ovarian reserve and exhibit even higher rates of aneuploidies in their oocytes. They are known to respond poorly to reproductive medicine, and represent as much as 9% of the infertile population treated in assisted reproduction centers.[48] Several possible mechanisms have been highlighted as being responsible for poor response in women of normal age and FSH:

- interference with FSH action as a result of low and high molecular weight proteins[49,50]
- the presence of autoantibodies or antibodies against granulosa cells[51,52]
- defective angiogenesis[53]
- autocrine/paracrine alterations, leading to decreased quantities of certain intraovarian peptides[54]
- altered signal transduction following ligand binding.[55]

However, none of these hypotheses has been demonstrated in low responders (LR). Conversely, logic suggests that these patients have a diminished ovarian reserve, which we proved by employing 3D ultrasound.[56] The possibility of developing an alternative source of follicles in this population is very attractive. If one can isolate, grow and divide these cells, it could constitute a new and more effective approach to poor responders in the future (Figure 4.2).

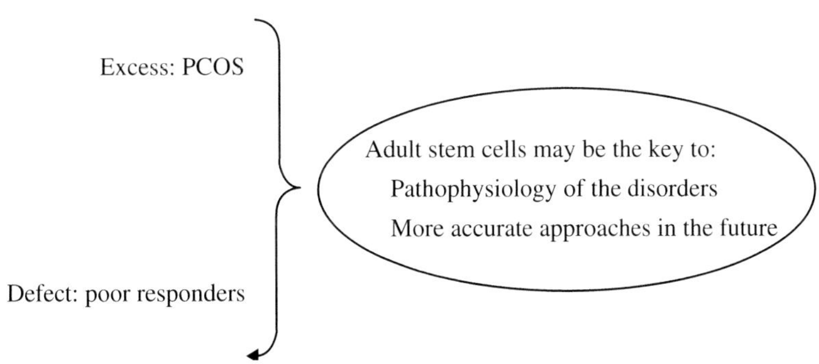

Figure 4.2 Adult stem cells as a solution to infertility problems in polycystic ovarian syndrome (PCOS) and poor responders

Another interesting group of infertile patients are those with polycystic ovarian syndrome (PCOS). The incidence of PCOS in normal subjects is as high as 23%,[57] but the coincidence of menstrual disorders and/or hyperandrogenism is present in 10% of women.[57]

The mechanism underlying the development of PCOS in women is only partially understood. A family grouping of the disease has recently been demonstrated.[58] Different hypotheses have been put forward, including dominant autosomic inheritance with variable penetrance,[59–61] X-related transmission[62] and polygenic inheritance. Various genes have been shown to be related to the disease, but there is no consensus regarding the real extent of each one, alone or in combination.[63,64]

The final common finding is the presence within the ovaries of a high number of antral follicles that only occasionally reach maturity and give place to anovulation. It has been said that a microambient rich in androgens is the cause of this accumulation of preantral follicles in the PCOS ovaries,[65] but an analysis of the presence of adult stem cells in women with PCOS would perhaps reveal the intrinsic mechanism of the large population of preantral follicles observed in this frequent disease. In this sense, it is a further important area to be explored in future trials.

CONCLUSIONS

Theory has it that, in most mammalian species, oocytes are formed before or shortly after birth, but never in adulthood. However, this dogma has recently been challenged by experiments performed in rodents that showed the presence of new germ cells and follicles in adult ovaries. These cells may originate in the bone marrow and are also present in peripheral blood. In humans, immunohistochemical studies have also described the presence of such cells in adult ovaries. These studies in animals and humans have been questioned due to methodological flaws, but they have awoken the curiosity of many scientists internationally. This new concept needs further confirmation, but acceptance that adult mammalian females are capable of producing new oocytes is slowly growing.

If this is true for humans, new approaches to treating infertility will undoubtedly be developed. Women defined within the field of assisted reproduction as 'poor responders' will benefit, as a new source of oocytes could be the key to reconstituting their fertility. The presence of adult stem cells in human ovaries may also be a marker of ovarian function in women treated with chemo- and/or radiotherapy for cancer. Similarly, it could explain the intrinsic mechanism involved in the pathogenesis of polycystic ovarian disease, since an increased number of preantral follicles has been described in this common condition.

REFERENCES

1. Zuckerman S. The number of oocytes in the mature ovary. Recent Prog Horm Res 1951; 6: 63–108.
2. Johnson J, Canning J, Kaneko T, Pru J, Tilly J. Germline stem cells and follicular renewal in the postnatal mammalian ovary. Nature 2004; 428: 145–50.
3. Johnson J, Bagley J, Skaznik-Wikiel M et al. Oocyte generation in adult mammalian ovaries by putative germ cells in bone marrow and peripheral blood. Cell 2005; 122: 303–15.
4. Faddy MJ. Follicle dynamics during ovarian ageing. Mol Cell Endocrinol 2000; 163: 43–8.
5. Pearl R, Schoppe WF. Studies on the physiology of reproduction in the domestic fowl. J Exp Zool 1921; 34: 101–18.
6. Allen E. Ovogenesis during sexual maturity. Am J Anat 1923; 31: 439–81.
7. Evans HM, Swezy O. Ovogenesis and the normal follicular cycle in adult mammalian. Mem Univ Calif 1931; 9: 119–224.
8. Duke KL. Ovogenetic activity of the fetal-type in the ovary of the adult slow loris, *Nycticebus coucang*. Folia Primatol (Basel) 1967; 7: 150–4.
9. David GF, Anand Kumar TC, Baker TG. Uptake of tritiated thymidine by primordial germinal cells in the ovaries of the adult slender loris. J Reprod Fertil 1974; 41: 447–51.
10. Castrillon DH, Quade BJ, Wang TY, Quigley C, Crum CP. The human VASA gene is specifically expressed in the germ cell lineage. Proc Natl Acad Sci USA 2000; 97: 9585–90.
11. Arai H. On the postnatal development of the ovary (albino rat), with special reference to the number of ova. Am J Anat 1920; 27: 405–62.
12. Allen E. Ovogenesis during sexual maturity. Am J Anat 1923; 31: 439–70.
13. Davenport CB. Regeneration of ovaries in mice. J Exp Zool 1925; 42: 1–12.
14. Butcher EO. The origin of the definitive ova in the white rat (*Mus norvegicus albinos*) Anat Rec 1927; 37: 13–29.

15. Parkes AS, Fielding U, Brambell WR. Ovarian regeneration in the mouse after complete double ovariectomy. Proc Roy Soc London Ser B 1927; 101: 328–54.
16. Pallot O. À propos de la régénération ovarienne et des modifications périodiques de l'épithélium vaginal chez le rat blanc. Comp Rend Soc Biol 1928; 99: 1333–4.
17. Morris MA. Pregnancy following removal of both ovaries and tubes. Boston Med Surg J 1901; 144: 86–7.
18. Herzog EL, Chai L, Krause DS. Plasticity of marrow-derived stem cells. Blood 2003; 102: 3483–93.
19. Grove JE, Bruscia E, Krause DS. Plasticity of bone marrow-derived stem cells. Stem Cells 2004; 22: 487–500.
20. Heike T, Nakahata T. Stem cells plasticity in the hematopoietic system. Int J Hematol 2004; 79: 7–14.
21. Jones EC, Krohn PL. The relationships between age, numbers of oocytes and fertility in virgin and multiparous mice. J Endocrinol 1961; 21, 469–95.
22. Byskov AG. Cell kinetic studies of follicular atresia in the mouse ovary. J Reprod Fertil 1974; 37: 277–85.
23. Gosden RG, Laing SC, Felicio LS, Nelson JF, Finch CE. Imminent oocyte exhaustion and reduced follicular recruitment mark the transition to acyclicity in aging C57BL/6J mice. Biol Reprod 1983; 28: 255–60.
24. Faddy MJ, Telfer E, Gosden RG. The kinetics of pre-antral follicle development in ovaries of CBA/Ca mice during the first 14 weeks of life. Cell Tiss Kinet 1983; 20: 551–60.
25. Gosden RG. Germline stem cells in the postnatal ovary: is the ovary more like a testis? Hum Reprod Update 2004; 10: 193–5.
26. Krarup T. Oocyte survival in the mouse ovary after treatment with 9,10-dimethyl-1,2-benzanthracene. J Endocrinol 1970; 46: 483–95.
27. Motta PM, Makabe S. Germ cells in the ovarian surface during fetal development in humans. A three-dimensional microanatomical study by scanning and transmission electron microscopy. J Submicrosc Cytol 1986; 18: 271–90.
28. Gosden RG. Restitution of fertility in sterilized mice by transferring primordial ovarian follicles. Hum Reprod 1990; 5: 499–504.
29. Eppig JJ, Wigglesworth K. Development of mouse and rat oocytes in chimeric reaggregated ovaries after interspecific exchange of somatic and germ cell components. Biol Reprod 2000; 63: 1014–23.
30. Spradling A. More like a man. Nature 2004; 428: 133–4.
31. Bukovsky A, Caudle MR, Svetlikova M, Upadhyaya NB. Origin of germ cells and formation of new primary follicles in adult human ovaries. Reprod Biol Endocrinol 2004; 2: 20.
32. Bukovsky A, Svetlikova M, Caudle M. Oogenesis in cultures derived from adult human ovaries. Reprod Biol Endocrinol 2005; 3: 17.
33. Dalle JH, Huot C, Duval M et al. Successful pregnancies after bone marrow transplantation for Fanconi anemia. Bone Marrow Transplant 2004; 34: 1099–1100.
34. Weir HK, Thun MJ, Hankey BF et al. Annual report to the nation on the status of cancer, 1975–2000, featuring the uses of surveillance data for cancer prevention and control. J Natl Cancer Inst 2003; 95: 1276–99.
35. Gatta G, Capocaccia R, Stiller C et al. EUROCARE Working Group. Childhood cancer survival trends in Europe: a EUROCARE Working Group study. J Clin Oncol 2005; 23: 3742–51.
36. Larsen EC, Muller J, Schmiegelow K, Rechnitzer C, Andersen AN. Reduced ovarian function in long-term survivors of radiation- and chemotherapy-treated childhood cancer. J Clin Endocrinol Metab 2003; 88: 5307–14.
37. Larsen EC, Muller J, Rechnitzer C, Schmiegelow K, Andersen AN. Diminished ovarian reserve in female childhood cancer survivors with regular menstrual cycles and basal FSH <10 IU/l. Hum Reprod 2003; 18: 417–22.
38. Stachecki JJ, Cohen J. An overview of oocyte cryopreservation. Reprod Biomed Online 2004; 9: 152–63.
39. Silber SJ, Lenahan KM, Levine DJ et al. Ovarian transplantation between monozygotic twins discordant for premature ovarian failure. N Engl J Med 2005; 353: 58–63.
40. Donnez J, Dolmans MM, Demylle D et al. Livebirth after orthotopic transplantation of cryopreserved ovarian tissue. Lancet 2004; 364: 1405–10.
41. Meirow D, Levron J, Eldar-Geva T et al. Pregnancy after transplantation of cryopreserved ovarian tissue in a patient with ovarian failure after chemotherapy. N Engl J Med 2005; 353: 318–21.
42. Blumenfeld Z, Avivi I, Ritter M, Rowe JM. Preservation of fertility and ovarian function and minimizing chemotherapy-induced gonadotoxicity in young women. J Soc Gynecol Investig 1999; 6(5): 229–39.
43. Oktay K. Spontaneous conceptions and live birth after heterotopic ovarian transplantation: is there a germline stem cell connection? Hum Reprod 2006; 21: 1345–8.
44. De Vet A, Laven JS, de Jong FH, Themmen AP, Fauser BC. Antimüllerian hormone serum levels: a putative marker for ovarian ageing. Fertil Steril 2002; 77: 357–62.
45. Van Rooij IA, Broekmans FJ, Te Velde ER et al. Serum anti-müllerian hormone levels: a novel measure of ovarian reserve. Hum Reprod 2002; 17: 3065–71.

46. Pastor CL, Vanderhoof VH, Lim LCL et al. Pilot study investigating the age-related decline in ovarian function of regularly menstruating normal women. Fertil Steril 2005; 84,1462–9.

47. Rubio MC, Simón C, Vidal F et al. Chromosomal abnormalities and embryo development in recurrent miscarriage couples. Hum Reprod 2003; 18: 182–8.

48. Pellicer A, Lightman A, Diamond MP, Russell JB, De Cherney AH. Outcome of in vitro fertilization in women with low response to ovarian stimulation. Fertil Steril 1987; 47: 812–15.

49. Sanzo MA, Reichert LE Jr. Gonadotropin receptor binding regulators in serum. Characterization and separation of follitropin binding inhibitor and utropin binding stimulator. J Biol Chem 1982; 257: 6033–40.

50. Lee DW, Grasso P, Dattatreyamurty B, Deziel MR, Reichert LE Jr. Purification of a high molecular weight follicle-stimulating hormone receptor-binding inhibitor from human follicular fluid. J Clin Endocrinol Metab 1993; 77: 160–8.

51. Pellicer A, Ballester MJ, Serrano MD et al. Aetiologic factors involved in the low response to gonadotrophins in infertile women with normal basal serum follicle stimulating hormone. Hum Reprod 1994; 9: 806–11.

52. Wheatcroft NJ, Rogers CA, Metcalfe RA et al. Is subclinical ovarian failure an autoimmune disease? Hum Reprod 1997; 12: 244–9.

53. Gaulden ME. Maternal age effect: the enigma of Downs' syndrome and other trisomic conditions. Mutat Res 1992; 296: 69–88.

54. Ling N, Ui M, Shimonaka M, Shimasaki S, Bicsak TA. An ICF-binding protein in ovarian follicular fluid blocks FSH-stimulated steroid production by ovarian granulosa cells. In: Yen SSC, Vale WW, eds. Neuroendocrine Regulation of Reproduction, Serono Symposia Series, Norwell, 1990: 207–15.

55. Fauser BCJ, Van Heusden AM. Manipulation of human ovarian function: physiological concepts and clinical consequences. Endocrine Rev 1997; 18: 71–106.

56. Pellicer A, Ardiles G, Neuspiller F et al. Evaluation of the ovarian reserve in young low responders with normal basal FSH levels using three-dimensional ultrasonography. Fertil Steril 1998; 70: 671–5.

57. Polson DW, Wadsworth J, Adams J, Franks S. Polycystic ovaries – a common finding in normal women. Lancet 1988; 1(8590): 870–2.

58. Strauss III JF. Some new thoughts on the pathophysiology and genetics of polycystic ovary syndrome. Ann NY Acad Sci 2003; 997: 42–7.

59. Cooper HE, Spellacy WN, Prem KA, Cohen WD. Hereditary factors in Stein–Leventhal syndrome. Am J Obstet Gynecol 1968; 100: 371–82.

60. Carey AH, Chan KL, Short F et al. Evidence of a single gene effect causing polycystic ovaries and male pattern baldness. Clin Endocrinol (Oxf) 1993; 386: 653–8.

61. Govind A, Obhrai MS, Clayton RN. Polycystic ovaries are inherited as an autosomal dominant trait: analysis of 29 polycystic ovary syndrome and 10 control families. J Clin Endocrinol Metab 1999; 811: 38–43.

62. Wild RA, Umstot ES, Andersen RN, Ranney GB, Givens JR. Androgen parameters and their correlation with body weight in one hundred thirty-eight women thought to have hyperandrogenism. Am J Obstet Gynecol 1983; 146: 602–6.

63. Urbanek M, Legro RS, Discroll DA et al. Thirty-seven candidate genes for polycystic ovary syndrome: strongest evidence for linkage is with follistatin. Proc Natl Acad Sci USA 1999; 9615: 8573–8.

64. Kahasar-Miller M, Boots LR, Bartolucci A, Azziz R. Role of a CYP17 polymorphism in the regulation of circulating dehydroepiandrosterone sulphate levels in women with polycystic ovary syndrome. Fertil Steril 2004; 82: 973–5.

65. Webber LJ, Stubbs S, Stark J et al. Formation and early development of follicles in the polycystic ovary. Lancet 2003; 362(9389): 1017–21.

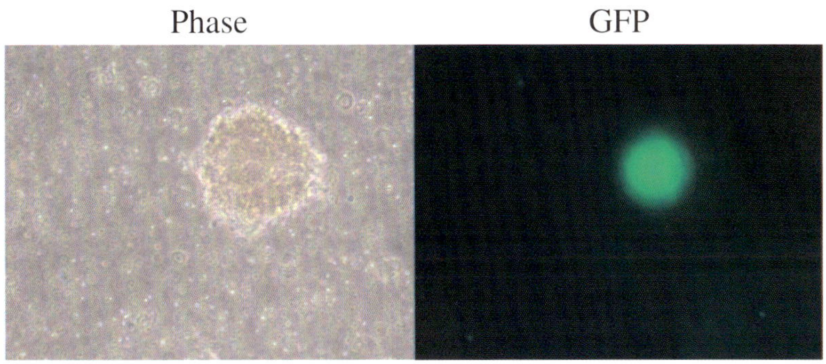

Figure 2.2 In-vivo expression of GFP in oocytes. Mouse ES cells transfected with a *Gdf9*/GFP plasmid were injected into blastocyst stage embryos, which were then subsequently transferred into host females. The mice that resulted were analyzed for agouti coat color and scored for percent of chimerism. Chimeric founders were then sacrificed and the oocyte–cumulus cell complexes were analyzed. This figure shows both GFP and phase-contrast images of such a complex.

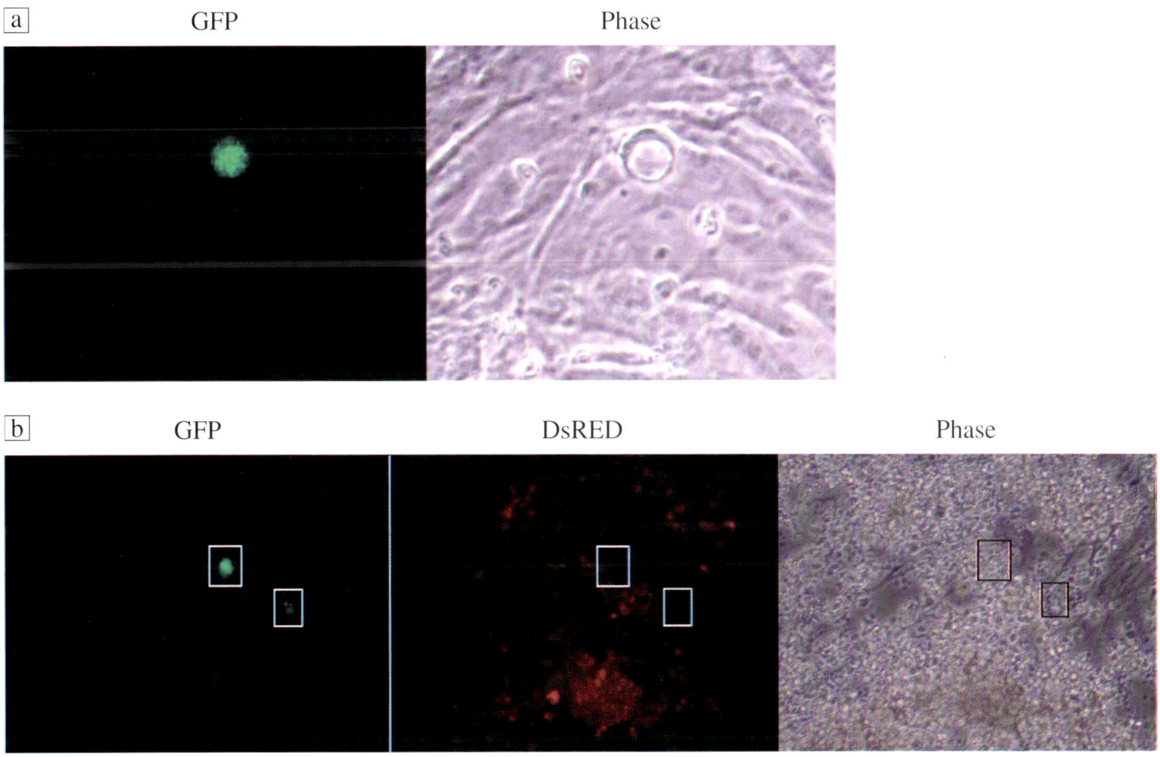

Figure 2.3 In-vitro expression of GFP and Ds-Red in transfected mouse ES cells. ES cells electroporated with *Gdf9*/GFP (M. Matzuk) and *Sf-1*/DsRed plasmids were selected for these constructs using G418 for 8 days. Screened clones were confirmed by PCR and Southern blot analysis. Positive ES cell clones were then cultured in the presence of LIF. Cells were examined for expression of GFP and DsRed by fluorescence microscopy. (a) GFP and phase contrast images on day 2 of culture. (b) GFP, DsRed and phase contrast images on day 8 of culture.

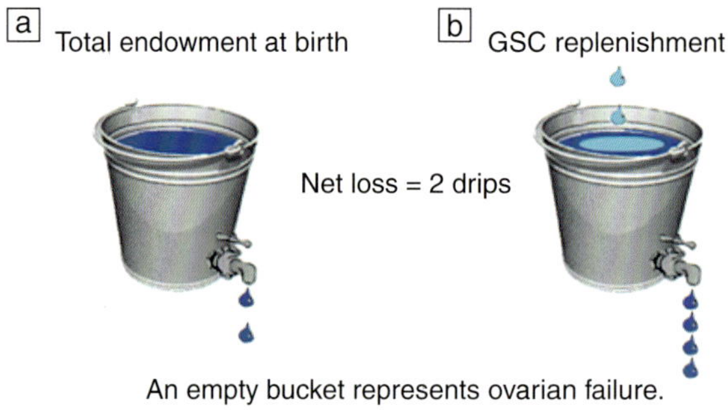

Figure 3.1 Simple cartoon representation of diminishing oocyte number over postnatal life in mammals. Here, oocyte number is represented by the level of water inside buckets. Drips of liquid from the bottom of the buckets represent oocyte loss via growth activation, ovulation, or atresia. (a) The dogma of a total endowment of oocytes at birth is represented; 2 drips have been lost. No input of new oocytes (input drips) exists. (b) A more rapid loss of oocytes (4 drips) is offset by the input of new drips. Here, input drips offset and slow the more rapid loss of liquid. Critically, the net loss of drips/oocytes is equal in both cases. Static histomorphometric analyses of oocytes within histological preparations over postnatal life (e.g. measuring the water level) would show the same trend of oocyte loss in either situation.

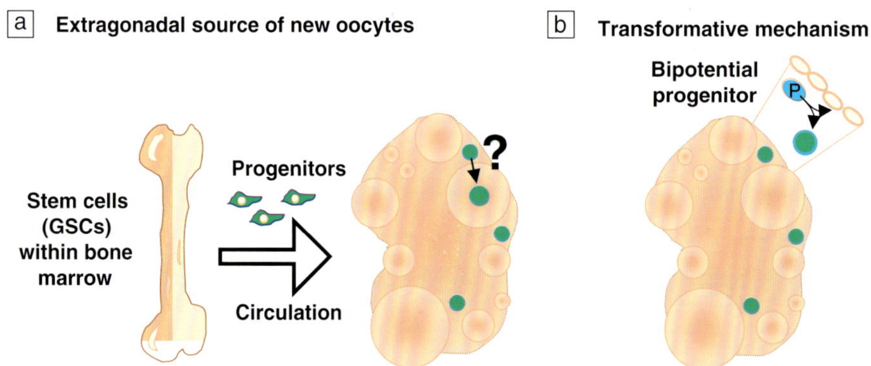

Figure 3.2 Two proposed mechanisms for the generation of new oocytes in postnatal mammals. (a) New oocytes are produced via germ stem cells that reside in an extragonadal location, the bone marrow.[4] Germ progenitor cells are released to the peripheral circulation, and these progenitors home to the ovary, where they may engraft as new oocytes (depicted in green) within new follicles. The question of the developmental potential of labeled oocytes after bone marrow transplantation remains unclear.[10] (b) New oocytes (green) are produced by a transformative mechanism. Bipotential progenitor cells (depicted in blue) produce both new oocytes and somatic cells within the ovary.[26,29,30]

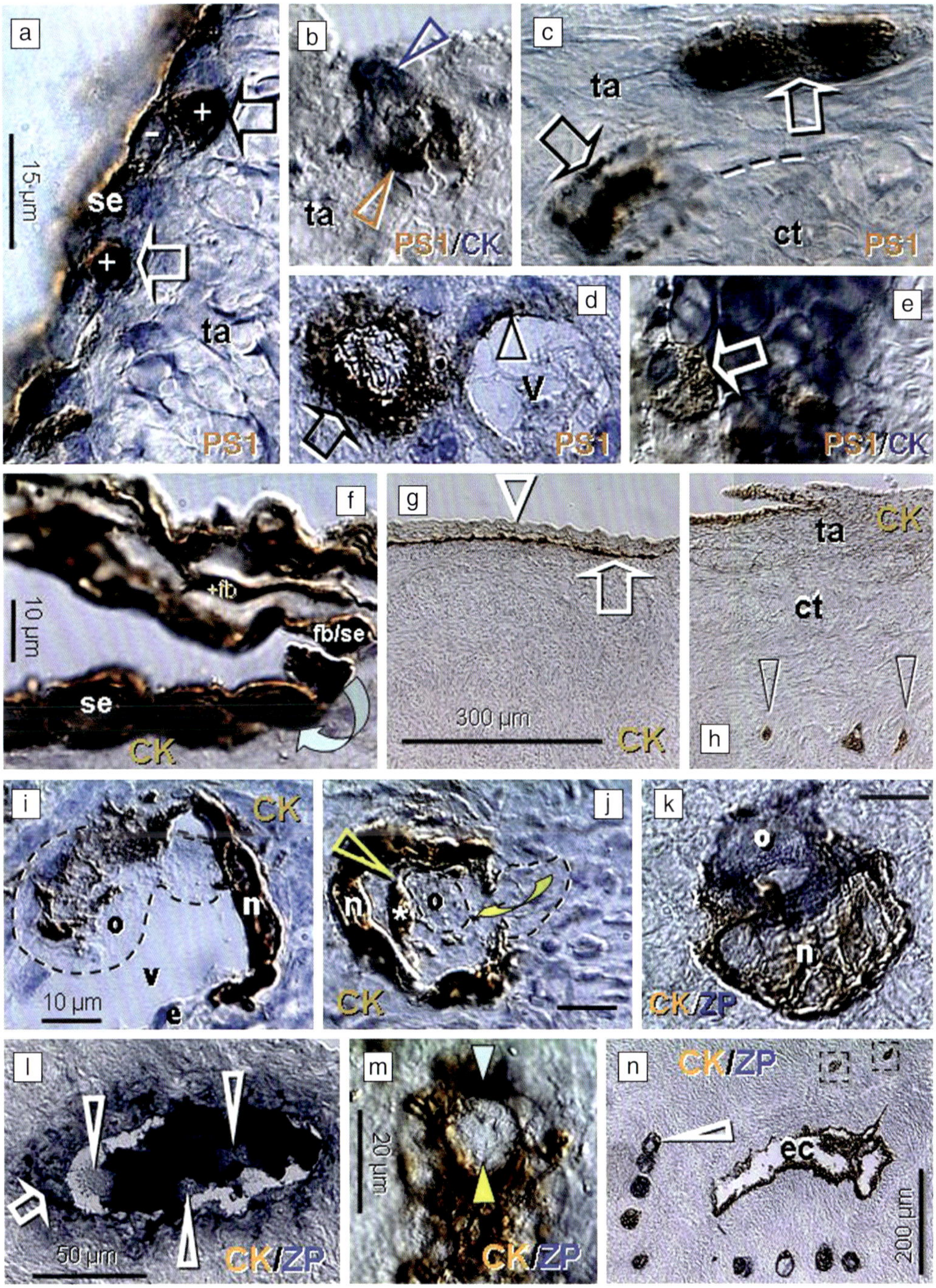

Figure 5.3 Differentiation of germ cells and primitive granulosa cells. (a) Segments of OSE show cytoplasmic PS1 (brown color) expression (se). Dividing OSE cells give rise to cells exhibiting nuclear PS1 immunostaining (+ nuclei, asymmetric division) and descending from the OSE (arrows) into tunica albuginea (ta). (b) Except asymmetrically divided OSE cell – note CK+ (blue color and arrowhead) and PS1+ (brown color and arrowhead) daughter cells, no PS1 or CK immunoexpression is apparent in this OSE segment. (c) In TA, the putative germ cells increase in size, but nuclear PS1 immunostaining persists. They show a symmetric division (white arrow) and exhibit development of cytoplasmic PS1 immunoexpression when entering (black arrow) the upper ovarian cortex (ct). (d) In the cortex, the cells show diminution of nuclear and increase of

▲ cytoplasmic PS1 staining (arrow), particularly when attached to the cortical vessels (v). In such cases, the PS1 immunoexpression appears to be extended toward endothelial cells (arrowhead). (e) In some instances, the asymmetric division giving rise to the putative PS1+ (brown color) germ cells could be observed at the periphery of CK+ (blue color) cortical epithelial crypts (arrow). (f) Shows association of CK+ (brown color) fibroblasts (+fb,) with the TA flap surface (arrowhead), and transition from mesenchymal to epithelial morphology (fb/se) and surface epithelium cells (se, arched arrow). (g) View of ovarian surface (arrowhead) and adjacent cortex. Arrow indicates bilaminar epithelial cord. (h) Ovarian tunica albuginea (ta) filled with CK18+ mesenchymal cells and exhibiting flap projection, and adjacent cortex (ct) with epithelial nests (arrowheads). (i) The CK+ (brown color) epithelial nest (n) inside of the cortical venule, which extends an arm to catch the oocyte (o, dashed line) from the blood circulation. (j) The nest body and closing 'gate'. A portion of the oocyte (dashed line) still lies outside of the complex, and is expected to move inside (arched arrow). The oocyte contains intraooplasmic CK+ (brown color) extensions from the nest wall (arrowhead), which contribute to the formation of CK+ paranuclear (Balbiani) body (asterisk). The oocyte nucleus is indicated by a dashed line. (k) Occupied 'bird's nest' type indicates a half-way oocyte–nest assembly. (l) Some medullary vessels show accumulation of ZP+ (blue color) degenerating oocytes with unstained nuclei (arrowheads). Arrow indicates ZP release. (m) Appearance of germ-like cell among CK+ cells (brown color) in epithelial crypt. Note ZP+ segment (blue color and white arrowhead) associated with unstained round cell (yellow arrowhead). (n) Association of primary follicles (arrowhead) with the cortical epithelial crypt (ec). Dashed boxes indicate unassembled epithelial nests. (Adapted from Bukovsky et al[29] – see http://www.rbej.com/content/2/1/20 for more details. © Antonin Bukovsky).

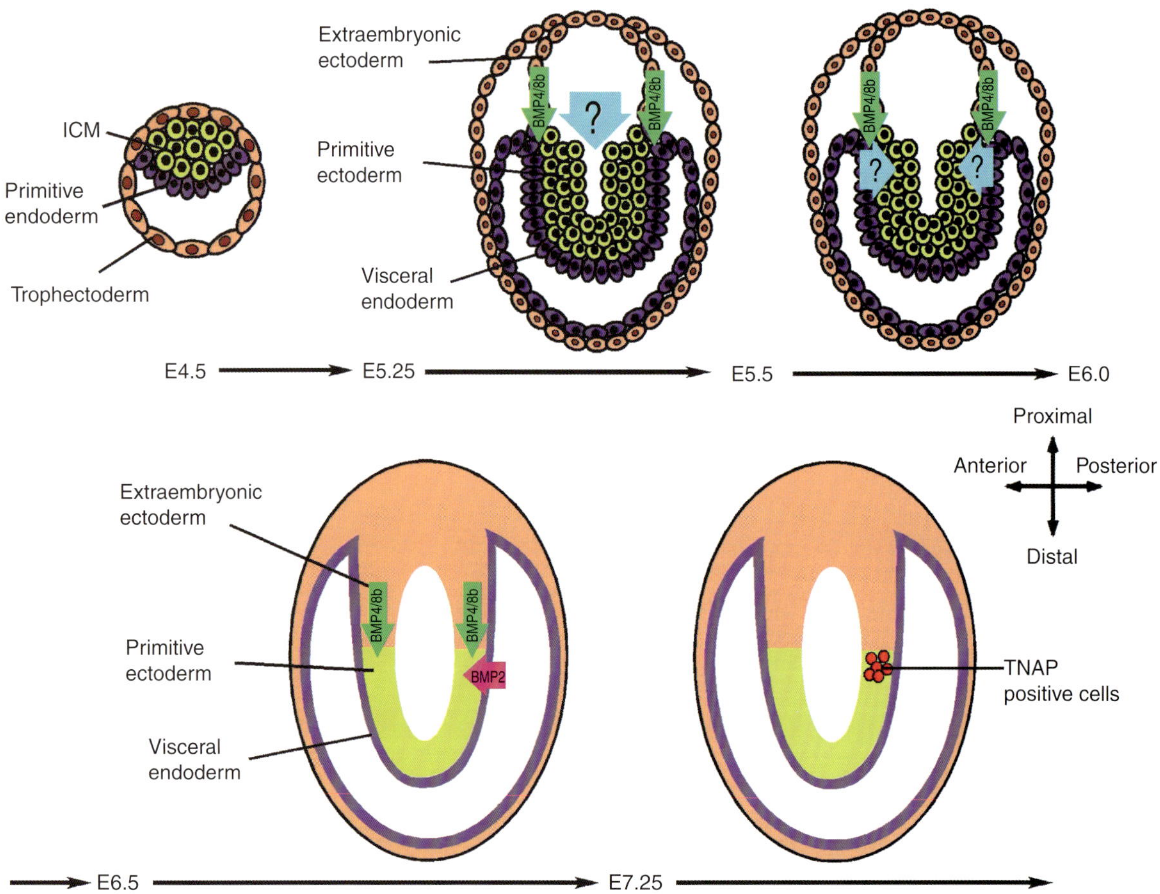

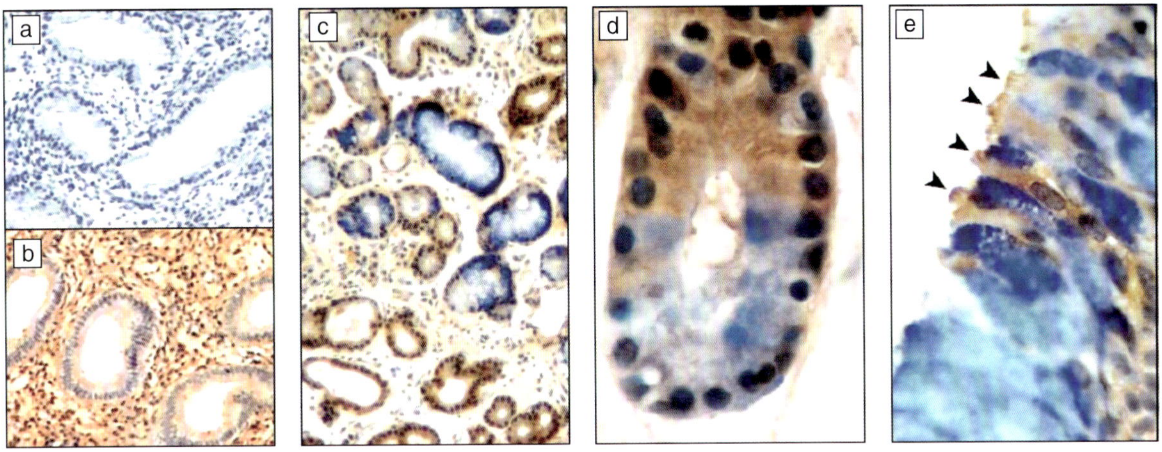

Figure 10.1 Donor-derived cells in the endometrium of an HLA-A11-mismatched bone marrow transplant recipient (patient 1). Immunohistochemistry using anti-HLA-A11 monoclonal antibody, biotin peroxidase detection system, diaminobenzidine as the chromogen (brown), and hematoxylin counterstain. (a) HLA-A11-negative control (original magnification ×200). (b) HLA-A11 immunopositivity (brown) in an HLA-A11-positive control (original magnification ×200). (c) HLA-A11 immunopositivity (brown) in patient 1. More than 50% of the cells were of donor origin (original magnification ×100). (d) Endometrial glands partially derived from cells of donor origin (brown; original magnification ×400). (e) Rare cells of donor origin (brown) in an endometrial gland. Functional differentiation is noted by characteristic cilia. Arrowheads identify the ciliated epithelial surface (original magnification ×600).

Figure 6.1 Signals required for PGC formation in mouse embryonic development. Primordial germ cell (PGC) specification requires multiple signals from different sources during mouse development. At E5.25–E5.5, a yet unknown signal generated by the extraembryonic ectoderm is needed to prime the cells for later BMP signals, presumably by up-regulating SMAD5 in selected cell populations. At E5.5–E6.0, a second unknown signal from the visceral endoderm is required. This signal is dependent on ALK2 signaling in the visceral endodermal cells, suggesting that the BMP4/8b from the extraembryonic ectoderm stimulate the production of this second unknown signal. The lineage restriction of PGCs occurs at E6.5–E7.25. At this last stage of PGC specification, both BMP4/8b signals from the extraembryonic ectoderm and BMP2 signal from the visceral endoderm are required; the BMP2 expression is the highest in the posterior region of the visceral endoderm. After E7.25, PGCs are detectable by alkaline phosphatase activity. ICM, inner cell mass; TNAP, tissue non-specific alkaline phosphatase. Blue block arrows denote unknown signals from extraembryonic ectoderm and visceral endoderm. Green arrows indicate BMP4 and BMP8b signals from extraembryonic ectoderm. Magenta arrow denotes BMP2 signal from visceral endoderm. Red ovals represent TNAP-positive primordial germ cells.

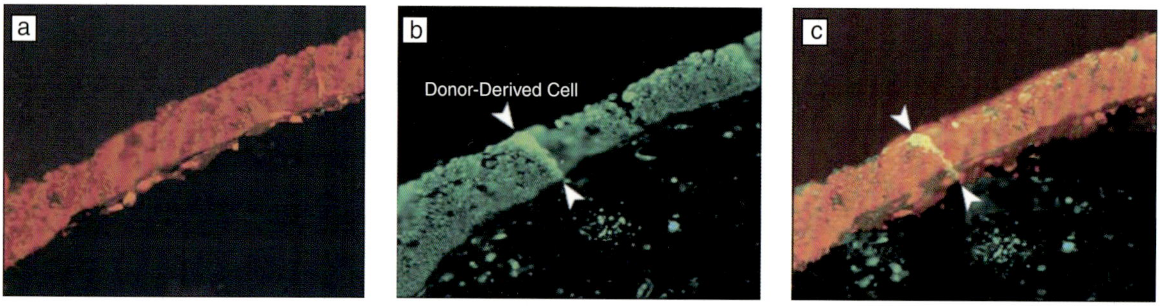

Figure 10.2 Differentiation shown by immunofluorescence in donor-derived cell in endometrial epithelial layer. Immunofluorescence using tetrarhodamine isothiocyanate for calcitonin expression (red) and fluorescein isothiocyanate for donor-derived cells (green) in endometrial epithelial cells of HLA-A11-negative transplant recipient (patient 1) who received bone marrow from an HLA-A11-positive donor. (a) Calcitonin expression in endometrial epithelium indicative of receptivity to blastocyst implantation. (b) Mismatched HLA-A11-positive endometrial epithelial cell of donor origin (arrowheads). (c) Merge demonstrating HLA-mismatched cell expressing calcitonin as a marker of functional differentiation (original magnification ×100).

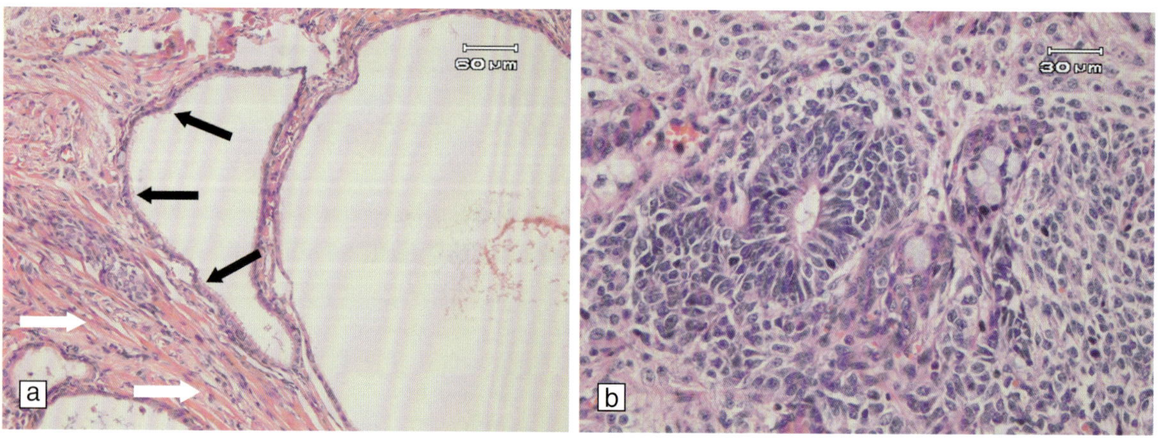

Figure 12.7 In-vivo differentiation assessment. Histological section of a teratoma tumor with representation of the endodermal (ciliated columnar epithelium; black arrows) and mesodermal (striated muscle; white arrows) differentiation (a), and ectodermal (neural rosette) differentiation (b)

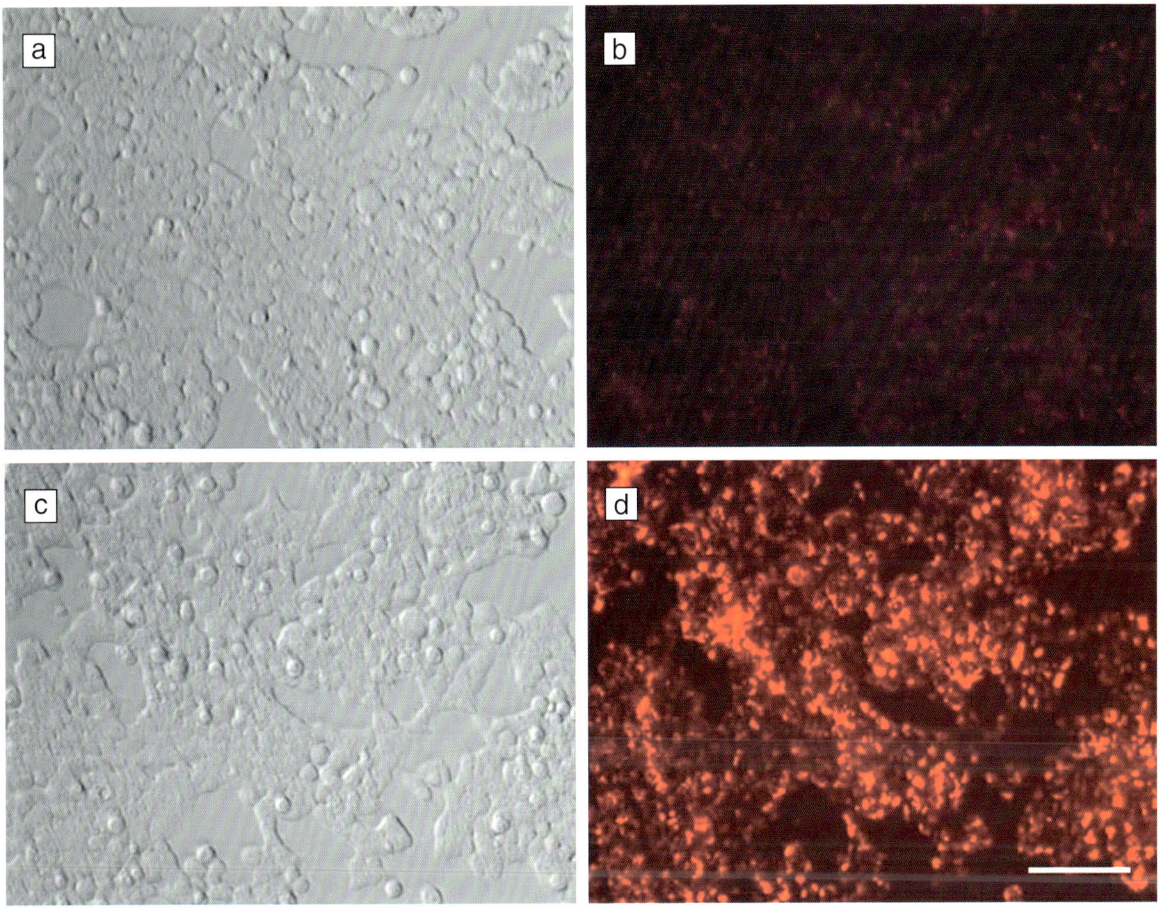

Figure 13.1 Uptake of rhodamine-albumin by unpermeabilized (a,b) and permeabilized (c,d) 293T cells in the presence of cell extracts: (a,c) phase contrast; (b,d) fluorescence. Scale bar, 100μm. (Images courtesy of Dr Sadhana Agarwal, Advanced Cell Technology, Inc.)

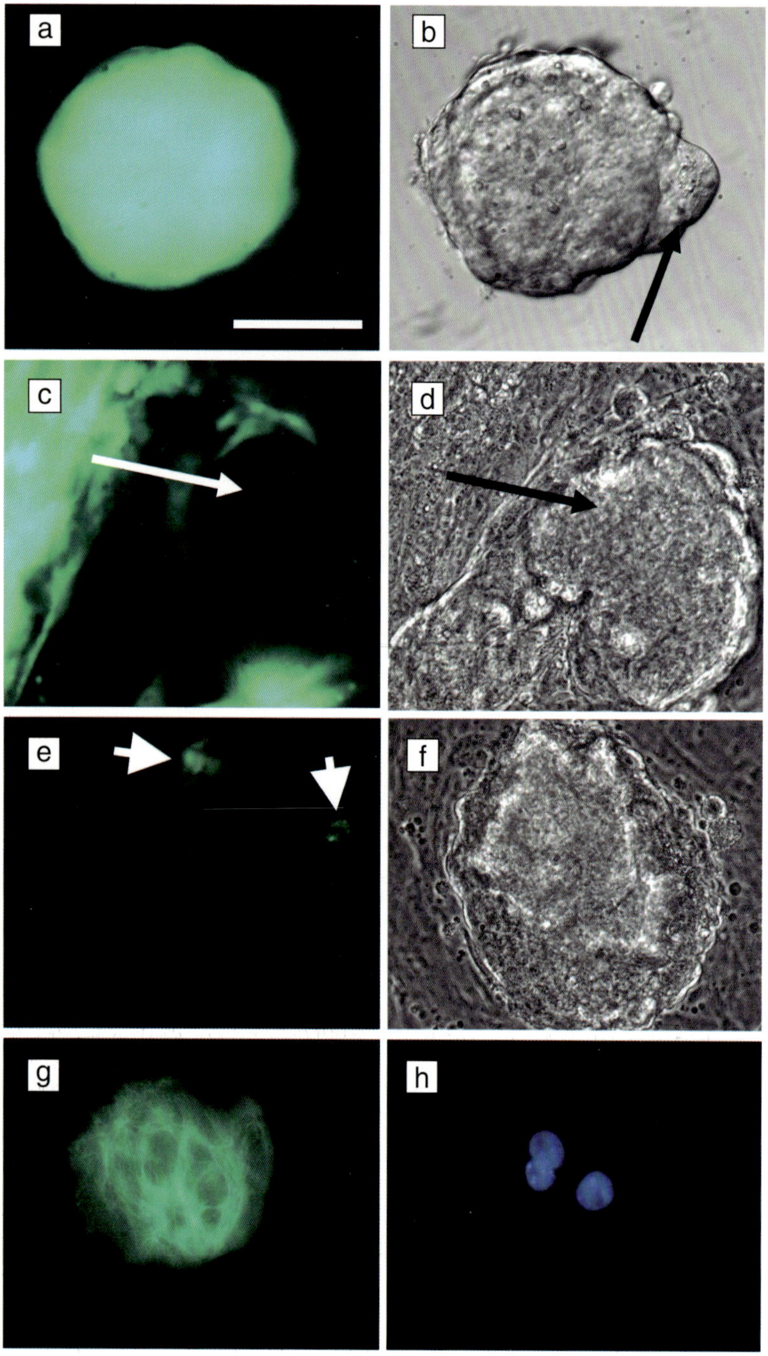

Figure 13.2 Stages of single blastomere growth in the presence (a–f) or absence (g,h) of mouse embryonic stem (mES) cells: (a,c,e) green fluorescence; (b) Hoffman modulation optics; (d,f) phase contrast. (a,b) Clump of GFP-positive mES cells 48 hours after aggregation with single blastomeres; arrow shows a protruding cluster of GFP-negative cells. (c,d) Outgrowth of GFP-negative cells aggregated with GFP^+ mES cells, after being plated on MEF; arrows point to GFP-negative cells. (e,f) Passage 1 of the outgrowth; arrows show remaining GFP^+ mES cells. (g,h) Single blastomere outgrowth on MEF for 4 days without ES cells, stained with Troma-1 and DAPI. Scale bar, 100 μm. (Reproduced from Chung et al,[23] with permission)

CHAPTER 5

Adult stem cells in the human ovary

Antonin Bukovsky and Irma Virant-Klun

INTRODUCTION

The existence of adult stem cells in the human ovary has been a matter of dispute for over 100 years. If they are totipotent, such stem cells may give rise to the two distinct cell types required for the formation of ovarian primary follicles, i.e. somatic granulosa cells and female germ cells differentiating into oocytes. They may already exist in fetal ovaries, and reappear during adulthood.

Nevertheless, it is still widely believed that the formation of new oocytes and primary follicles does not occur in adult mammalian ovaries. However, from a Darwinian viewpoint on the evolution of species, it seems contradictory that in contrast to adult amphibians with persisting oogenesis, mammalian females, including humans, would evolve a uniquely retrogressive reproductive mechanism whereby they are required to preserve their gametes from the fetal period for up to several decades.

By the end of the 19th century, and during the first half of the 20th century, two opinions concerning oogenesis were discussed. The first view was introduced by Waldeyer[1] and elaborated by Kingery,[2] who proposed that new oocytes were formed from the germinal (surface) epithelium of adult ovaries. The second view was based on the studies of Beard[3] and paper of Pearl and Schoppe,[4] who suggested that all oocytes present in adult mammalian individuals originate from the period when the ovaries were formed and are stored and utilized until menopause.

During the 1950s and 1960s, the belief that all primary follicles in adult mammalian females were formed during the fetal period[5,6] prevailed, primarily because of the overall diminution of primary follicle numbers with age reported by Block in the early 1950s.[7] Nevertheless, Erik Block wrote: 'In the age range eighteen to thirty-eight, the relation between the patient's age and the number of primary follicles cannot be established statistically'.[7] This suggests that during the 20 years of the human female prime reproductive period, there is no significant change in the number of primary follicles. However, this important part of Block's conclusions has not been appreciated by interpreters.[5,6]

PRIMORDIAL MAMMALIAN GERM CELLS ORIGINATE FROM EMBRYONIC SOMATIC STEM CELLS

Until recently, the origin of primordial germ cells in mammalian females was attributed to Weissmann's theory of the continuity of the germ plasm.[8] This theory assumed that during the earliest stages of embryonic development, before embryonic cells become committed along specific pathways, a set of germ cells is set aside, which are destined to give rise to the gametes.

Utilization of newer techniques has shown that Weissmann's theory may fit invertebrates (*Caenorhabditis elegans* and *Drosophila*) and some lower vertebrates (zebrafish and frogs), but not mice, and possibly not mammals in general.[9,10] Studies of mouse embryos, in which genetically marked cells were introduced at the 4- and 8-cell stage blastomere, have shown that such cells can either become germ cells or somatic cells.[11] This suggests that no specific germ cell commitment exists prior to implantation. During the postimplantation period, mouse germ cells are not identifiable before about 7 days after fertilization,[12] suggesting that germ cells differentiate from somatic lineage.[13] It has also been shown that cellular differentiation of grafted embryonic cells does not depend on where the grafts were taken, but rather where they were placed.[14] In other words, the stem cells for primordial germ cells are totipotent embryonic stem cells.

In human embryos, primordial germ cells arise outside the urogenital ridge, in the dorsal endoderm of the yolk sac at 24 days of age. They migrate by ameboid movements to indifferent gonadal primordia at 28–35 days.[15] Differentiation of the indifferent gonad into an ovary or a testis takes place during the second fetal month.[16] After the primordial germ cells enter the developing embryonic gonad, they commit to a developmental pathway that will lead them to become either eggs or sperm, depending not on their own sex chromosome constitution, but on whether the gonad has begun to develop into an ovary or a testis, respectively. The sex chromosomes in the gonadal somatic cells determine which type of the gonad will develop, as a single *Sry* gene on the Y chromosome can redirect a female embryo to become a male (reviewed in Reference 10). Hence, gonadal somatic cells play an important role in the development of germ cells.

FETAL OVARIAN STEM CELLS (FIGURE 5.1)

Ovarian surface epithelial cells differentiate into fetal oocytes and granulosa cells (Figure 5.1a–d)

The surface of the ovary is covered by a serous membrane made of ovarian surface epithelium (OSE), which is continuous with the peritoneal mesothelium. During the early stages of ovarian development there is a rapid proliferation of OSE cells, resulting in cellular stratification, nuclear pleomorphism and nuclear irregularities. Toward the end of intrauterine life the OSE is reduced to a single layer of cells, exhibited in the adult ovary in a cuboidal, columnar or squamous pattern. Many cells from the OSE enter the cortex in fetal ovaries and become associated with oocytes.[15]

The OSE cells have been suggested to be a source of germ cells in mammalian species,[1,2,17–19] including human fetuses.[16,20] Scanning and transmission electron microscopy have revealed numerous germ cells (10 μm in diameter) within the ovarian OSE of human fetuses from 7 to 24 weeks of intrauterine life. Germ cells are easily distinguished from smaller OSE cells by their rounded contour, smooth surface and, in some instances, large ameboid evaginations.[21] Using differential interference contrast and immunohistochemistry, we previously reported the occurrence of similar putative germ cells within the OSE and cortex of adult human ovaries.[22] These data indicate that germ cells are present in the OSE. They may either invade the OSE from adjacent structures and are extruded from the ovary,[21] originate in the OSE and invade the ovarian cortex, or both.[22]

The presence of oocytes in the OSE is usually interpreted as an extrusion of superfluous gametes from the ovary.[21] It may occasionally happen that the germ cells within the OSE enlarge into oocytes, which are sequestered, but most germ cells leave the OSE to enter ovarian tunica albuginea (TA) and the cortex.[22] In midpregnancy human ovaries, which lack the TA layer, the OSE contained small germ cells (asterisks, Figure 5.1a), contrasting larger cells in the adjacent and distant cortex (white and black arrowheads, respectively).

The germ cells originated from OSE stem cells by asymmetric division (white arrowhead, Figure 5.1b), during which the OSE daughter cell kept (white asterisk) and daughter germ cell was devoid of the

Figure 5.1 Oocytes and granulosa cells originate from OSE stem cells in midpregnancy human fetuses. (a) Papanicolaou's staining (PAP) shows OSE (se) containing small germ cells (asterisks), exhibiting increase in size in the adjacent (white arrowhead) and distant cortex (black arrowhead). nc, nuclear cluster; mcc, mesenchymal cell cord. (b) Major histocompatibility complex class I (MHC-I) staining, no hematoxylin counterstain. Asymmetric division (white arrowhead) gives rise to MHC-I+ OSE (white asterisk) and MHC-I– germ (black asterisk) daughter cells. Symmetric division (black arrowhead) produces two MHC– germ cells (crossing over). Larger (tadpole-like) germ cell (dashed line) enters the ovarian cortex (arched arrow). (c) CK18 staining

Continued

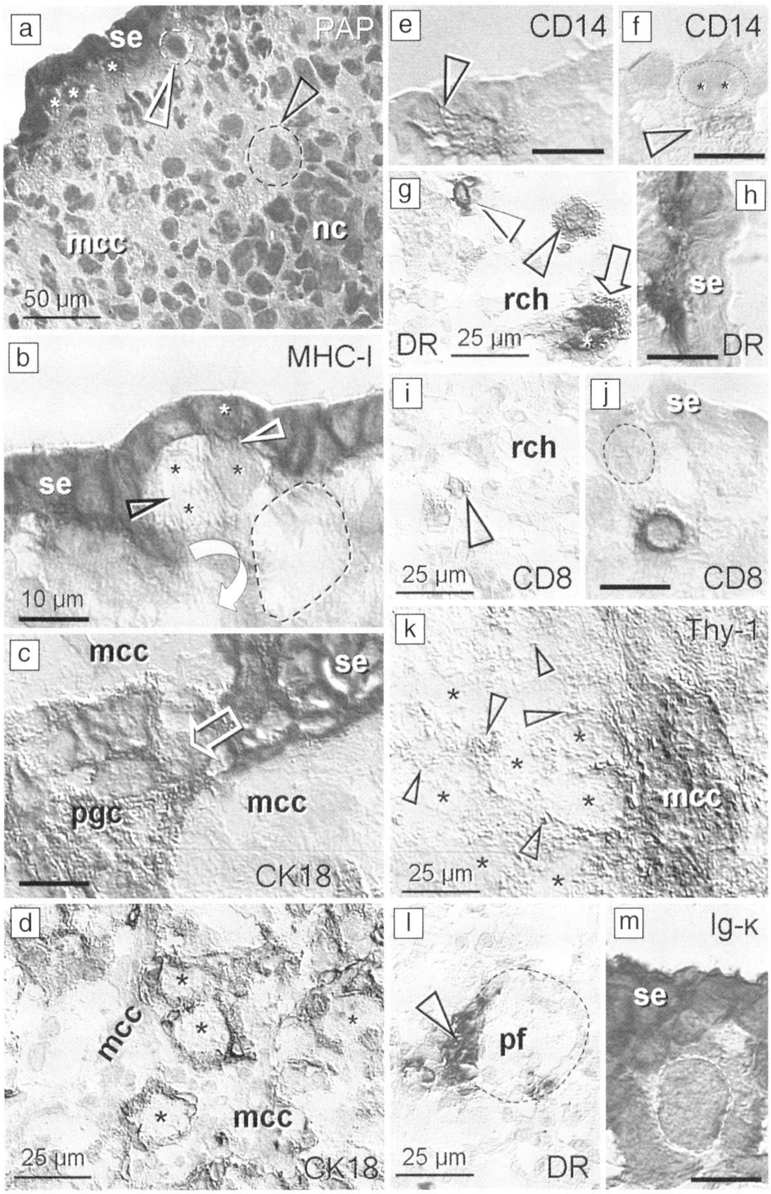

of a cluster of primitive granulosa cells (pgc) descending from the OSE (se; arrow) between mesenchymal cell cords (mcc). (d) Small (primordial) follicles (asterisks) in the lower cortex, without CK18+ Balbiani bodies in oocytes. (e and f) CD14 primitive monocyte-derived cells (MDC; tissue macrophages) associate with OSE (arrowheads) and developing germ-like cells; dashed line and asterisks in (f) indicates symmetric division of germ cells. Hematoxylin counterstain. (g) HLA-DR+ (activated) lymphocyte (white arrowhead) and monocyte type cells (black arrowhead) migrate through the rete channels (rch) and interact (arrow) with resident MDC (asterisk). (h) Association of activated MDC with the OSE. (i) CD8 T cells in rete channels (arrowhead) and beneath the OSE (j) with emerging germ cell (dashed line; no hematoxylin counterstain). (k) Thy-1 differentiation protein is secreted (arrowheads) from the Thy-1+ mesenchymal cell cord among primordial follicles (asterisks). (l) HLA-DR cells intimately associate with larger (primary) follicles (pf). (m) Immunoglobulins (Ig-κ) have a low affinity for germ-like cells (dashed line) but heavily bind to OSE cells. The measurement bar in b for c, e, f, h, j and m. (Adapted from Bukovsky et al,[28] with permission of Humana Press Inc.)

major histocompatibility complex class I (MHC-I) expression (black asterisk). This appears to be followed by a symmetric division (black arrowhead), resulting in two daughter germ cells lacking MHC class I (black asterisks), which may serve for the crossing over. Next, the germ cells increased in size and exhibited a tadpole-like shape (dashed line; note a lack of nuclear counterstain in this panel), when entering the ovarian cortex (arched arrow).

A second potential of the OSE stem cells in the same fetal ovaries was to differentiate into the sprouts of primitive granulosa cells (arrow, Figure 5.1c) between mesenchymal cell cords (mcc) rich in Thy-1 differentiation protein (see mcc, Figure 5.1k). The emerging primitive granulosa cells (pgc, Figure 5.1c) showed lower cytokeratin expression than the OSE cells (se). The primitive granulosa cells associated with oocytes descended into the deeper cortex and formed primordial follicles (asterisks, Figure 5.1d).

Immune system-related cells and molecules influence commitment of stem cells in fetal ovaries (Figure 5.1e–m)

Immune system-related cells – monocyte-derived cells (MDC; tissue macrophages) and T and B lymphocytes and their products (immunoglobulins, growth factors and cytokines) – are not only involved in the immune surveillance but also in the regulation of differentiation of epithelial and other tissue cell types throughout the body (see Reference 23 for data and review). In addition, the immune system components can also be involved in the determination of the commitment of pluripotent or totipotent stem cells in vivo. For instance, the stem cells represented by OSE may either differentiate into the germ or granulosa cells in fetal ovaries (Figure 5.1a–c). Although systemic hormonal influences may be involved in fetal oogenesis, only some OSE cells will produce daughter germ cells (Figure 5.1b). This indicates that some kind of local signaling may be required.

Association of monocyte-derived cells with fetal ovarian surface epithelium

Monocyte-derived cells expressing CD14 (primitive MDC) show cytoplasmic extensions among OSE cells in fetal ovaries (Figure 5.1e), and accompany appearance of germ cells (Figure 5.1f). This indicates that certain MDC may be determined to induce transformation of OSE stem cells into the germ cells. How, however, can such determination be achieved?

A role of rete ovarii

Ovarian differentiation begins before follicles form, and it is characterized by the development of oocytes, organization of the rete ovarii and evolution of the OSE. At the embryonic age of 9 weeks, human female gonads show a marked development of rete cords with lumen formation, and the rete reaches the center of the ovary at 12 weeks. The first follicles are formed after the 4th fetal month, and follicle formation always begins in the innermost part of the cortex, close to the rete ovarii.[15] This structure is essential for follicular development, since if it is removed before formation of follicles has started, follicles will not form.[24] However, how this structure influences the development of fetal ovaries is not well understood.

Rete is a simple structure consisting of rete channels lined by a labyrinth of mesenchymal rete cords containing resident MDC (asterisk, Figure 5.1g). Rete cords, and their extensions toward the ovarian surface (mesenchymal cell cord, Figure 5.1k), are rich in Thy-1 differentiation protein (Thy-1 dp). Thy-1 dp is an ancestral member of the immunoglobulin gene superfamily of molecules,[25] and appears to play an important role in the stimulation of early steps in cellular differentiation of distinct tissues, including ovaries.[23,26,27] Rete channels contain MDC and T lymphocytes (arrowheads, Figure 5.1g, i), which interact with resident MDC (arrow, Figure 5.1g), and such cells interact with OSE (Figure 5.1h, j).

We speculated that the resident MDC in rete ovarii carry a memory on the primordial germ cells, which populated the embryonic gonad, and this memory could be transferred to MDC and T cells migrating through the rete channels.[28] The migrating cells reaching the OSE may stimulate a transformation of OSE cells into new (secondary) germ cells. In this way only a limited number of OSE cells will produce new germ cells.

Primordial vs primary follicles

The OSE stem cells differentiate into granulosa and germ cells, which eventually assemble to form ovarian primordial or primary follicles. However, throughout the literature, there is a misconception between the terms primordial and primary follicle.

Cleveland Silvester Simkins was the first to distinguish two types of follicles in human fetal ovaries: the smaller (about 20 μm in diameter), which he called 'primordial' follicles, and the larger (about 50 μm), which he designated as 'primary' follicles[16] (see also Figure 5.1d and k vs Figure 5.1l).The primordial follicles consist of oocytes with often altered nuclei, which are surrounded by an inconstant and incomplete layer of small ellipsoid granulosa cells. These follicles are found only in the cortex of the fetal and infant ovaries, where they constitute the most conspicuous part of the gland. The primary follicles are found only in the peripheral margin of the ovarian medulla. Their oocytes take deeper stain and are always surrounded by at least one row of large, round and regular granulosa cells. Primary follicles are the follicles that grow and develop into definitive structures, while the primordial follicles gradually disappear during childhood and are not detected in adult human ovaries.[16]

The formation of primordial follicles (asterisks, Figure 5.1k) is accompanied by Thy-1 dp (arrowheads) released from mesenchymal cell cords (mcc). Some fetal primordial follicles may reach the primary follicle stage, which shows an intimate association of activated MDC (arrowhead, Figure 5.1l). The OSE also shows strong binding of immunoglobulin (Ig)-κ chain (possibly IgM), which is depleted in developing germ cells (dashed line, Figure 5.1m).

Altogether, the differentiation of OSE stem cells into ovarian granulosa and germ cells and follicular development in human fetal ovaries appear to be under the control of immune system-related cells and molecules.

ADULT OVARIAN STEM CELLS (FIGURES 5.2, 5.3 AND 5.4)

Like in fetal ovaries the OSE stem cells in adult human female gonads differentiate either into the germ cells or primitive granulosa cells.[29] In contrast to the fetal period, however, the process of formation of new primary follicles is much more complex.[28] This may be why the follicular renewal in humans during adulthood was difficult to explore. For instance, Simkins believed that the formation of new follicles occurs in human fetuses and persists during adulthood, and indicated that oocytes in fetal ovaries originate from OSE stem cells (like in adult mice[17]) but suggested that committed precursors of germ cells persist deep in the cortex (close to medulla) in adult women.[16]

Tunica albuginea contains progenitors of adult human ovarian stem cells

In functional human ovaries the OSE is found in certain areas only, but in women with anovulatory cycles, or patients with polycystic or sclerotic ovaries, the ovarian surface is completely covered with OSE.[30] The adult OSE is attached to the basal lamina continuous with the subjacent TA by means of collagenous fibrils. Except in the ovaries of newborns, mitoses are essentially absent in OSE.[31] This raises the question of where the OSE cells in adult ovaries come from. A possibility exists that adult OSE stem cells differentiate from mesenchymal progenitors in ovarian TA.

Mesenchymal–epithelial transition of adult human OSE stem cells

In culture, OSE cells undergo an epithelio–mesenchymal transition. The resulting mesenchymal type cells can be stimulated to differentiate back into the epithelial phenotype.[32,33] Ovarian surface epithelium cells undergoing this epithelio–mesenchymal conversion are initially cytokeratin (CK) positive, but lose CK expression with time and passages in cultures.[34]

The TA is absent in fetal ovaries covered by proliferating OSE, and differentiates during the perinatal period.[16,21] Even then, it is not a true membrane, but merely a collection of loose mesenchymal cells.[16] Like in OSE culture, the ovarian TA can evolve perinatally from epithelio–mesenchymal transition of OSE cells. During adulthood, the TA mesenchymal cells may express CK and differentiate back into OSE stem cells.[22,29]

It may be expected that mesenchymal cells of the TA are more resistant to the endogenously and environmentally induced genetic alterations than more sensitive oocytes. If so, the follicular renewal during the prime reproductive period will ensure that fresh eggs are always available for the generation of healthy progeny. However, with the termination of new follicle formation between 35–40 years of age, the number of genetic alterations progressively increases with maternal age advancement (reviewed in Reference 31). Hence, TA progenitors of OSE stem cells may represent endogenously and environmentally resistant progenitors of new oocytes.

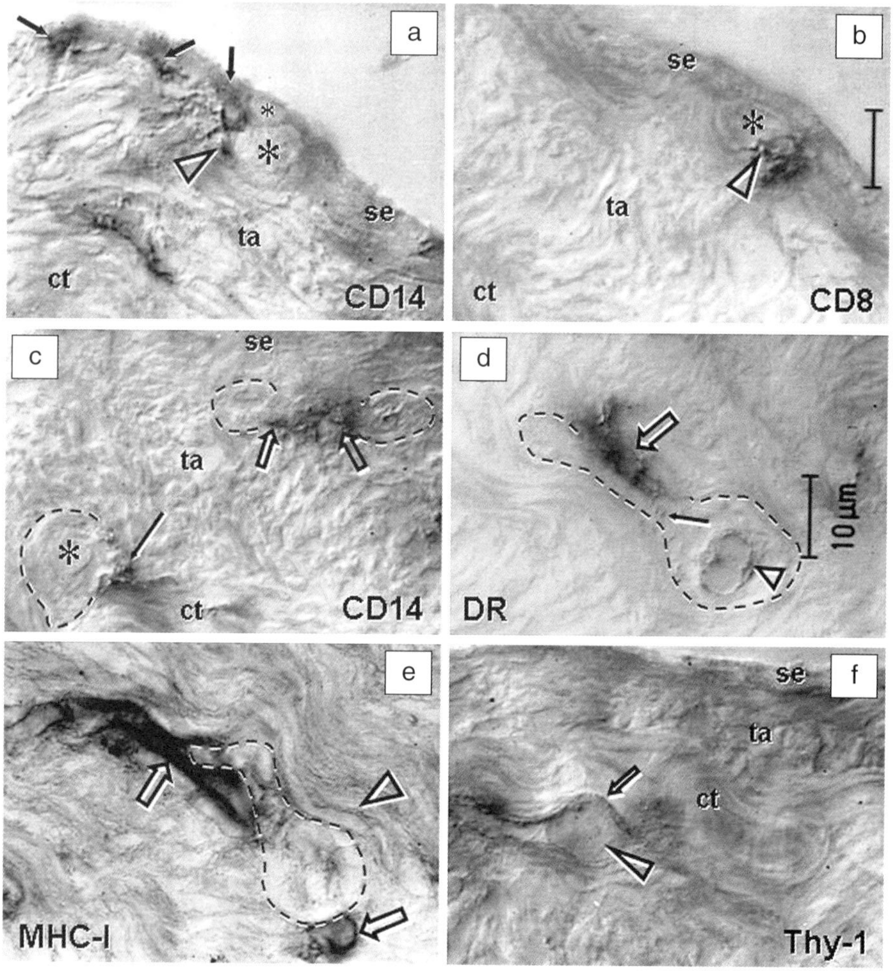

Figure 5.2 Immune cells influence commitment of OSE stem cells. Staining of the adult human OSE (se), tunica albuginea (ta) and adjacent cortex (ct) for CD14 of primitive MDC and HLA-DR of activated MDC, CD8 of cytotoxic/suppressor T cells, MHC class I heavy chain, and Thy-1 glycoprotein of pericytes, as indicated in panels. Large asterisks and dashed lines indicate putative germ cells. For other symbols and description see text. (Adapted from Bukovsky,[22] with permission of Blackwell Publishing, Oxford, UK.)

Immune system-related cells influence commitment of stem cells in adult ovaries

Like in fetal ovaries, not all OSE cells during a certain period differentiate into germ cells. Our observations[22] indicate that such a transition is associated with the presence of primitive MDC within OSE (arrows, Figure 5.2a) accompanying (arrowhead) developing germ cell (large asterisk), and occurrence of CD8 T cells (arrowhead, Figure 5.2b). Primitive MDC also accompany germ cells in TA (open arrows, Figure 5.2c) and those entering the ovarian cortex (asterisk and solid arrow). The activated MDC (HLA-DR+) accompany (arrow, Figure 5.2d) tadpole-like germ cells (dashed line) migrating through the adjacent ovarian cortex and exhibiting DR+ nuclear envelope (arrowhead).

These observations indicate that immune system-related cells play an important role in the commitment of OSE stem cells to differentiate into germ cells. In adult human ovaries the germ cells appear to differentiate during midcycle, associated with elevated estrogen and gonadotropin levels, and similar conditions exist in midpregnancy fetuses. Although midcycle

Table 5.1 Working model of age-associated changes of ovary-specific mesenchymal cells (SMC) and hormonal signals (LH/hCG and E2) required for the initiation and resumption of oogenesis in human ovaries

Period of life	*SMC*[c]	*LH/hCG*[d]	E_2[e]	*Oogenesis*
First trimester–midpregnancy	Yes	Yes	Yes	Yes[f]
Last trimester–newborn	Yes	No	Yes	No[f]
Postnatal–menarche	Yes	No	No	No[g]
Reproductive period[a]	Yes	Yes	Yes	Yes[f]
Premenopause[b]	No	Yes	Yes	No[g]
Postmenopause	No	Yes	No	No[f]

[a]From menarche until 38 ± 2 years old
[b]From 38 ± 2 years old until menopause
[c]Specialized mesenchymal cells (tissue macrophages and T cells) with commitment for stimulation of OSE to germ cell transformation
[d]LH/hCG, luteinizing hormone/human chorionic gonodotropin. Levels corresponding to the midcycle LH peak, or more (hCG levels should be 10× more, since it has a 10% affinity to the LH receptor compared with that of LH[62])
[e]Levels corresponding to the preovulatory E_2 peak, or more
[f]Confirmed
[g]Predicted
Reprinted from Bukovsky et al,[28] with permission of Humana Press Inc.

elevation may persist during the premenopausal period, certain immune system-related cells may not be available, owing to the onset of the immune senescence. On the other hand, while proper immune system cells are expected to be available perinatally and during childhood, the hormonal signals are absent (reviewed in Reference 28). Hence, there may be two periods suitable for formation of new follicles in human females: the midpregnancy fetal period and the prime reproductive period (Table 5.1).

Germ cells originate from asymmetric division of ovarian surface epithelial stem cells

Markers of germ cells and oocytes are zona pellucida (ZP) glycoproteins, which may also be expressed by OSE and granulosa cells (reviewed in Reference 29). Most of the OSE cells show characteristic CK immunoexpression, but immunoexpression of ZP is restricted to certain OSE segments. The oocyte ZP marker PS1 is a meiotically expressed porcine oocyte carbohydrate antigen.[35]

Immunoexpression of PS1 in human OSE cells is cytoplasmic. Cells descending from the OSE into TA showed nuclear PS1 (brown) staining (arrows, Figure 5.3a). The dividing OSE cells show an asymmetric distribution of meiotically expressed nuclear PS1 (+ signs), suggesting meiotic activity. Double-color immunostaining for PS1 (brown) and CK (blue) also revealed an asymmetric distribution of PS1 in germ cells descending from the OSE (Figure 5.3b) – note CK+ (blue arrowhead) and PS1+ (brown arrowhead) daughter cells. Larger germ-like cells with nuclear PS1 staining were detected in TA (Figure 5.3c). Such cells divided symmetrically (white arrow) and entered the adjacent ovarian cortex (black arrow).

These observations indicate that, like in fetal ovaries, the germ cells may originate by asymmetric division of OSE stem cells, followed by a single symmetric division of germ cells (crossing over). In this way, the germ cells are able to differentiate further into oocytes and form primary follicles by assembly with granulosa cells.

Intravascular transport of germ cells in adult ovaries

As already indicated by Simkins, formation of new primary follicles in adult human ovaries occurs in

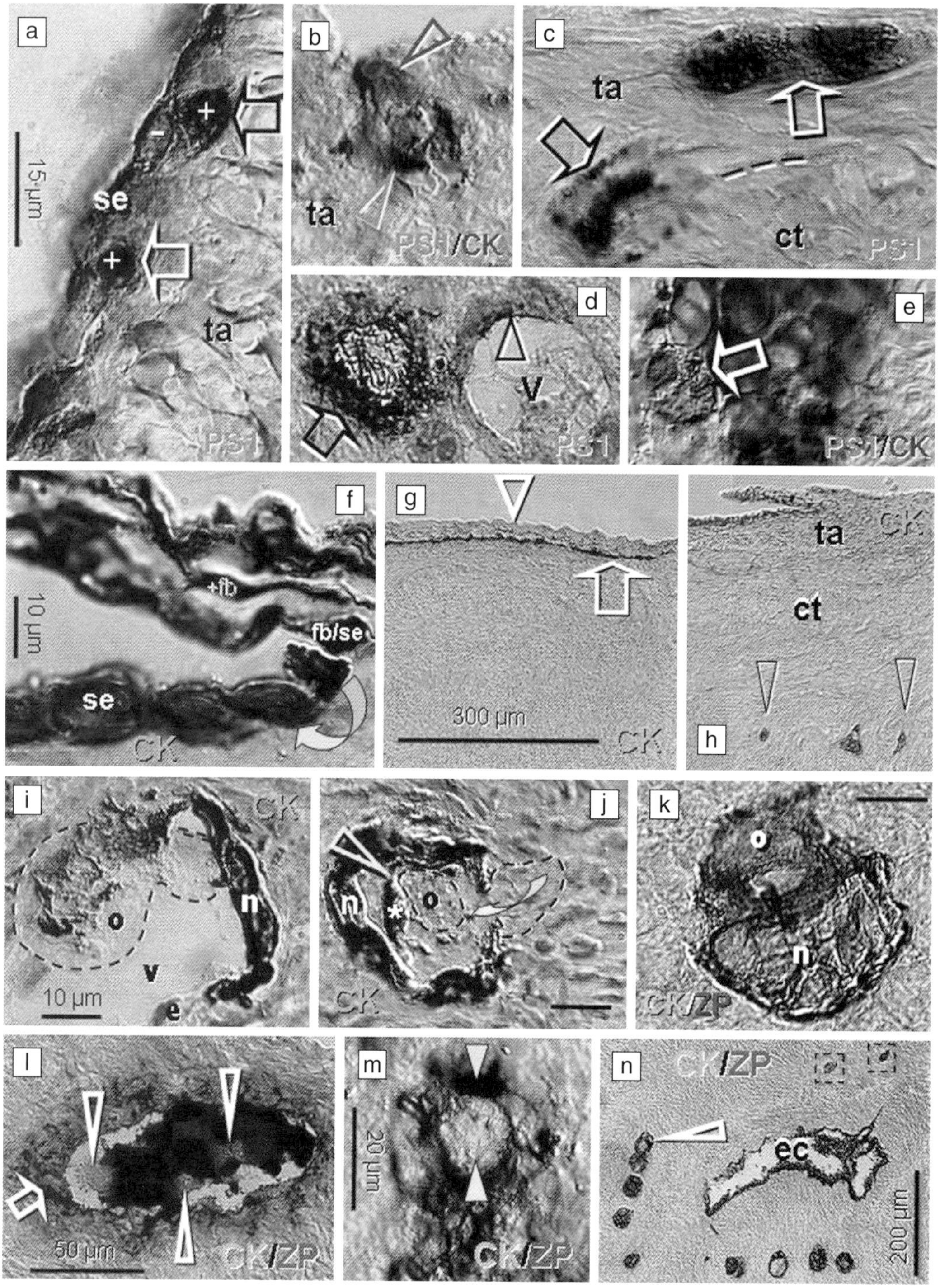

Figure 5.3 Differentiation of germ cells and primitive granulosa cells. (a) Segments of OSE show cytoplasmic PS1 (brown color) expression (se). Dividing OSE cells give rise to cells exhibiting nuclear PS1 immunostaining (+ nuclei, asymmetric division) and descending from the OSE (arrows) into tunica albuginea (ta).

Continued

the deep ovarian cortex, an area close to the medulla and distant from the ovarian surface. Although the germ cells show a tadpole-like pattern enabling them to migrate by ameboid movements to certain distance (about 100–150 μm – see below), the formation of new follicles in adult human ovaries occurs about six times deeper from the surface (about 1000 μm). To pass such a distance, the germ cells may utilize vascular transport, which has also been described in fetal ovaries of some large mammals.[6,36] When entering cortex, the putative germ cells show a translocation of nuclear PS1 immunoexpression to cytoplasmic staining (arrow, Figure 5.3d), and an association with cortical vasculature (v) showing minute amounts of PS1 immunoexpression in adjacent endothelial cells (arrowhead).

Figure 5.2e shows an association of a tadpole-like cell (dashed line) with endothelial cells strongly expressing major histocompatibility complex class I (MHC-I) antigens (arrows). Staining for Thy-1 differentiation protein of pericytes (Thy-1, arrow in Figure 5.2f) shows a germ cell migrating through the vessel in the cortex (ct) adjacent to the TA (ta).

Hence, in contrast to fetal ovaries, where the germ cells enter cortex, differentiate into oocytes and assemble with generally available granulosa cells to form new follicles, the large size of adult human ovaries may require germ cells to utilize vascular transport for formation of primary follicles. There is also a possibility that germ cells may develop in one ovary only, and after entering systemic circulation, they may assemble with primitive granulosa cells in both gonads. The granulosa cells are not generally available, as in human fetal ovaries (or adult ovaries of small laboratory rodents[28]), but they are available as small nests of epithelial cells originating from OSE stem cells.[22,29]

Origin of granulosa cell nests from adult ovarian surface epithelial stem cells

In human fetal ovaries, the OSE stem cells can differentiate either into germ cells or granulosa cells at the same time (see Figure 5.1). However, during adulthood, these processes seem to be divided. The nests of primitive granulosa cells should be formed first and moved by stromal rearrangements into the deeper

(b) Except asymmetrically divided OSE cell – note CK+ (blue color and arrowhead) and PS1+ (brown color and arrowhead) daughter cells, no PS1 or CK immunoexpression is apparent in this OSE segment. (c) In TA, the putative germ cells increase in size, but nuclear PS1 immunostaining persists. They show a symmetric division (white arrow) and exhibit development of cytoplasmic PS1 immunoexpression when entering (black arrow) the upper ovarian cortex (ct). (d) In the cortex, the cells show diminution of nuclear and increase of cytoplasmic PS1 staining (arrow), particularly when attached to the cortical vessels (v). In such cases, the PS1 immunoexpression appears to be extended toward endothelial cells (arrowhead). (e) In some instances, the asymmetric division giving rise to the putative PS1+ (brown color) germ cells could be observed at the periphery of CK+ (blue color) cortical epithelial crypts (arrow). (f) Shows association of CK+ (brown color) fibroblasts (+fb,) with the TA flap surface (arrowhead), and transition from mesenchymal to epithelial morphology (fb/se) and surface epithelium cells (se, arched arrow). (g) View of ovarian surface (arrowhead) and adjacent cortex. Arrow indicates bilaminar epithelial cord. (h) Ovarian tunica albuginea (ta) filled with CK18+ mesenchymal cells and exhibiting flap projection, and adjacent cortex (ct) with epithelial nests (arrowheads). (i) The CK+ (brown color) epithelial nest (n) inside of the cortical venule, which extends an arm to catch the oocyte (o, dashed line) from the blood circulation. (j) The nest body and closing 'gate'. A portion of the oocyte (dashed line) still lies outside of the complex, and is expected to move inside (arched arrow). The oocyte contains intraooplasmic CK+ (brown color) extensions from the nest wall (arrowhead), which contribute to the formation of CK+ paranuclear (Balbiani) body (asterisk). The oocyte nucleus is indicated by a dashed line. (k) Occupied 'bird's nest' type indicates a half-way oocyte–nest assembly. (l) Some medullary vessels show accumulation of ZP+ (blue color) degenerating oocytes with unstained nuclei (arrowheads). Arrow indicates ZP release. (m) Appearance of germ-like cell among CK+ cells (brown color) in epithelial crypt. Note ZP+ segment (blue color and white arrowhead) associated with unstained round cell (yellow arrowhead). (n) Association of primary follicles (arrowhead) with the cortical epithelial crypt (ec). Dashed boxes indicate unassembled epithelial nests. (Adapted from Bukovsky et al[29] – see http://www.rbej.com/content/2/1/20 for more details. © Antonin Bukovsky). (See also color plate) cortex, where they should associate with vessels to be ready to assemble with circulating germ cells.

In scanning electron microscopy and submicroscopic studies of human OSE during ovulatory cycles, it has been reported that the ovarian surface is frequently evaginated into a series of villous-like projections or papillae, which may vary widely in the number, size and distribution (reviewed in Reference 37). The OSE also invaginates into the ovarian cortex throughout the entire organ. Cortical invaginations appear as small elongated clefts, subsurface channel-like crypts and solid cords of epithelial cells. Crypts are hollow, tubular invaginations lined by cells possessing the same general features as OSE cells. However, the cord cells are very similar to some of the granulosa cells. In some areas of the ovary, cords fragment and appear as small 'nests' of epithelial cells. Typically, these epithelial nests (fragmented cords) lie in proximity to primary follicles.[31,37]

In adult ovaries, the OSE retains a relatively embryonic structure.[38] The OSE-derived cords are in contact or penetrated by nerve terminals, and fragmented cords (nests) are suggested to contribute epithelial elements to ovarian follicles.[31]

Hence there are two distinct structures derived from OSE stem cells in the cortex of adult human ovaries:

- epithelial crypts lined by OSE cells retaining embryonic (stem cell) structure
- epithelial nests, which may contribute epithelial (granulosa) cells to ovarian follicles.

Our observations indicate that formation of epithelial nests is initiated by evagination of TA over the ovarian surface, like an envelope flap (Figure 5.3f; see also top of Figure 5.3h). The TA fibroblasts (precursors of OSE stem cells) show expression of cytokeratin (+fb, Figure 5.3f). After reaching the surface, they exhibit mesenchymal–epithelial transition (fb/se) and differentiate into OSE stem cells (se) covering the inner side of the flap and ovarian cortex. When a certain segment of the cortex is covered, the 'envelope' flap is closed. This results in the formation of a bilaminar layer of OSE cells (arrow, Figure 5.3g), covered by TA without OSE (arrowhead). This OSE layer descends into the cortex and forms solid OSE cords, which fragment into epithelial nests (arrowheads, Figure 5.3h). The nests of primitive granulosa cells created in this way are moved by stromal rearrangements to the deeper ovarian cortex (close to medulla), where they are ready to assemble with oocytes and form primary follicles.

Assembly of germ cells with granulosa cell nests

The nests of primitive granulosa cells eventually associate with ovarian vessels in the deep cortex to pick up oocytes from circulation. Such nests (n, Figure 5.3i) enter the vessel (v) and replace endothelial cells (e), and may show an extension to catch the oocyte (o).

The primitive oocyte does not have enough organelles, and mitochondria in particular. An important part of the oocyte–nest assembly is formation of the Balbiani body. Oocytes in primary (resting) follicles show a single Balbiani body in the cytoplasmic region near the nucleus, where the majority of oocyte organelles are concentrated (reviewed in Reference 39). The Balbiani body contains aggregated mitochondria.[40–42] In a study of turkey hens, no Balbiani body was detected in stage I oocytes, appeared in stage II oocytes and diminished in the oocytes of growing follicles, coinciding with the dispersion of mitochondria throughout the ooplasm.[40] Similar observations were reported in human oocytes.[41] Balbiani bodies show immunostaining for CK 8, 18 and 19.[22,43] In primary follicles of fetal and adult human ovaries, follicular (granulosa) cell extensions penetrate deep into the ooplasm, much like a sword in its sheath. There may be as many as 3–5 'intraooplasmic processes', even in one scanning microscopy plane. These intraoocytic invaginations are closely associated with a variety of organelles. They are close to the nuclear zone, and may help activate growth of the oocyte.[44]

In adult human ovaries, the Balbiani body (asterisk, Figure 5.3j) shows CK expression, and is apparently formed during the oocyte–nest assembly by intraooplasmic projections from granulosa cells (arrowhead). Figure 5.3k shows the oocyte (blue, ZP protein)–nest (brown, CK staining) assembly in dual-color immunohistochemistry.

These observations indicate that formation of primary follicles is a complex process, requiring epithelial nests and germ cells to develop from OSE stem cells by distinct pathways and attract assemble with each other in the deep layers of the ovarian cortex.

An 'ovary-within-the ovary' pattern of Thy-1 differentiation protein distribution (Figure 5.4)

It is important to discover why the new primary follicles in adult human ovaries are formed in the area

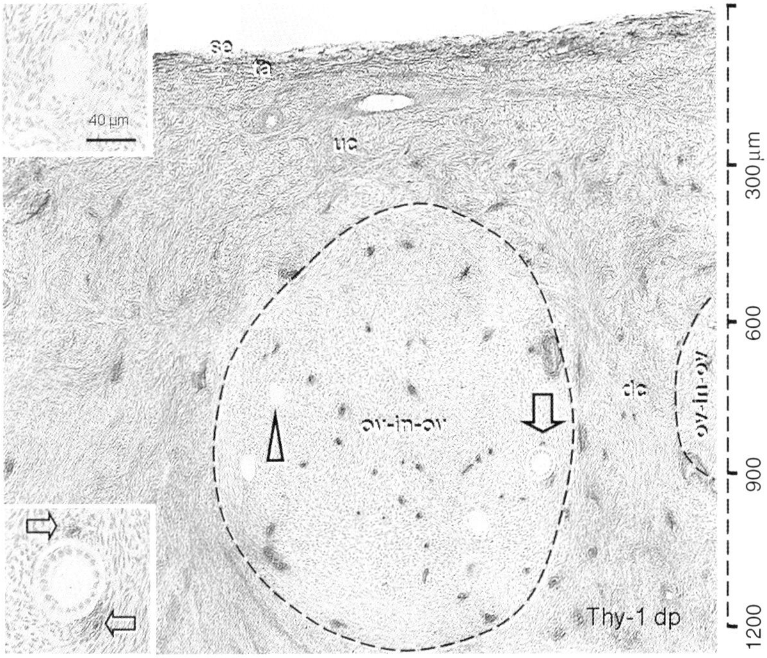

Figure 5.4 Ovarian primary follicles and Thy-1 dp. Thy-1 dp was strongly expressed by TA fibroblasts (ta), and moderately in the upper (uc) and deeper ovarian cortex (dc), excluding areas showing an 'ovary-within-the-ovary' pattern (ov-in-ov) with virtually no Thy-1 dp immunoexpression except for vascular pericytes. These areas characteristically contained primary follicles (arrowhead and upper inset), some of which showed an increase in size accompanied by Thy-1 dp+ pericytes (arrow and lower inset). (Adapted from Bukovsky et al,[29] http://www.rbej.com/content/2/1/20. © Antonin Bukovsky)

distant from the origin of germ cells and granulosa cell nests. We have reported previously that groups of follicles (cohorts) lie in isolated areas of the cortex, exhibiting an oval arrangement of stromal elements.[22] In a more recent study,[29] staining for Thy-1 dp revealed that groups of primary follicles reside in the center of rounded areas, extending about 400–1200 µm from the ovarian surface, exhibiting low stromal Thy-1 dp immunoexpression and showing an ovary-within-the-ovary pattern (ov-in-ov, Figure 5.4). In addition, growth of some follicles in a given cohort is associated with Thy-1 dp+ vasculature (lower vs upper inset). Hence, a lack of Thy-1 dp may be required to maintain primary follicles in the resting state, and the presence of Thy-1 dp may stimulate follicular growth. Note strong Thy 1 immuno staining of the TA fibroblasts (ta).

Superfluous oocytes

Another important issue is to find out if the number of newly formed follicles in adult human ovaries is determined by the number of OSE-derived epithelial nests or the number of generated germ cells. In the first instance, the isolated nests will either persist or degenerate; in the second, the degenerating oocytes not utilized in new follicle formation might be detected.

We utilized double-color immunohistochemistry to search for ZP+ (blue color) oocytes not assembled with CK+ (brown) structures. Our observations (Figure 5.3l) show multiple oocytes accumulated in some medullary vessels.[29] Note a lack of CK+ structures, strong ZP cytoplasmic immunoexpression, spread of ZP immunostaining in the adjacent stroma (arrow) and a lack of staining in the oocyte nuclei (arrowheads).

The detection of degenerating oocytes in ovarian medullary vessels may document an ongoing differentiation of new oocytes, since these oocyte remnants have been observed only in ovaries exhibiting the formation of new primary follicles. It is believed that the total number of oocytes produced within a given time in adult ovaries exceeds by several-fold the number of oocytes successfully forming primary follicles.

Stem cells in epithelial crypts – an alternative source of germ cells

The layer of OSE cells, which differentiates on the ovarian surface, may also exhibit deep invaginations into the ovarian cortex and form crypts lined by cells possessing the same general features as OSE cells.[31,37,38] We observed that such crypts could be an alternative source of germ cells expressing PS1 (arrow, Figure 5.3e), losing CK expression (yellow arrowhead, Figure 5.3m) and showing ZP+ intermediate segment (white arrowhead, Figure 5.3m). After reaching the tadpole-like shape, such germ cells can saturate approaching epithelial nests (dashed boxes, Figure 5.3n) and form neighboring primary follicles (arrowhead). That may be why the primary follicles are found in adult human ovaries in the neighborhood of OSE-derived epithelial crypts (ec, Figure 5.3n).[29]

HUMAN OVARIAN SURFACE EPITHELIAL CELLS MAY REPRESENT A TOTIPOTENT ADULT STEM CELL

Multipotential progenitor cells exhibiting a mesenchymal phenotype and capable of differentiation into distinct cells types have been derived from various adult tissues.[45–49] They exhibit mesenchymal–epithelial and epithelial–mesenchymal transitions (like OSE cells and TA progenitors in adult ovaries and OSE cells *in vitro* and possibly during TA formation), which may reflect a plasticity of progenitor cells in a particular microenvironment. They may occur sequentially (epithelial > mesenchymal followed by mesenchymal > epithelial transitions e.g. OSE > TA > OSE) under the influence of the extracellular matrix, cytokines, adhesion molecules, membrane receptors, intercellular junctions, signaling pathways or transcription factors, commonly produced in the embryo and less frequently in adult organisms. Such transitions are examples of manifestations of cell plasticity and subsequent dramatic changes resulting in lineage commitments into certain cell types (reviewed in Reference 50).

It is possible that the OSE stem cells with preserved embryonic character, which are capable of differentiating within the ovary into two distinct cell types – the primitive granulosa and germ cells – have a character of totipotent stem cells.

Differentiation of oocytes from OSE cells in vitro

Early in 2005, we established primary OSE cultures and observed that OSE cells have a capacity to differentiate into distinct somatic cell types (epithelial cells, fibroblasts, granulosa, and neural type cells) and also oocytes.[51] Although OSE cells originate from fetal mesothelial cells covering peritoneal cavity, the adult peritoneal mesothelial cells do not have a character of stem cells since they persist unchanged in the culture (unpublished observations). Therefore, the OSE cells may represent a new adult stem cell type with unique totipotent features.

Potential treatment of ovarian infertility

Late in 2005, the criteria for the utilization of OSE cultures in the treatment of the female ovarian infertility have been elaborated[52] as follows.

Suitability of patients for clinical trial

Patients with diagnosis of premature ovarian failure (POF) could be included in the clinical trial. Optimally, these patients would have failed to conceive due to lack of own functional oocytes during previous standard IVF therapy, or such therapy was impossible due to the lack of oocytes within ovaries, and they would be considering new options to have a genetically related child before undergoing conventional IVF with donated oocytes. Patients should provide detailed medical history and available laboratory results for consideration for the trial. Ultrasound or MRI images of ovaries may be requested, and patients may be advised to utilize certain hormonal therapy, including replacement of the existing one, several weeks prior to admission.

Prospective patients and their partners should not carry any genetical alterations that can be transmitted to the child. Of particular importance is the exclusion of POF with fragile X premutation (>200 CGG trinucleotide repeats of FMR1 gene), since the birth of a child in such women may result in mental retardation of the progeny.[53] Genetic alterations are detected in a proportion of patients with POF, particularly those with primary amenorrhea,[54] and fragile X premutation was detected in 4.8% of patients with POF.[55]

Therefore, evidence on the lack of genetic abnormality should be provided, or the patients will be tested.

If needed, additional laboratory investigation from blood and urine, as well as imaging procedures would be done after admission. All considered women should have a male partner with normal semen quality. Women with infertile partners (i.e. with azoospermia) should be excluded.

Therapy of ovarian infertility with cultured ovarian stem cells should be explained to the patient by a specialist in gynecology and obstetrics, who is familiar with the new technique. The medical documentation of each patient and her male partner should be evaluated by an interdisciplinary committee for in vitro fertilization, which would decide inclusion into the trial.

Collection of ovarian stem cells and utilization of oocytes

Ovarian surface epithelium cells and small ovarian biopsy are collected during laparoscopy. The OSE cells and cells collected by scraping of tissue biopsy are cultured for 5 to 10 days to determine whether or not they can produce new oocytes. If oocytes develop, they can be fertilized by classical IVF, or by intracytoplasmic sperm injection (ICSI) with the partner's semen. Embryos can be cultured to the blastocyst stage, and before transfer into the uterus, evaluated by preimplantation genetic diagnosis. At most two normal blastocysts are transferred into the uterus and supernumerary blastocysts are cryopreserved for a potential later need of the patient. In case of a pregnancy, amniocentesis should be performed (genetic evaluation of embryo/fetus).

Potential pitfalls

During the clinical trial, the following complications of cultured cells could occur: Oocytes will not develop, oocytes will not be appropriate for fertilization, oocytes will not be fertilized, fertilized oocytes will not develop into embryos, or embryos will not be transferred into the uterus because they will be genetically abnormal. If the oocyte culture is not successful, the infertility treatment could be continued by usual treatment with donated oocytes.

Initiation of the first clinical trial

Criteria for initiation of clinical trial have been found appropriate and its initiation in IVF laboratory, Department of Obstetrics and Gynecology, University Medical Center Ljubljana, approved by the Slovenian Committee for the Medical Ethic. Early in 2006, both authors met in the IVF laboratory, Ljubljana, Slovenia, to initiate the trial. The objective was to evaluate if there are OSE stem cells in infertile women with POF, and if they can develop into oocytes capable of fertilization *in vitro*. After informed consent process, three patients with POF and no oocytes in ovaries, ages 30, 38 and 40, and their normospermic partners were selected.

The OSE cells were collected during diagnostic laparoscopy by scratching ovarian surface and ovarian biopsies were collected from both ovaries. From the half of each biopsy and collected OSE, the cell cultures were set up in DMEM/F12 medium with phenol red (weak estrogenic action), supplemented with antibiotics and 20% comprehensively heat-inactivated serum (59°C, 60 minutes) of the corresponding patient. The culture was daily monitored.

Ovarian cells attached to the bottom of a dish began to differentiate into epithelial and fibroblast cell types, and some of them into oocytes. On day 3 of culture, the initial medium was replaced with *in vitro* maturation medium (Medicult IVM, Copenhagen, Denmark) supplemented with FSH (75 mIU/ml), hCG (5 IU/ml) and 10% heat-inactivated patient's serum. Prepared male partner's sperm were added several hours later.

Embryo-like structures developed in the OSE cultures of two POF women on the next day. They detached spontaneously and were transferred into the wells with standard medium for *in vitro* fertilization, where they developed progressively to the morula-, preblastocyst- (Figure 5.5) and blastocyst-like structures. They were frozen to be later genetically analyzed and transferred into the uterus, if normal.

Remaining material from biopsies was investigated by immunohistochemistry for the presence of OSE and granulosa cells of primary follicles (cytokeratin expression). No primary or other follicle types were found and development of oocyte-like cells and embryo-like structures after *in vitro* insemination of cultures correlated with the presence of the OSE in the biopsies. In one woman with no OSE in both biopsies no oocyte-like cells developed and embryo-like structures were absent after utilization of IVM and sperm (manuscript submitted).

Results of this research confirm the presence of OSE stem cells in some infertile women with POF,

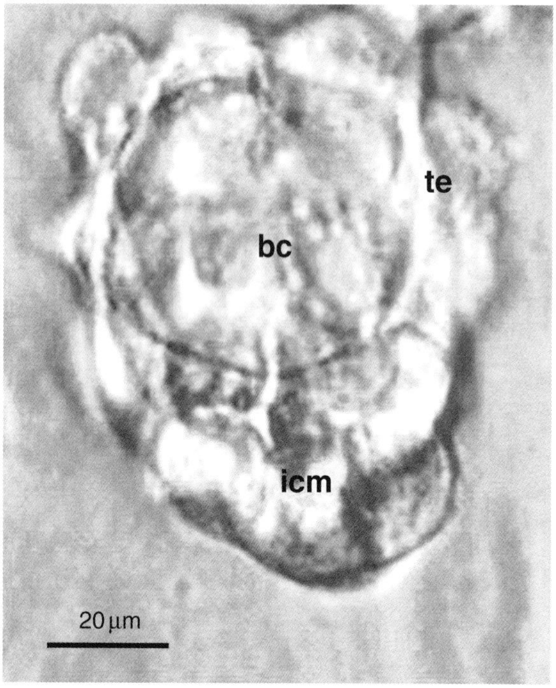

Figure 5.5 Ovarian surface epithelium culture from POF patient after *in vitro* insemination. Optical section through preblastocyst like structure with early formation of blastocoele (bc), trophectoderm (te), and inner cell mass (icm). The image was not published or submitted elsewhere

which are capable to develop into oocytes and be fertilized. These observations indicate that adult human ovaries are capable to produce new oocytes for follicular renewal, which, however, fails to occur *in vivo* in the POF patients. The OSE cultures offer new chances for infertile women with POF to have a genetically related offspring, and are worthy to be investigated further.

Autologous ovarian stem cells and treatment of degenerative diseases

Our observations also indicate that OSE stem cells are capable of fast differentiation into distinct cell types under the influence of already committed cells.[51] We also observed that human sera from some individuals cause fast (within one hour) differentiation of cultured OSE cells into neural type cells (unpublished observations). This supports the idea that uncommitted totipotent stem cells injected into the blood stream will differentiate into cell types required in different tissues, or into a single cell type required most in the given individual.

Hence, in contrast to males, human females with preserved ovaries have the advantage of totipotent adult ovarian stem cells persisting until advanced age, which can be utilized for autologous stem cell therapy without involvement of allogeneic embryonic stem cells and somatic cell nuclear transfer with questionable therapeutic outcome.[56]

CONCLUSION

Our observations indicate that in adult human females, the bipotent OSE stem cells derived from the tunica albuginea differentiate into granulosa cells and oocytes forming new primary follicles for follicular renewal. Mammalian oogenesis during adulthood was not only described by several investigators in mice, but also in the ovaries of much more developed species, the prosimian primates (reviewed in Reference 57). The number of primary follicles in human ovaries does not show a significant change during the prime reproductive period,[7] and similar observations were reported in middle aged rats and mice.[58,59] The existence of follicular renewal during the prime reproductive period, and its termination thereafter, is strongly supported by the evidence that the incidence of trisomic human fetuses is low (0.5%) until ~38 years of maternal age, and rises 40 fold during next several years, along with a diminution of persisting primary follicles in aging ovaries (Fig. 5.6; reviewed in Reference 29).

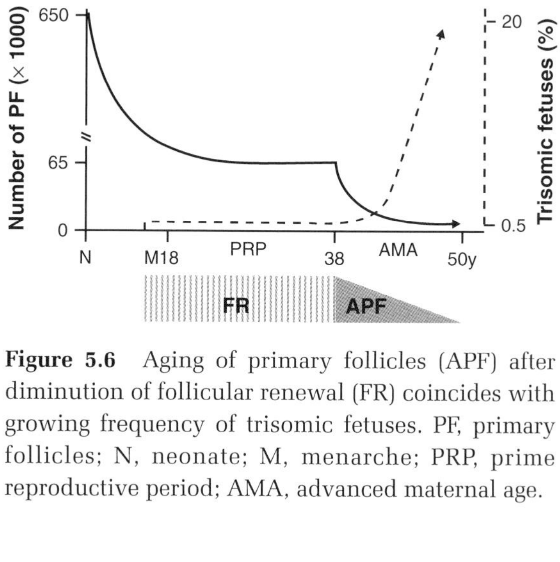

Figure 5.6 Aging of primary follicles (APF) after diminution of follicular renewal (FR) coincides with growing frequency of trisomic fetuses. PF, primary follicles; N, neonate; M, menarche; PRP, prime reproductive period; AMA, advanced maternal age.

Survey of human oogenesis and a role of bipotential OSE stem cells in the formation of fetal primary follicles and in follicular renewal during adulthood could be summarized as follows:

- It is now evident that extragonadal primordial germ cells migrate into developing mammalian gonads, and their sex commitment is determined by the gonadal somatic cells.
- In mid pregnancy human fetuses, the secondary female germ cells differentiate from the OSE under the influence of MDC (tissue macrophages) and T cells. Pegs of OSE cells descending into the cortex become primitive granulosa cells. Association of oocytes with primitive granulosa cells results in the formation of fetal primary follicles.
- Formation of new primary follicles ceases during the third trimester and the TA, consisting of progenitors of adult OSE stem cells, develops by epithelial–mesenchymal transition of OSE cells in perinatal ovaries.
- Formation of new primary follicles may not occur until menarche, when persisting fetal primary follicles are expected to degenerate.
- In adult ovaries, the TA is a source of OSE cells (mesenchymal–epithelial transition). After menarche and during prime reproductive period the OSE cells under the influence of MDC and T cells sequentially differentiate into nests of primitive granulosa cells and germ cells. Germ cells differentiate into oocytes, which associate with granulosa cell nests to form new primary follicles replacing older follicles undergoing atresia. This follicular renewal ensures that fresh eggs are always available for ovulation and healthy progeny.
- Follicular renewal ceases physiologically between 35 and 40 years of age, or earlier in premature ovarian failure. Persisting primary follicles may accumulate genetic alterations in oocytes.
- Onset of postmenopause (or premature ovarian failure) is a result of the exhaustion of the pool of functional primary follicles remaining after diminution of follicular renewal.

In vitro, the OSE stem cells differentiate into distinct cell types (fibroblasts, epithelial, granulosa, and neural type cells) and oocytes. This suggests that OSE cells represent a new type of totipotent adult stem cells, which could be considered for autologous IVF treatment of premature or natural ovarian failure, and possibly for the local or systemic applications in distinct approaches of autologous regenerative medicine (reviewed in References 52, 60).

It has been recently suggested that since the oogenic capability of OSE stem cells has been proven, the term "germinal epithelium" might reasonably be reinstated.[61]

Acknowledgments

Supported by the Physicians' Medical Education and Research Foundation, Knoxville, TN. Authors thank Drs. Helena Meden-Vrtovec, Tomaž Tomaževič, Jasna Šinkovec, and Andrej Vogler of the Department of Obstetrics and Gynecology, University of Ljubljana Medical Center, for stimulating suggestions and support, as well as excellent laparoscopic collection of OSE cells and ovarian biopsies by Dr. Andrej Vogler. The technical skills and assistance of Marta Svetlikova, M.S. and Isabelle Willson, B.S. are highly appreciated and acknowledged, as well as proof reading of the manuscript by Isabelle Willson and Rachel S White BS.

REFERENCES

1. Waldeyer W. Eierstock und Ei. Leipzig: Engelmann, 1870.
2. Kingery HM. Oogenesis in the white mouse. J Morphol 1917; 30: 261–315.
3. Beard J. The morphological continuity of the germ cells in *Raja batis*. Anat Anz 1900; 18: 465–85.
4. Pearl R, Schoppe WF. Studies on the physiology of reproduction in the domestic fowl. XVIII. Further observations on the anatomical basis of fecundity. J Exp Zool 1921; 34: 101–18.
5. Franchi LL, Mandl AM, Zuckerman S. The development of the ovary and the process of oogenesis. In Zuckerman S, ed. The Ovary. London: Academic Press, 1962: 1–88.
6. Baker TG. Oogenesis and ovarian development. In Balin H, Glasser S, eds. Reproductive Biology. Amsterdam: Excerpta Medica, 1972: 398–437.
7. Block E. Quantitative morphological investigations of the follicular system in women. Variations at different ages. Acta Anat (Basel) 1952; 14: 108–23.

8. Weissmann A. Die Continuitat des Keimplasmas als Grundlage einer Theorie der Vererbung. Jena: Fischer-Verlag, 1885.
9. McLaren A. Signaling for germ cells. Genes Dev 1999; 13: 373–6.
10. Alberts B, Johnson A, Lewis J et al. Molecular Biology of the Cell. New York: Garland Science, 2002.
11. Kelly SJ. Studies of the developmental potential of 4- and 8-cell stage mouse blastomeres. J Exp Zool 1977; 200: 365–76.
12. Ginsburg M, Snow MH, McLaren A. Primordial germ cells in the mouse embryo during gastrulation. Development 1990; 110: 521–8.
13. Lawson KA, Hage WJ. Clonal analysis of the origin of primordial germ cells in the mouse. Ciba Found Symp 1994; 182: 68–84.
14. Tam PP, Zhou SX. The allocation of epiblast cells to ectodermal and germ-line lineages is influenced by the position of the cells in the gastrulating mouse embryo. Dev Biol 1996; 178: 124–32.
15. Peters H, McNatty KP. The Ovary. A Correlation of Structure and Function in Mammals. Berkeley and Los Angeles, California: University of California Press, 1980.
16. Simkins CS. Development of the human ovary from birth to sexual maturity. J Anat 1932; 51: 465–505.
17. Allen E. Ovogenesis during sexual maturity. Am J Anat 1923; 31: 439–81.
18. Evans HM, Swezy O. Ovogenesis and the normal follicular cycle in adult mammalia. Mem Univ Calif 1931; 9: 119–224.
19. Everett NB. Observational and experimental evidences relating to the origin and differentiation of the definite germ cells in mice. J Exp Zool 1943; 92: 49–91.
20. Simkins CS. Origin of the sex cells in man. Am J Anat 1928; 41: 249–53.
21. Motta PM, Makabe S. Germ cells in the ovarian surface during fetal development in humans. A three-dimensional microanatomical study by scanning and transmission electron microscopy. J Submicrosc Cytol 1986; 18: 271–90.
22. Bukovsky A, Keenan JA, Caudle MR et al. Immunohistochemical studies of the adult human ovary: possible contribution of immune and epithelial factors to folliculogenesis. Am J Reprod Immunol 1995; 33: 323–40.
23. Bukovsky A, Caudle MR, Keenan JA et al. Association of mesenchymal cells and immunoglobulins with differentiating epithelial cells. BMC Dev Biol 2001; 1: 11. http://www.biomedcentral.com/1471-213X/1/11
24. Byskov AG, Skakkebaek NE, Stafanger G et al. Influence of ovarian surface epithelium and rete ovarii on follicle formation. J Anat 1977; 123: 77–86.
25. Williams AF, Barclay AN. The immunoglobulin superfamily – domains for cell surface recognition. Annu Rev Immunol 1988; 6: 381–405.
26. Williams AF. Immunoglobulin-related domains for cell surface recognition. Nature 1985; 314: 579–80.
27. Bukovsky A, Caudle MR, Keenan JA et al. Quantitative evaluation of the cell cycle-related retinoblastoma protein and localization of Thy-1 differentiation protein and macrophages during follicular development and atresia, and in human corpora lutea. Biol Reprod 1995; 52: 776–92.
28. Bukovsky A, Caudle MR, Svetlikova M et al. Oogenesis in adult mammals, including humans: a review. Endocrine 2005; 26: 301–16.
29. Bukovsky A, Caudle MR, Svetlikova M et al. Origin of germ cells and formation of new primary follicles in adult human ovaries. Reprod Biol Endocrinol 2004; 2: 20. http://www.rbej.com/content/2/1/20
30. Makabe S, Iwaki A, Hafez ESE et al. Physiomorphology of fertile and infertile human ovaries. In Motta PM, Hafez ESE, eds. Biology of the Ovary. The Hague: Martinus Nijhoff Publishers, 1980: 279–90.
31. Motta PM, Van Blerkom J, Makabe S. Changes in the surface morphology of ovarian 'germinal' epithelium during the reproductive cycle and in some pathological conditions. J Submicrosc Cytol 1980; 12: 407–25.
32. Dyck HG, Hamilton TC, Godwin AK et al. Autonomy of the epithelial phenotype in human ovarian surface epithelium: changes with neoplastic progression and with a family history of ovarian cancer. Int J Cancer 1996; 69: 429–36.
33. Auersperg N, Pan J, Grove BD et al. E-cadherin induces mesenchymal-to-epithelial transition in human ovarian surface epithelium. Proc Natl Acad Sci USA 1999; 96: 6249–54.
34. Auersperg N, Wong AS, Choi KC et al. Ovarian surface epithelium: biology, endocrinology, and pathology. Endocr Rev 2001; 22: 255–88.
35. Skinner SM, Kieback DG, Chunn J et al. Identification of a meiotically expressed carbohydrate antigen in ovarian carcinoma: II. Association with proteins in tumors and peritoneal fluid. Anticancer Res 1997; 17: 907–11.
36. Wartenberg H. Germ cell migration induced and guided by somatic cell interaction. Bibl Anat 1983; 24: 67–76.
37. Van Blerkom J, Motta PM. The Cellular Basis of Mammalian Reproduction. Baltimore–Munich: Urban & Schwarzenberg 1979.
38. Mossman HW, Duke KL. Some comparative aspects of the mammalian ovary. In Greep RO, ed. Handbook of Physiology, Sect. 7: Endocrinology. Washington: Am Physiol Soc 1973: 389–402.

39. Zamboni L. Ultrastructure of mammalian oocytes and ova. Biol Reprod Suppl 1970; 2: 44–63.

40. Carlson JL, Bakst MR, Ottinger MA. Developmental stages of primary oocytes in turkeys. Poult Sci 1996; 75: 1569–78.

41. Motta PM, Nottola SA, Makabe S et al. Mitochondrial morphology in human fetal and adult female germ cells. Hum Reprod 2000; 15(Suppl 2): 129–47.

42. Cox RT, Spradling AC. A Balbiani body and the fusome mediate mitochondrial inheritance during Drosophila oogenesis. Development 2003; 130: 1579–90.

43. Santini D, Ceccarelli C, Mazzoleni G et al. Demonstration of cytokeratin intermediate filaments in oocytes of the developing and adult human ovary. Histochemistry 1993; 99: 311–19.

44. Motta PM, Makabe S, Naguro T et al. Oocyte follicle cells association during development of human ovarian follicle. A study by high resolution scanning and transmission electron microscopy. Arch Histol Cytol 1994; 57: 369–94.

45. Jiang Y, Vaessen B, Lenvik T et al. Multipotent progenitor cells can be isolated from postnatal murine bone marrow, muscle, and brain. Exp Hematol 2002; 30: 896–904.

46. Reyes M, Dudek A, Jahagirdar B et al. Origin of endothelial progenitors in human postnatal bone marrow. J Clin Invest 2002; 109: 337–46.

47. Van Damme A, Vanden Driessche T, Collen D, Chauh MK. Bone marrow stromal cells as targets for gene therapy. Curr Gene Ther 2002; 2: 195–209.

48. Keene CD, Ortiz-Gonzalez XR, Jiang Y et al. Neural differentiation and incorporation of bone marrow-derived multipotent adult progenitor cells after single cell transplantation into blastocyst stage mouse embryos. Cell Transplant 2003; 12: 201–13.

49. Muguruma Y, Reyes M, Nakamura Y et al. In vivo and in vitro differentiation of myocytes from human bone marrow-derived multipotent progenitor cells. Exp Hematol 2003; 31: 1323–30.

50. Prindull G, Zipori D. Environmental guidance of normal and tumor cell plasticity: epithelial mesenchymal transitions as a paradigm. Blood 2004; 103: 2892–9.

51. Bukovsky A, Svetlikova M, Caudle MR. Oogenesis in cultures derived from adult human ovaries. Reprod Biol Endocrinol 2005; 3: 17. http://www.rbej.com/content/3/1/17

52. Bukovsky A, Copas P, Virant-Klun I. Potential new strategies for the treatment of ovarian infertility and degenerative diseases with autologous ovarian stem cells. Expert Opin Biol Ther 2006; 6(4): 341–65.

53. Corrigan EC, Raygada MJ, Vanderhoof VH et al. A woman with spontaneous premature ovarian failure gives birth to a child with fragile X syndrome. Fertil Steril 2005; 84: 1508.

54. Rebar RW. Premature ovarian failure. In Lobo RA, Kesley J, Marcus R, eds. Menopause Biology and Pathobiology. San Diego: Academic Press 2000: 135–46.

55. Gersak K, Meden-Vrtovec H, Peterlin B. Fragile X premutation in women with sporadic premature ovarian failure in Slovenia. Hum Reprod 2003; 18: 1637–40.

56. Prentice DA. Adult stem cells. Issues Law Med 2004; 19: 265–94.

57. Telfer EE. Germline stem cells in the postnatal mammalian ovary: A phenomenon of prosimian primates and mice? Reprod Biol Endocrinol 2004; 2: 24.

58. Nikolic Z, Blagojevic Z, Mrvic V et al. Effect on neonatal oestrogen and hCG treatment on the genital organs of adult female rats. Acta Vet Hung 1999; 47: 109–15.

59. Kerr JB, Duckett R, Myers M et al. Quantification of healthy follicles in the neonatal and adult mouse ovary: evidence for maintenance of primordial follicle supply. Reproduction 2006; 132: 95–109.

60. Bukovsky A. Oogenesis from human somatic stem cells and a role of immune adaptation in premature ovarian failure. Curr Stem Cell Res Ther 2006; 1: 289–303.

61. Nishida T, Nishida N. Reinstatement of "germinal epithelium" of the ovary. Reprod Biol Endocrinol 2006; 4: 42.

62. Bousfield GR, Butnev VY, Gotschall RR et al. Structural features of mammalian gonadotropins. Mol Cell Endocrinol 1996; 125: 3–19.

CHAPTER 6

Signaling germline commitment

Hsu-Hsin Chen and Niels Geijsen

INTRODUCTION

The critical importance of germ cells in the propagation of a species has long inspired research into the origin of these cells. It was August Weismann who in 1893 for the first time proposed a mechanism by which the germline would distinguish itself from the soma through the inheritance of what he called germ plasm. In Weismann's theory, the inheritance of germ plasm components by a small subset of cells determines the germline fate of these cells. Indeed, in many lower organisms germ plasm has been demonstrated to exist as a maternally inherited complex of proteins and RNA that controls germ cell fate determination. But while homologues of germ plasm components have been identified, and have been shown to play a role during mammalian germline differentiation, no higher-order germ plasm complexes have been identified in the fertilized mammalian egg. In fact, in mammals germline determination appears to occur later in development and is a more plastic process that is mainly triggered by extracellular signaling events, a process called epigenesis. This was elegantly demonstrated by Lawson and Hage, who injected lineage tracer into single proximal epiblast cells of day 6.5 murine embryos and analyzed the cell fate of these labeled cells after a period of explant culture. These experiments demonstrated that while some labeled cells gave rise to primordial germ cells (PGCs), they never did so exclusively, suggesting that at day 6.5 lineage determination has not yet occurred. This was further corroborated by Tam and Zhou who performed a series of experiments in which they transplanted cells of the distal epiblast, which would normally give rise to neuroectoderm, to the proximal epiblast where the founder germ cells are located. Relocation of distal epiblast cells to the germ cell microenvironment redirected the differentiation of these cells toward the germline, suggesting that at day 6.5 of murine development, germline fate determination is plastic and depends largely on signaling cues from the microenvironment. However, the nature and role of these signals is largely unknown. Here we take a look at possible candidate signaling pathways and review their possible role in germline fate determination.

THE TGF-β SUPERFAMILY

The transforming growth factor-β (TGF-β) family is a large group of cytokines playing pivotal roles in various aspects of embryonic development (reviewed in Reference 1). The cytokines consist of homo- or heterodimers, which bind and activate specific type I and type II receptor serine/threonine kinases at the cell membrane. Upon ligand stimulation, the type II receptor phosphorylates and thereby activates the type I receptor kinase, which in turn phosphorylates the downstream R-SMAD proteins. Phosphorylation of the R-SMADs by the receptor kinases promotes their nuclear localization and dimer/trimer formation with SMAD4 (reviewed in Reference 2); the R-SMAD–SMAD4 oligomers then directly bind to DNA and other transcription factors.

TGF-β cytokines are divided into two subgroups: the TGF-β/activin/Nodal subfamily and the BMP/GDF/MIS subfamily, each of which activates distinct combinations of receptors and downstream effectors.[1]

As discussed below, members of both subfamilies are implicated in the establishment of germ cell fate in the mouse embryo, but the specific roles of these cytokines and the interaction among these signaling pathways are still unclear.

BMP4, BMP8b AND BMP2

BMP4 expression becomes detectable at E5.5 in the extraembryonic ectoderm adjacent to the epiblast[3] (Figure 6.1). Its expression in this region continues throughout gastrulation, spanning the window of PGC lineage restriction (E6.5–E7.25, early midstreak stage). In-situ hybridization showed that BMP8b transcript is also expressed in the extraembryonic ectoderm during this period.[4] BMP2, on the other hand, is detected in the posterior visceral endoderm (VE) at E5.0–E6.5 by in-situ hybridization.[5] The proximal epiblast cells that will soon become founders of the PGCs would then be receiving multiple BMP signals emanating from different sources. The multiple sources of signals in vivo may determine the spatial confinement of PGCs in their specific location; however, the requirement of each BMP signal for the induction of PGC fate in vitro is still controversial. Knockout studies have shown that mouse embryos lacking BMP4 fail to form any primordial germ cells, whereas BMP4+/– embryos show an ~50% reduction in PGC number compared with wild type, regardless of the genetic background,[3] demonstrating a critical role for BMP4 signaling in germline fate determination. BMP8b knockout embryos display a similar phenotype in the C57Bl/6 background, but the phenotype is much less severe in other genetic backgrounds.[4] Thus, although both BMP4 and BMP8b are essential for PGC development, the former appears to be the more dominant signal. In addition, BMP4+/– BMP8+/– double heterozygotes did not differ in PGC number from the BMP4 heterozygotes, suggesting that BMP4 and BMP8b may function as heterodimers as well as homodimers in vivo.[4] BMP2 is highly homologous to BMP4 in primary sequence. BMP2-null embryos also showed a reduction in PGC number at early developmental stages; however, its effect is much smaller than BMP4 and BMP8b.[5] It has been suggested that BMP2 homodimers may function in the same fashion as BMP4 homodimers, while the source and timing of these signals are different (see below). In addition to the knockout studies described above, explant cultures of murine embryos have further elucidated the mechanism by which different BMP signals contribute to PGC specification and suggest that BMP signals need to reach a critical threshold for PGC induction to occur. In one study, PGC formation was induced in epiblasts deprived of the extraembryonic ectoderm at E5.5–E5.75 by exogenous stimulation with high concentrations of recombinant BMP4,[6] suggesting that in-vitro BMP8b is dispensable for PGC induction. However, explant culture of E6.0–6.25 epiblasts on COS cells expressing either BMP4 or BMP8b alone or in combination demonstrated that PGC formation was only supported when both BMPs were expressed.[7] These seemingly contradictory results can be reconciled when we consider that BMP4 and BMP8b can form heterodimers, which potentiates the action of these growth factors. Thus, while at low concentration, only the BMP4–BMP8b heterodimer can overcome the signaling threshold required for PGC specification; at high concentration, BMP4 alone is sufficient.[8]

BMP RECEPTORS

Of the type I BMP receptors, both ALK2 and ALK3 expression have been detected in the early epiblast.[9–11] ALK3 null embryos die at E8.0 due to the lack of mesoderm development.[12] The effect of ALK3 null mutation on PGC formation has not been investigated and such studies are difficult to perform in vivo due to the profound effect of ALK3 mutation on epiblast development. The genetic study on ALK2 revealed another level of complexity of BMP signaling in PGC lineage restriction. ALK2 is not detected in the epiblast but is expressed in the VE surrounding the boundaries of the epiblast and the extraembryonic tissues. Interestingly, deletion of ALK2 also resulted in total ablation of PGCs in the mouse embryos, and this effect is dose-dependent, as the numbers of PGCs are reduced in ALK2+/– embryos.[13] Furthermore, expression of constitutively active ALK2 in the visceral endoderm could partially rescue PGC formation in the BMP4–/– embryo,[13] demonstrating that the effect of BMP4 on PGC formation is at least partially indirect, acting through the induction of a yet unknown signal in the VE.

There are three type II receptors for BMPs: BMP type II receptor (BMPRII) and activin type II

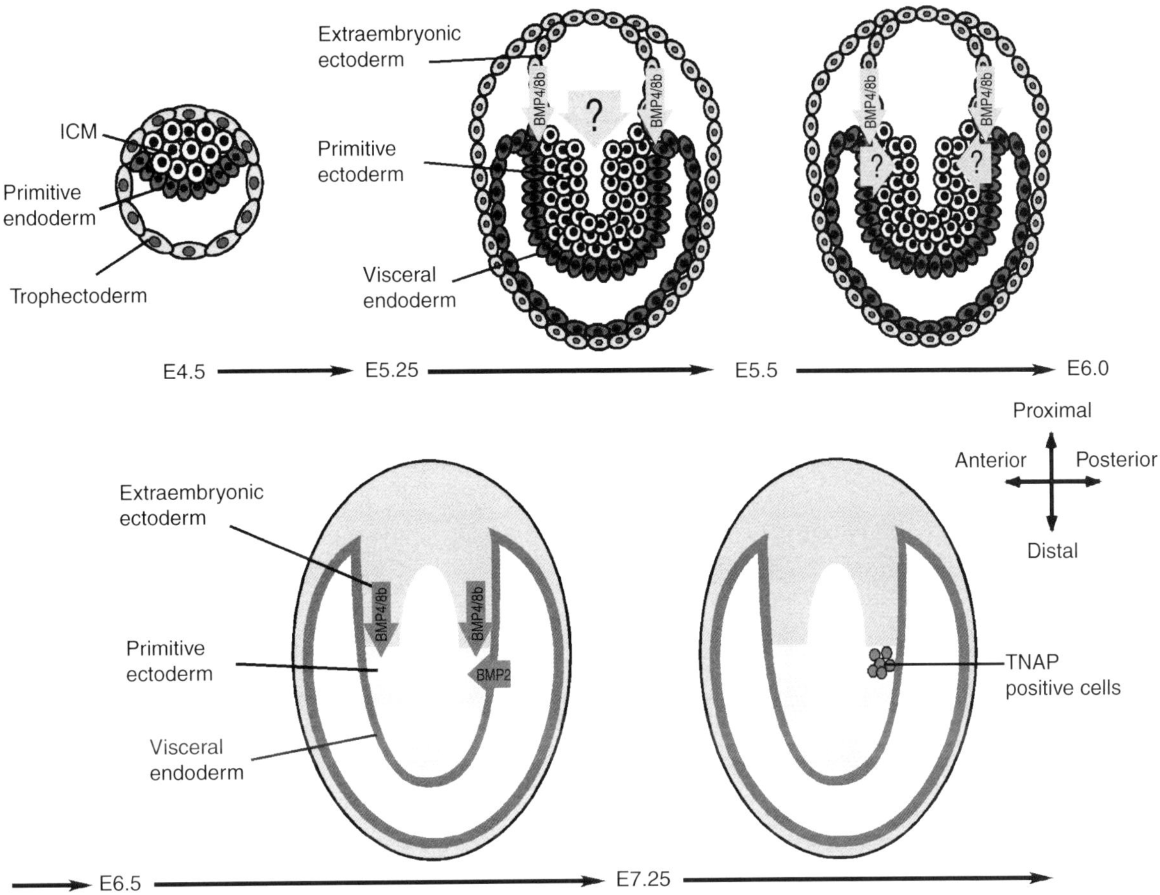

Figure 6.1 Signals required for PGC formation in mouse embryonic development. Primordial germ cell (PGC) specification requires multiple signals from different sources during mouse development. At E5.25–E5.5, a yet unknown signal generated by the extraembryonic ectoderm is needed to prime the cells for later BMP signals, presumably by up-regulating SMAD5 in selected cell populations. At E5.5–E6.0, a second unknown signal from the visceral endoderm is required. This signal is dependent on ALK2 signaling in the visceral endodermal cells, suggesting that the BMP4/8b from the extraembryonic ectoderm stimulate the production of this second unknown signal. The lineage restriction of PGCs occurs at E6.5–E7.25. At this last stage of PGC specification, both BMP4/8b signals from the extraembryonic ectoderm and BMP2 signal from the visceral endoderm are required; the BMP2 expression is the highest in the posterior region of the visceral endoderm. After E7.25, PGCs are detectable by alkaline phosphatase activity. ICM, inner cell mass; TNAP, tissue non-specific alkaline phosphatase. Blue block arrows denote unknown signals from extraembryonic ectoderm and visceral endoderm. Green arrows indicate BMP4 and BMP8b signals from extraembryonic ectoderm. Magenta arrow denotes BMP2 signal from visceral endoderm. Red ovals represent TNAP-positive primordial germ cells. (See also color plate)

receptors A and B (ActRII, ActRIIB).[1] The effect of knocking out these receptors on PGC formation has not been documented, but since BMPRII mutant embryos displayed a phenotype similar to the ALK3 knockouts, the effect of BMPRII null mutation on PGC formation is confounded by a profound effect on mesoderm development. However, BMPRII transcript is expressed ubiquitously in the early embryo, suggesting it might be the relevant type II receptor for BMP signaling in PGC formation.[10] Single mutations of the ActRII and ActRIIB receptors result in less-dramatic phenotypes. ActRII knockout mice are viable and fertile, while ActRIIB knockout mice survive until birth.[14] However, ActRII/IIB double knockouts are arrested before gastrulation.[15] Since the transcripts for both activin type II receptors are detected at E5.5–E7.5, they may also play a role in mediating the BMP signaling in germ cell fate determination. However, the phenotypes associated with the disruption of activin type II receptor genes are probably due to inactivation of the Nodal signaling pathways, which we discuss below.

INTRACELLULAR EFFECTORS OF BMP SIGNALING

The main downstream effectors of the BMP signaling pathways are SMAD1, SMAD5 and SMAD8,[2] all of which are expressed in the pregastrulation epiblast. Total phosphorylation of these three SMADs is up-regulated in the epiblast upon recombinant BMP4 treatment.[16] SMAD1–/– embryos could form virtually no PGCs as judged by alkaline phosphatase activity, evidently indicating the requirement of SMAD1 in the BMP pathways.[16,17] SMAD5 deletion also resulted in a major reduction in PGC number, and the effect is dose-dependent as in the case of the BMPs discussed above.[18] The role of SMAD8 in PGC formation has not yet been explored.

When the extraembryonic ectoderm is dissected away from the epiblast at E5.25, BMP4 treatment fails to induce PGC formation as it would in epiblast from embryos at E5.5.[6] The identity of this required signal from the extraembryonic ectoderm during this period is still unknown. In this time window, SMAD5 is up-regulated in the proximal but down-regulated in the distal epiblast, and its expression in the specific cell populations may account for the change in their responsiveness to BMP4.[6] Interestingly, in a separate study, the expression patterns of SMADs 1, 5 and 8 at E6.25 were found to be heterogeneous by single-cell reverse transcription polymerase chain reaction (RT-PCR) from the proximal epiblast.[17] It is thus possible that the earlier signals from the extraembryonic ectoderm determine the SMAD signature of individual epiblast cell, which in turn dictates the potential of each cell to commit to the PGC lineage.

Dissection of embryos had demonstrated that a pre-determination signal from another source is also essential for PGC specification.[13] This unidentified signal may be dependent on ALK2 expression in the VE, since the time point and the resulting phenotype are similar between ALK2 null embryos and explants without VE, and in both cases their phenotype can be partially rescued by co-culture with STO feeder cells.[13] The identity of this VE-derived signal remains unknown.

In summary, the PGC founder cells in the proximal epiblast require a combination of BMP signals that are both spatially and temporally regulated to attain germ cell fate. We have summarized current data and models in Figure 6.1. At E5.25–E5.5, the extraembryonic ectoderm induces a change in responsiveness to BMP in the proximal epiblast, possibly by up-regulating SMAD5. Later, at E5.5–E6.0, the visceral endoderm releases another unknown signal to the proximal epiblast, possibly following the activation of the BMP4–ALK2 pathway in the VE. During the window of PGC lineage restriction (E6.5–E7.25), BMP4 and BMP8b from the extraembryonic ectoderm and BMP2 from the VE activate the ALK3/BMPRII receptors in the PGC founder cells, which are primed for germ cell fate commitment by the earlier sequence of signals.

NODAL SIGNALING

Nodal is a chordate-specific cytokine that belongs to the same subfamily as TGF-β and activin (reviewed in Reference 19). Nodal signaling establishes the anterior–posterior axis, induces mesoderm and endoderm formation, and sets up the left–right asymmetry in early embryogenesis. Homozygous deletion of Nodal results in the loss of primitive streak and early embryonic lethality.[20–22] The role of Nodal signaling in PGC fate decision has not been looked into; however, there is sufficient circumstantial evidence to suggest that this pathway may also be involved in germline determination.

Nodal is distinct from other TGF-β family members in that it requires a co-receptor in order to activate the type I/type II receptor complex (reviewed in Reference 23). There are two co-receptor genes in humans and mice: Cripto and Cryptic. Cripto expression is required for gastrulation,[24] whereas Cryptic is important in the later process of setting up the left–right axis.[25] The known type I receptor for Nodal is ALK4, although ALK7 may also be a potential receptor, and the type II receptors are likely to be ActRIIB and ActRII.[15] Activation by Nodal/Cripto induces phosphorylation of SMAD2 and possibly SMAD3 as well. Nevertheless, other SMAD-independent pathways are also involved, since deletion of either SMAD2[26] or SMAD4 does not incur all of the phenotypes observed in Nodal knockouts.

The expression of Nodal mRNA is detected throughout the primitive ectoderm and VE at E5.5. By E6.5, Nodal expression is lost from the VE, and becomes localized in the proximal-posterior region of the epiblast.[20] Cripto is also expressed uniformly in the primitive ectoderm, and its expression pattern in the epiblast follows that of Nodal in the pregastrulation and gastrulation stages.[23] In fact, Cripto transcription in the epiblast is dependent on Nodal signaling.[22] Thus, the posterior-proximal epiblast, which contains the founder cells of PGCs, expresses the highest level of both Nodal and Cripto before and during the time window of germ cell fate specification.

The expression of Nodal and other components of the Nodal signaling pathway seems to be closely associated with areas of the embryo in which pluripotent cells exist. At E6.0, pluripotent (oct-4 expressing) cells can be found throughout the epiblast and likewise Nodal is broadly expressed at this point. Shortly thereafter, Nodal expression is concentrated in the primitive streak region and at this point pluripotency becomes restricted to the germ cell precursors in this area. It is tempting to speculate that Nodal signaling plays a role in the maintenance of pluripotency in the early embryo and perhaps is a critical mediator of germline specification.

GERM CELLS AND EMBRYONIC STEM CELLS

In addition to the *in vivo* expression profiles, recent studies also hint at a critical role for Nodal signaling in the maintenance of pluripotency in human embryonic stem cells (ES cells). Human ES cells and mouse inner cell mass outgrowth from blastocysts both require SMAD2/3 phosphorylation, which is downstream of Nodal/activin, to maintain pluripotency.[27,28] In the human ES cells, conditions that preserve pluripotency correlate with activation of SMAD2/3 and inhibition of SMAD1/5,[27] suggesting an antagonistic relationship of the Nodal pathway and the BMP pathways. Interestingly SMAD2/3 activation is not required for the maintenance of mouse ES cell pluripotency, suggesting a fundamental difference in the nature of murine and human ES cells. Recently, Zwaka and Thompson suggested that ES cells have in fact a germline origin.[29] While this may indeed be true for human ES cells, the dependency of murine ES cells on the presence of LIF in the culture medium suggests that murine ES cells are a reflection of embryonic diapause, a state of suspended development that allows the occurrence of multiple simultaneous pregnancies.[30] LIF acts as an anti-differentiation factor for cells of the inner cell mass, which can then be propagated as ES cells in what is arguably a fortuitous artefact of cell culture. Because humans do not have diapause, it is perhaps not surprising that LIF does not play a role in hES maintenance.

The differences in growth factor requirements between human and murine ES cells could reflect a different origin of these cells, but alternatively, could reflect the existence of two pluripotent states. A state of diapause-like maintenance of pluripotency, which is unique to the murine cells. And a state of germcell like pluripotency that is currently employed to maintain human ES cells in culture. Attempts to maintain murine ES cells under such conditions have not been reported but the outcome of such experiments may provide novel insight in the nature and identity of ES cells.

FGF SIGNALING

Of the 22 fibroblast growth factors (FGFs) in the mammalian genome, FGF2 (bFGF) and FGF7 have been shown to be important in the postgastrula migration of the PGCs to the genital ridges.[31] FGF2 has also been shown to promote PGC proliferation in vitro (reviewed in Reference 32). However, mice lacking FGF2 are viable and fertile,[33–35] suggesting possible redundancy in signaling between different FGFs. Whether the FGFs are also involved in the early events that determine PGC fate is not yet clear, but several FGF pathways have been shown to be essential for early embryonic development.[36,37]

In human ES cells, FGF signaling pathways have been found to cooperate with Nodal signaling[28] and to suppress BMP signaling[38] in maintaining pluripotency. A recent report demonstrates that activation of the Nodal signaling pathway in human ES cells increases the expression of Oct4, Nanog, Nodal, Wnt3, basic FGF and FGF8, and demonstrates a cooperative effect of Nodal and FGF signals in maintaining human ES cell pluripotency. Given the importance of TGF-β signals in PGC development, and the requirement of FGF in the in-vitro culture of PGCs, it is probable that the FGFs and Nodal signals cooperate in a similar manner in specifying the germline.

At the egg cylinder stage, FGF4 is expressed in the epiblast and its receptor FGFR2 is expressed in the epiblast and at a higher level in the extraembryonic ectoderm. Both FGF4- and FGFR2-null embryos do not survive past the egg cylinder stage, due to defects in ICM proliferation and trophoblast proliferation.[37,39] The temporal and spatial expression patterns of FGF4 and FGFR2 thus support a putative role in PGC specification. Furthermore, FGF4 is required, along with FGF8, for cell movement from the primitive streak during gastrulation,[40] and the expression pattern of FGF8 is intriguing from the viewpoint of germline development. Just before gastrulation, FGF8 is first detected in a group of cells in the posterior epiblast, which overlaps with an area of PGC formation, and also in the VE. Redundancy in signaling between the various members of the FGF family and possible cross-talk with other signaling pathways, including BMP and Nodal signaling, may make it difficult to dissect the possible roles of individual members of this large family of growth factors in PGC specification and migration. Embryo explant cultures and studies of in-vitro PGC formation may, in this case, provide tractable tools for future analyses.

REFERENCES

1. Shi Y, Massague J. Mechanisms of TGF-beta signaling from cell membrane to the nucleus. Cell 2003; 113: 685–700.
2. Massague J, Seoane J, Wotton D. Smad transcription factors. Genes Dev 2005; 19: 2783–810.
3. Lawson KA, Dunn NR, Roelen BA et al. Bmp4 is required for the generation of primordial germ cells in the mouse embryo. Genes Dev 1999; 13: 424–36.
4. Ying Y, Liu XM, Marble A, Lawson KA, Zhao GQ. Requirement of Bmp8b for the generation of primordial germ cells in the mouse. Mol Endocrinol 2000; 14: 1053–63.
5. Ying Y, Zhao GQ. Cooperation of endoderm-derived BMP2 and extraembryonic ectoderm-derived BMP4 in primordial germ cell generation in the mouse. Dev Biol 2001; 232: 494–92.
6. Okamura D, Hayashi K, Matsui Y. Mouse epiblasts change responsiveness to BMP4 signal required for PGC formation through functions of extraembryonic ectoderm. Mol Reprod Dev 2005; 70: 20–9.
7. Ying Y, Qi X, Zhao GQ. Induction of primordial germ cells from murine epiblasts by synergistic action of BMP4 and BMP8B signaling pathways. Proc Natl Acad Sci USA 2001; 98: 7858–62.
8. Matsui Y, Okamura D. Mechanisms of germ-cell specification in mouse embryos. Bioessays. 2005; 27: 136–43.
9. Gu Z, Nomura M, Simpson BB et al. The type I activin receptor ActRIB is required for egg cylindetr organization and gastrulation in the mouse. Genes Dev 1998; 12: 844–57.
10. Beppu H, Kawabata M, Hamamoto T et al. BMP type II receptor is required for gastrulation and early development of mouse embryos. Dev Biol 2000; 221: 249–58.
11. Gu Z, Reynolds EM, Song J et al. The type I serine/threonine kinase receptor ActRIA (ALK2) is required for gastrulation of the mouse embryo. Development 1999; 126: 2551–61.
12. Mishina Y, Suzuki A, Ueno N, Behringer RR. Bmpr encodes a type I bone morphogenetic protein receptor that is essential for gastrulation during mouse embryogenesis. Genes Dev 1995; 9: 3027–37.
13. De Sousa Lopes SM, Roelen BA, Monteiro RM et al. BMP signaling mediated by ALK2 in the visceral endoderm is necessary for the generation of primordial germ cells in the mouse embryo. Genes Dev 2004; 18: 1838–49.
14. Matzuk MM, Kumar TR, Bradley A. Different phenotypes for mice deficient in either activins or activin receptor type II. Nature 1995; 374: 356–60.
15. Song J, Oh SP, Schrewe H et al. The type II activin receptors are essential for egg cylinder growth, gastrulation, and rostral head development in mice. Dev Biol 1999; 213: 157–69.
16. Tremblay KD, Dunn NR, Robertson EJ. Mouse embryos lacking Smad1 signals display defects in extra-embryonic tissues and germ cell formation. Development 2001; 128: 3609–21.
17. Hayashi K, Kobayashi T, Umino T et al. SMAD1 signaling is critical for initial commitment of germ cell lineage from mouse epiblast. Mech Dev 2002; 118: 99–109.
18. Chang H, Matzuk MM. Smad5 is required for mouse primordial germ cell development. Mech Dev 2001; 104: 61–7.
19. Schier AF. Nodal signaling in vertebrate development. Annu Rev Cell Dev Biol 2003; 19: 589–621.

20. Conlon FL, Lyons KM, Takaesu N et al. A primary requirement for nodal in the formation and maintenance of the primitive streak in the mouse. Development 1994; 120: 1919–28.

21. Conlon FL, Barth KS, Robertson EJ. A novel retrovirally induced embryonic lethal mutation in the mouse: assessment of the developmental fate of embryonic stem cells homozygous for the 413.d proviral integration. Development 1991; 111: 969–81.

22. Brennan J, Lu CC, Norris DP et al. Nodal signaling in the epiblast patterns the early mouse embryo. Nature 2001; 411: 965–9.

23. Shen MM, Schier AF. The EGF-CFC gene family in vertebrate development. Trends Genet 2000; 16: 303–9.

24. Ding J, Yang L, Yan YT et al. Cripto is required for correct orientation of the anterior-posterior axis in the mouse embryo. Nature 1998; 395: 702–7.

25. Gaio U, Schweickert A, Fischer A et al. A role of the cryptic gene in the correct establishment of the left-right axis. Curr Biol 1999; 9: 1339–42.

26. Heyer J, Escalante-Alcalde D, Lia M et al. Postgastrulation Smad2-deficient embryos show defects in embryo turning and anterior morphogenesis. Proc Natl Acad Sci USA 1999; 96: 12595–600.

27. James D, Levine AJ, Besser D, Hemmati-Brivanlou A. TGFbeta/activin/nodal signaling is necessary for the maintenance of pluripotency in human embryonic stem cells. Development 2005; 132: 1273–82.

28. Vallier L, Alexander M, Pedersen RA. Activin/Nodal and FGF pathways cooperate to maintain pluripotency of human embryonic stem cells. J Cell Sci 2005; 118: 4495–509.

29. Zwaka TP, Thomson JA. A germ cell origin of embryonic stem cells? Development 2006; 132: 227–33.

30. Nichols J, Chambers I, Taga T, Smith A. Physiological rationale for responsiveness of mouse embryonic stem cells to gp130 cytokines. Development 2001; 128: 2333–9.

31. Takeuchi Y, Molyneaux K, Runyan C, Schaible K, Wylie C. The roles of FGF signaling in germ cell migration in the mouse. Development 2005; 132: 5399–409.

32. Donovan PJ. Growth factor regulation of mouse primordial germ cell development. Curr Top Dev Biol 1994; 29: 189–225.

33. Dono R, Texido G, Dussel R, Ehmke H, Zeller R. Impaired cerebral cortex development and blood pressure regulation in FGF-2-deficient mice. EMBO J 1998; 17: 4213–25.

34. Ortega S, Ittmann M, Tsang SH, Ehrlich M, Basilico C. Neuronal defects and delayed wound healing in mice lacking fibroblast growth factor 2. Proc Natl Acad Sci USA 1998; 95: 5672–7.

35. Zhou M, Sutliffe RL, Paul RJ et al. Fibroblast growth factor 2 control of vascular tone. Nat Med 1998; 4: 201–7.

36. Yamaguchi TP, Harpal K, Henkemeyer M, Rossant J. fgfr-1 is required for embryonic growth and mesodermal patterning during mouse gastrulation. Genes Dev 1994; 8: 3032–44.

37. Arman E, Haffner-Krausz R, Chen Y, Heath JK, Lonai P. Targeted disruption of fibroblast growth factor (FGF) receptor 2 suggests a role for FGF signaling in pregastrulation mammalian development. Proc Natl Acad Sci USA 1998; 95: 5082–7.

38. Xu RH, Peck RM, Li DS et al. Basic FGF and suppression of BMP signaling sustain undifferentiated proliferation of human ES cells. Nat Methods 2005; 2: 185–90.

39. Feldman B, Poueymirou W, Papaioannou VE, DeChiara TM, Goldfarb M. Requirement of FGF-4 for postimplantation mouse development. Science 1995; 267: 246–9.

40. Sun X, Meyers EN, Lewandoski M, Martin GR. Targeted disruption of Fgf8 causes failure of cell migration in the gastrulation mouse embryo. Genes Dev 1999; 13: 1834–46.

CHAPTER 7

Adult stem cell population in the testis

Herman Tournaye and Ellen Goossens

INTRODUCTION

The preservation of spermatogenesis throughout a man's adult reproductive life depends on one cell type only: the adult testicular stem cell. Testicular stem cells are undifferentiated cells that give rise to the spermatogenic cells and, finally, the spermatozoa. Even though there is a continual loss of differentiated cells, the spermatogenic cell lineage maintains its cell number thanks to the adult testicular stem cells, which produce both new stem cells (self-renewal) and differentiating cells.

Maintaining the genetic integrity of testicular stem cells is important in order to preserve the quality and function of the differentiated cells, but also to guarantee a correct transmission of genetic information from one generation to the next. Adult testicular stem cells are thus essential for both the production of gametes and the continuation of the species. This chapter gives an overview of the theoretical aspects of testicular stem cells as well as of the current research on potential clinical applications.

THEORETICAL ASPECTS OF TESTICULAR STEM CELLS

Where do testicular stem cells come from?

Testicular stem cells originate from the primordial germ cells, which derive from pluripotent cells of the epiblast.[1] The mechanisms responsible for the differentiation of germ cells in the epiblast involve several factors, including bone morphogenetic protein 2 (BMP2), BMP4 and BMP8B. Germ cells move, at a very early stage of embryonic life, through the primitive streak into the extraembryonic region at the base of the allantois. In the 4th week, some cells present in the yolk sac, near the base of the allantois, differentiate into primordial germ cells, which can be identified by their expression of alkaline phosphatase, Oct4, VASA, SSEA1, EMA1, F9 and the tyrosine kinase receptor c-kit. In the 5th week, primordial germ cells become embedded in the wall of the hindgut and migrate through the dorsal mesentery to reach the gonadal ridges where they proliferate and increase in number.[2] The migration, cell proliferation and survival of primordial germ cells is driven by signaling between stem cell factor (SCF) which is expressed in somatic cells along the pathway of primordial germ cell migration, and its receptor c-kit, expressed in germ cells.[3] During migration, primordial germ cells proliferate actively, but do not differentiate. The differentiation into gonocytes starts when the primordial germ cells become enclosed by their niche cells, i.e. Sertoli cells. These germ cells differ morphologically from the migratory primordial germ cells and are therefore called gonocytes.[4] The gonocytes are positioned in the center of the seminiferous tubule. Gonocytes proliferate for a few days and then become quiescent in the G_0/G_1 phase of the cell cycle. In mice and rats, these cells resume proliferation about 2 days after birth. By day 6 all gonocytes have migrated to the basement membrane and become A_s-spermatogonia.[5,6] This event marks the initiation of spermatogenesis and is mainly directed by the Sertoli cells. In mice, Sertoli cells express only a soluble SCF until day 7 after birth. Between the 7th and the 11th day, the Sertoli cells switch their production from a soluble into a membrane-bound SCF. This switch is accompanied by the start of testicular stem cell differentiation, assuming that the membrane-bound form is more important in spermatogenesis than the soluble form.[7] C-kit negative testicular stem cells acquire sensitivity for SCF thanks to another factor that is secreted by Sertoli cells very early in postnatal life and down-regulated in adult life, i.e. BMP4. Its receptor Alk3 is expressed in postnatal spermatogonia. Stimulation of the Alk3 receptor with BMP4 triggers a cascade of actions that results in the expression of the c-kit receptor.[8]

How to identify testicular stem cells?

Testicular stem cells are single triangular cells located on the basement membrane of the seminiferous tubules in close contact with the Sertoli cells. They have an ovoid nucleus and a dense cytoplasm. The nucleoli, which lack heterochromatin, are positioned close to the nuclear membrane. The cytoplasm contains a small Golgi apparatus, few mitochondria and many free ribosomes.[9]

Testicular stem cells can be distinguished from pluripotent stem cells by their expression of Oct4 (Table 7.1). This transcription factor is down-regulated in multipotent and unipotent stem cells. Adult testicular stem cells can also be identified by the absence of the tyrosine kinase receptor c-kit. Pluripotent stem cells, primordial germ cells and neonatal testicular stem cells express this receptor, whereas in the adult testis, the c-kit-receptor is expressed in all differentiating spermatogonia but not in the undifferentiated spermatogonia.[10] A reciprocal relationship exists between c-kit and Thy1 expression; when c-kit expression is established, Thy1 expression is down-regulated. Thy1 is also a differentiation marker for thymocytes, T cells and some neuronal cells, but it was also found to be expressed on hematopoietic stem cells. C-kit negative testicular stem cells were

Table 7.1 Differential expression of testicular stem cell markers

Marker	*Expression site*	*Cell types that express the marker*
Oct4	Nucleus	ESCs (high expression) Undifferentiated spg (moderate expression)
c-kit	Surface	ESCs, PGCs, neonatal TSCs, differentiated spg
Thy1	Surface	TSCs
α_6-integrin	Surface	Undifferentiated spg, ESCs
β_1-integrin	Surface	Undifferentiated spg
CD9	Surface	spg, ESCs
MHC-I	Surface	Nucleated cells, except TSCs and ESCs
GFRα1	Surface	Type A spg
c-ret	Transmembrane	TSCs
Daz(l)	Nucleus Cytoplasm	ESCs, PGCs, spg Postmeiotic germ cells
Plzf	Nucleus	TSCs
Stra8	Cytoplasm	Premeiotic germ cells
TAF4b	Nucleus	spg

ESC, embryonic stem cell; PGC, primordial germ cell; spg, spermatogonia; TSC, testicular stem cell found to express β_1- and α_6-integrins on their surface.[11] These integrins are also found on stem cells from other tissues. Recently, Kanatsu-Shinohara et al found that CD9, a β_1-integrin-associated transmembrane protein that is involved in cell adhesion and cell motility events, and which is expressed on stem cells of other tissues, is also expressed in testicular stem cells. Expression of CD9, however, is not specific to testicular stem cells. The CD9-selected cells showed a significant amount of c-kit, which is expressed on differentiating spermatogonia.[12] Other markers to identify spermatogonia in a testicular cell suspension are the major histocompatibility (MHC)-I molecules. Although MHC-I molecules are expressed on virtually all nucleated somatic cells, the expression is very limited in spermatogonia. Recently, it was shown that undifferentiated spermatogonia express the receptor for glial cell line-derived neurotrophic factor (GDNF), the GDNF-family receptor α1 (GFRα1) and the associated tyrosine kinase receptor (REarranged during Transfection [c-Ret]). GDNF, which is produced by the Sertoli cells, is required for testicular stem cell renewal and spermatogenesis.[13] Another family of markers for undifferentiated spermatogonia is the Daz (deleted in azoospermia) family. Daz is a Y-chromosome-linked protein in humans and Dazl (Daz-like) is an autosomal homolog expressed in humans and mice. These proteins were found to be located in the nucleus of spermatogonia. During male meiosis, however, the proteins are transferred from the nucleus to the cytoplasm.[14] A factor that is required for self-renewal and maintenance of the testicular stem cell population is the promyelocytic leukemia zinc finger (Plzf). Plzf is co-expressed with Oct4 in undifferentiated spermatogonia and functions as a transcriptional repressor regulating the epigenetic state of undifferentiated cells.[15,16] Another protein that is expressed exclusively in the premeiotic germ cells is the cytoplasmic stimulated by retinoic acid-protein (Stra8).[17] The expression of stem cell-specific molecules, such as Plzf, c-Ret and Stra8, requires the expression of the gonad-specific TAF4b component of TFIID, a transcriptional regulator expressed in mouse testes.[18] Other genes that are expressed in spermatogonia, but not in somatic cells, are Mage, Ube1y, Usp9y, Rbmy, Ott, Ddx4, Tex14, Usp26, Piwil2, Pramel1.

Although, at present, there is no specific marker to exclusively select testicular stem cells, the use of a combination of differentially expressed markers can result in a highly enriched stem cell population. Such a combination of factors was used by Kubota et al. They found an enrichment of stem cells after flow cytometric cell sorting in the fraction containing (MHC-I)$^-$, Thy1$^+$, c-kit$^-$ cells. The (MHC-I)$^-$, Thy1$^+$, c-kit$^-$ cells also showed α_6-integrin and CD24 expression, but were negative for α_V-integrin, Sca1 and CD34.[19]

Testicular stem cell lines

Two groups have reported the establishment of testicular stem cell lines.[20,21] In both studies, type A spermatogonia were immortalized by using the Simian virus large T antigen. The cell lines were characterized and found to express Oct4, a marker for undifferentiated spermatogonia. Expression of c-kit, normally expressed in type A spermatogonia from late A_{al} spermatogonia onwards, could not be detected.

Moreover, Hofmann et al found detectable levels of some more protein markers specific for germ cells such as Dazl, GFRα1, Piwil2 and Pramel1.[21] The establishment of these cell lines is a great step forward in the study of spermatogonial gene expression and regulation.

Recent studies showed that neonatal as well as adult testicular stem cells can retain the ability to generate pluripotent cells and are able to differentiate into derivatives of the three embryonic germ layers in vitro.[22,23]

Testicular stem cell renewal

Testicular stem cells have, like stem cells in other tissues, the capacity to self-renew or to differentiate. Two models exist for stem cell renewal and spermatogonial proliferation in non-primate mammals: the A_s-model and the slightly different A_0/A_1-model.

The mechanism of proliferation for primates is somewhat different. Since most of the research focuses on rodent spermatogenesis, the proliferation schemes of both non-primate and primate mammals are presented.

Two models for non-primate mammalian testicular stem cell proliferation

The A_s-model, originally proposed in 1971 by Huckins[24] and Oakberg,[25] is still the most widely accepted. This model is a one-compartment stem cell model. At the onset of spermatogenesis, a compartment of undifferentiated type A spermatogonia is subdivided into A_{single} (A_s), A_{paired} (A_{pr}) and $A_{aligned}$ (A_{al}) spermatogonia. These type A spermatogonia have the same morphology and can only be distinguished according to their topographical arrangement on the basement membrane of the seminiferous tubules. The A_s spermatogonia are considered to be the true population of testicular stem cells. It was found that A_s spermatogonia have a longer cell cycle than A_{pr} and A_{al} spermatogonia, resulting in a lower proliferation rate and thus less accumulation of replication errors.[26] When A_s spermatogonia divide, they either produce two A_s daughter cells or they produce two type A_{pr} or paired spermatogonia. When A_s spermatogonia divide into two A_s cells, they usually migrate separately. If cytokinesis is incomplete, the daughter cells stay together and become A_{pr} spermatogonia, connected to each other by an intercellular cytoplasmic bridge. The production of type A_{pr} spermatogonia is the first step towards differentiation. Normally, about 50% of the testicular stem cells divide to form A_{pr} spermatogonia, while the other 50% goes through self-renewing divisions, thereby maintaining the size of the testicular stem cell population. The type A_{pr} spermatogonia that are formed divide once again to produce groups of four type A_{al} spermatogonia, also connected to one another. The A_{al} cells proliferate, resulting in chains of 8, 16 and occasionally 32 A_{al} cells, all interconnected by cytoplasmic bridges. Most of the A_{al} spermatogonia will undergo a morphological change and transform into type A_1 spermatogonia, which are the first generation of differentiated spermatogonia (Figure 7.1). These differentiated spermatogonia subsequently divide into A_2, A_3, A_4, In and B spermatogonia to form the primary spermatocytes.

In mice, spermatogenesis occurs in a cyclic manner and can be divided into 12 stages (I–XII). At stage VIII, A_s, A_{pr} and a few A_{al} spermatogonia are present. It takes until stage X before these cells start to proliferate. The proliferation stops at stage II–III, and cells become arrested in the G_1/G_0 phase. At stage VII–VIII, A_{al} cells undergo morphological changes and become A_1 spermatogonia, which enter the S phase. At stage IX, these cells divide into A_2 spermatogonia. At stage XI, A_3 spermatogonia are formed and A_4 spermatogonia first appear at stage I. A_4 cells divide into In spermatogonia at stage II and these form B spermatogonia at stage IV. The final spermatogonial division occurs at stage VI with the formation of primary spermatocytes.

The A_0/A_1-model by Clermont and Bustos-Obregon[27] and Clermont and Hermo[28] is based on a slightly different identification scheme for type A spermatogonia. This is a two-compartment stem cell model. In the normal adult testis, the A_s and the A_{pr} spermatogonia are quiescent and are called A_0 spermatogonia in this model. These cells will only divide after cell loss and are therefore also called 'reserve stem cells'.[29] The differentiating spermatogonia A_1, A_2, A_3 and A_4 of the A_s-model are considered cells with stem cell properties in this model. A_4 spermatogonia can divide into A_1 or In spermatogonia. The proliferating A_{al} cells are not considered a distinct class and are called A_3 and A_4 cells, which can retransform into type A_1 spermatogonia. Thus, according to this alternative model, two stem cell compartments exist, i.e. the type A_0 compartment or 'reserve stem cells' and the compartment consisting of type A_1 through A_4 spermatogonia, also referred to as 'renewing stem cells' (Figure 7.2).

This model has been the subject of controversy, because of some experimental findings:

(1) The A_s and A_{pr} spermatogonia are not quiescent in the adult testis.

(2) A_{al} cell cycles bear more resemblance to the cell cycles from A_s and A_{pr} spermatogonia than to those from A_1–A_4 spermatogonia.

(3) In the absence of A_1 spermatogonia, A_{al} spermatogonia can still be formed.

(4) A_{al} and A_1–A_4 spermatogonia do not have the same radiosensitivity, suggesting that A_{al} and A_1–A_4 spermatogonia are different cell types.

(5) The length of A_1–A_4 chains is longer than that of A_{al} spermatogonia.

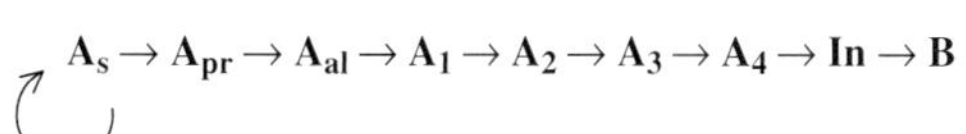

Figure 7.1 The A_s-model for non-primate spermatogonial differentiation

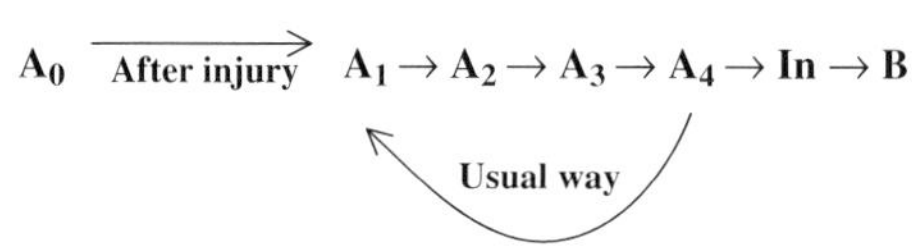

Figure 7.2 The A_0/A_1-model for non-primate spermatogonial differentiation

The A_p/A_d-model for primates

In primates, two morphologically different classes of type A spermatogonia are observed: the dark (A_d) and the pale (A_p) spermatogonia, named after their staining intensity with hematoxylin. It is generally accepted that in primates there is a dual stem cell compartment, as in the A_0/A_1-model. Clermont applied his rodent theory to the primates, with the A_d in the role of the A_0 (reserve stem cells) and the A_p as the A_1 through A_4 (renewing stem cells).[30] In general, there are equal numbers of A_d and A_p spermatogonia. A_p spermatogonia divide once every cycle, whereas A_d spermatogonia normally do not divide. The self-renewal of the type A_p spermatogonia is analogous to that in the A_s-model, because most of the type A_p spermatogonia appear in clones of 2, 4 and 8 cells, but single A_p cells may also exist. Furthermore, the A_d and A_p cells can transform into each other. A_d spermatogonia are often found in clusters. Such a cluster of A_d cells could be a result of a transformation of A_p into A_d at low renewal frequency. Conversely, after cytotoxic injury, the A_d spermatogonia may become active again and transform into A_p spermatogonia, which can start to proliferate and form type B spermatogonia. In monkeys, there are four generations of B spermatogonia (B_1–B_4), whereas in humans, there is only one. Very recently, new information about this model was reported by Ehmcke et al. They concluded that the population of A_p spermatogonia cycle continuously and initiate spermatogenesis by an equal spermatogonial self-renewing division at stage VII. Subsequently, the clones of A_p spermatogonia will separate and initiate a second division at stage IX, which leads to clones of B spermatogonia as well as pairs or quadruplets of A_p cells. These latter cells are responsible for the maintenance of the original size of the A population. Because the A_p, which are found in clones of 2 or 4 cells, cycle continuously, the true stem cells are probably the seldom-dividing single A_p and A_d spermatogonia[31] (Figure 7.3).

The process of spermatogenesis results in a large number of sperm cells. It is estimated that a mouse testis contains about 35 000 A_s spermatogonia. One single A_s cell is theoretically able to give rise to 4096 spermatids. In the human, this number is lower because of fewer mitotic divisions, apoptosis and the low effectiveness of the process.[32,33]

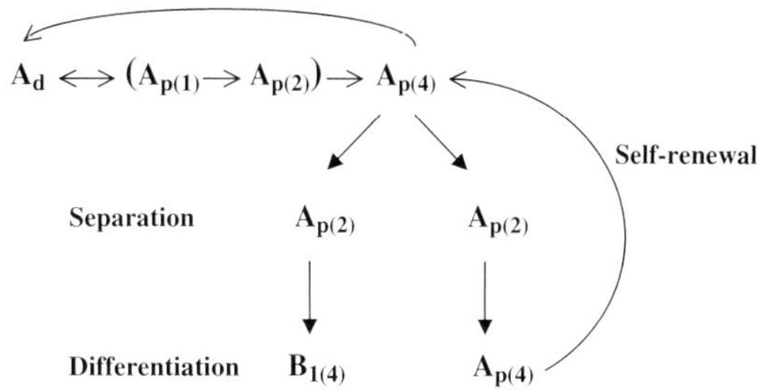

Figure 7.3 The A_d/A_p-model for primate spermatogonial differentiation

Regulation of the size of the stem cell population

Testicular stem cells can develop in three different ways: they can renew themselves, they can differentiate or they can go into apoptosis. The mechanism determining which pathway will be followed is the subject of a great deal of investigation. The only cells in direct contact with the stem cells are the Sertoli cells; hence, the regulation of the germ cell pool will probably occur through the Sertoli cell. Sertoli cells have large contact areas with the germ cells through desmosome–gap junction complexes. However, these intercellular contacts are rarely seen on type A spermatogonia. Therefore, it is assumed that Sertoli cells regulate spermatogonial proliferation by secreting paracrine factors. In addition, Sertoli cells limit the expansion of testicular stem cells, since it is assumed that each Sertoli cell can only support a defined number of testicular stem cells.

The spermatogonia are also in contact with the basement membrane of the seminiferous tubules and may therefore also respond to diffusing paracrine factors secreted by Leydig cells or myoid cells in the interstitial space.

Regulation of stem cell renewal

In normal seminiferous epithelium, the ratio between self-renewal and differentiation should be about 1.0. More self-renewal than differentiation would reduce the seminiferous epithelium to only testicular stem cells and a tumor might be formed. In the other case, if there is more differentiation than self-renewal, the testis would become depleted of testicular stem cells. However, in rodents, it was observed that during a period of active proliferation of the testicular stem cells, the number of these cells slowly decreases, indicating that more than half of the daughter cells become A_{pr} spermatogonia. The cell density in the seminiferous tubules is kept constant by density-dependent degeneration of differentiating spermatogonia.[34]

On the other hand, when the seminiferous epithelium is depleted by cytotoxic agents or irradiation, the restoration of spermatogenesis must occur from testicular stem cells. Indeed, testicular stem cells are less sensitive than differentiating spermatogonia, but they can still be lost. Surviving testicular stem cells may start repopulating the seminiferous tubules by forming colonies that grow along the length of the tubules. Moreover, in this situation, the percentage of A_{pr} daughter cells was much lower than in the normal testis, which indicates that testicular stem cells prefer self-renewal above differentiation.[35]

These last few years, a number of factors have been characterized that influence testicular stem cell survival and proliferation in vitro. Testicular stem cell self-renewal and differentiation depend on GDNF, a factor produced by Sertoli cells.[15,36] Loss of GDNF expression results in depletion of testicular stem cell reserves and overexpression leads to an accumulation of undifferentiated spermatogonia. Stem cell self-renewal is also regulated by the pituitary gland. In neonatal testes, gonadotropins stimulate self-renewal, but in the adult, they have the opposite effect.

Regulation of differentiation

A crucial phase during non-primate spermatogenesis is thought to be the transition from A_{al} to A_1 spermatogonia. Different factors and/or mechanisms have been reported that cause an arrest in spermatogonial differentiation and therefore an increase in the stem cell population in the seminiferous tubules (Table 7.2).

A first mechanism is cryptorchidism, developed by Nishimune and Haneji. The higher temperature in the mouse testis causes infertility owing to the disruption of spermatogenesis, including the reduction of germ cells. Sertoli cells also appear to be temperature-sensitive, although the mechanisms involved are not clear. In mice that were made cryptorchid, only type A spermatogonia remained after 2 months. Despite the fact that these cells were still proliferating, they were unable to give rise to more differentiated cells. However, when the testis was transferred back into the scrotum, spermatogenesis could be re-established.[37]

Table 7.2 Mechanisms causing an arrest in spermatogonial differentiation

Model	*Deficiency*
Cryptorchidy	Temperature too high
Steel or W mutation	No SCF or c-kit expression
Vitamin A deficiency	No retinoic acid production
Jsd mutation	Intratubular defect
2,5-hexanedione	Sertoli cell damage
LBNF1 rats	Irradiation

SCF, stem cell factor; LBNF, Lewis × Brown Norway F1

Secondly, as mentioned before, c-kit receptor and its ligand SCF play an important role in the differentiation of type A spermatogonia. This can be illustrated by the following two mutant mouse models: the dominant White spotting (W) mutation that hampers the expression of the c-kit receptor and the Steel (Sl) mutation that blocks the transcription of stem cell factor. Males that are heterozygous for mutations in one of the genes encoding for these proteins show an arrest of spermatogenesis on the spermatogonial level.[38,39]

A third mechanism is vitamin A deficiency by which only type A spermatogonia which are unable to differentiate, will remain.[40] However, after vitamin A supplementation or continuous administration of retinoic acid, spermatogenesis can be restored.[41]

A fourth mechanism has been described in adult male mice homozygous for the mutant gene juvenile spermatogonial depletion (jsd). These animals are sterile and have small testes.[42] Even though type A spermatogonia are found, they are not able to differentiate. In a study by Mizunuma et al it was concluded that the defect must be intratubular, since the intertubular environment of jsd/jsd-mice was normal.[43]

In rats, a fifth mechanism has been described. When rats were given 2,5-hexanedione, a Sertoli cell toxicant, spermatogonial differentiation was found to be irreversibly impaired. The only cell type that remained were type A spermatogonia, which were able to actively proliferate.[44]

A final mechanism has been reported in LBNF1 rats. These rats were X-irradiated with doses of 3.5–6 Gy, which caused a depletion of the seminiferous epithelium.[45] Yet, 4–6 weeks after irradiation, the seminiferous epithelium recovered. Unexpectedly, spermatogenesis subsequently slowed down until only undifferentiated spermatogonia were present. These cells were incapable of differentiating, unless the rats were treated with either gonadotropin-releasing hormone agonist or testosterone.[46] Since no hormone receptors are as yet known to exist on spermatogonia, this finding suggests that the Sertoli cells, rather than the spermatogonia, were damaged by irradiation and that these hormones could induce these cells to regain their function.

At present, it is still not understood how the differentiation of undifferentiated spermatogonia is regulated. Sertoli cells probably play the most important role. In all mechanisms of arrested differentiation described above, Sertoli cell function is impaired, which results in deficient spermatogenesis. Only in the W/W mice, which lack the c-kit receptor, is the problem located within the spermatogonia, which are unable to respond to SCF secreted by the Sertoli cells.

Regulation of apoptosis

One of the proteins involved in stem cell apoptosis is p53, which has important functions in cell growth and differentiation. Although p53 is not expressed in normal spermatogonia, high levels of p53 have been observed after an irradiation dose of 4 Gy in mice, resulting in apoptosis of the spermatogonia.[47]

The B-cell CLL/lymphoma 2 (Bcl2)-protein family is another group of apoptosis regulators. During normal spermatogenesis, large numbers of differentiated spermatogonia go into apoptosis as a result of the density regulation. When Bcl2 or Bcl-x_L is overexpressed, apoptosis is suppressed and this density regulation does not occur. As a consequence, spermatogonia will accumulate and, finally, both the spermatogonia and spermatocytes will enter into apoptosis.[48] Bcl-w is another prosurvival factor that participates in the regulation of apoptosis by binding the proapoptotic factors Bax and Bak. It is suggested that the ratios of Bax/Bcl-w and Bak/Bcl-w are decisive for the survival of spermatogonia.[49]

CURRENT RESEARCH ON POTENTIAL CLINICAL APPLICATIONS

The importance of the testicular stem cell is reflected in a variety of research fields. The study of fundamental aspects of germ cell development has become possible thanks to the introduction of the testicular stem cell transplantation technique[33,50] and germ cell culture.[51] In the future, these techniques may also have clinical applications. Indeed, the preservation of spermatogonial stem cells may prove an important strategy in preserving fertility in young cancer patients.[52] Another field of research with clinical potential is the introduction of transgenes into the germ line by the transfection of spermatogonia.[53] Although ethically very challenging, this application might one day pave the way for transgenerational gene therapy. We shall focus on some of the recent scientific breakthroughs and potential future use of spermatogonia.

Testicular stem cell transplantation

The technique of testicular stem cell transplantation, introduced by Brinster's group in 1994, involves the introduction of a germ cell suspension from a fertile donor testis into the seminiferous tubules of an infertile recipient mouse.[33] Testicular stem cells were able to relocate onto the basement membrane and colonize the tubules in the first month after transplantation. From that moment on, stem cells started to proliferate and initiated spermatogenesis. Spermatozoa obtained by this method were capable of fertilization.[50] Currently, two research models for stem cell transplantation are in use. A first model involves the transplantation of testicular cell suspensions from a fertile donor into the tubules of a sterile W/W^V mutant mouse. A mutation in the dominant white spotting gene hampers the expression of the c-kit receptor, resulting in testes with the appearance of a Sertoli cell only syndrome (germ cell aplasia). A second model uses busulphan-treated recipient mice. Busulphan is a cytotoxic drug that eliminates most germ cells from the testis. Since some endogenous spermatogenesis may remain, it is necessary to use testicular cells from a donor with a genetic marker in order to distinguish donor spermatogenesis from endogenous (recipient) spermatogenesis. One popular marker is lac-Z, a gene transcribing for the β-galactosidase protein. Transgenic cells can be visualized after staining with 5-bromo-4-chloro-3-indolyl-β-D-galactopyranoside (X-gal). Another popular marker is green fluorescent protein (GFP), which enables cells to be visualized under UV light.

Although healthy live offspring can be obtained from transplanted mice, it has recently been shown that the fertilizing capacity of post-transplantation spermatozoa may be diminished. Also blastocyst[55] and postimplantation[56] development were hampered. A few years after the introduction of the testicular stem cell transplantation technique, it was shown that the testis of one species can provide support for spermatogenesis from another species. França et al found that it is the transplanted stem cells themselves that impose the duration of the cell cycle and not the Sertoli cells. A cell suspension from a rat testis was transplanted into an immunodeficient mouse which eventually resulted in rat spermatozoa being produced. The duration of spermatogenesis was comparable to that of the rat and not to that of the mouse.[57] Xenogeneic transplantations to the mouse testis were also performed with testicular cell suspensions from hamster, rabbit, dog, primate and even human. Hamster cells were able to colonize and to produce spermatozoa. However, these spermatozoa developed abnormally and were lower in number compared with mouse-to-mouse and rat-to-mouse transplants.[58] Rabbit and dog cell suspensions could colonize seminiferous tubules in which they formed chains of cells; however, they failed to produce mature spermatozoa.[32] Primate cell suspensions were also able to colonize but not to proliferate in the recipient's tubules.[59] Finally, human cell suspensions were not able to colonize the murine seminiferous tubules, probably because of non-compatible cellular interactions and immunological rejection.[60] Two years later, proliferation of human stem cells was reported after transplantation into mouse seminiferous tubules. These stem cells could survive for 6 months in the murine testis.[61] These observations demonstrate the relationship of the transplantation success with the phylogenetical distance between donor and recipient species.

Selection of testicular stem cells

It has been estimated that, in the adult mouse, a testis contains only one stem cell in 5000 testicular cells. Since the number of stem cells is crucial for the success of testicular stem cell transplantation, enriching the proportion of stem cells may improve colonization efficiency and bring clinical applications closer. Shinohara et al selected testicular stem cells based on the ability of these cells to adhere to laminin, a component of the basement membrane of the seminiferous tubules. It was found that testicular stem cells could be enriched 5- to 10-fold with magnetic beads and antibodies against β_1- and α_6-integrins, which are expressed on the surface of the testicular stem cells.[11] In addition, stem cells have little or no c-kit and α_V-expression, and can therefore be negatively selected by fluorescence-activated cell sorting (FACS). By combining these two selection methods, a 166-fold enrichment of testicular stem cells was obtained.[62] Highly enriched stem cell populations were also obtained with FACS using the following selection criteria: (MHC-I)$^-$, Thy-1$^+$ and c-kit$^-$.[19]

Magnetic activated cell sorting (MACS) is another technique that may be used to enrich spermatogonia. Von Schonfeldt and colleagues reported the isolation of c-kit-positive spermatogonia via MACS. A total of 25–55% of the isolated magnetically labelled cells were c-kit positive.[63]

Sedimentation velocity and differential adhesion were used by Dirami et al to obtain a population of 95–98% porcine type A spermatogonia.[64] Using adhesion to laminin, the isolation of testicular stem cells has been found to increase three to fourfold.[11] Morena et al used sedimentation velocity in conjunction with differential adhesion to achieve a suspension with 85% of the cells being type A, c-kit-positive spermatogonia.[65]

Culture of testicular stem cells

The development of testicular stem cell transplantation has provided a functional assay for the evaluation of testicular stem cell culture. Nagano et al reported the first long-term survival, for approximately 4 months, of testicular stem cells on STO cell feeder layers.[51] In addition, suppressing the differentiation of testicular stem cells improves their in-vitro maintenance.[66] Testicular stem cells were kept in culture for more than 5 months, when GDNF, epithelial derived growth factor, basic fibroblast growth factor and leukemia inhibitory factor were added to the culture medium.[67] The same group has recently shown that in the absence of any feeder layers or serum, stem cells could survive for more than 6 months.[68] However, it was found that culture outcome is dependent on the age of the isolated tissue. Prepubertal cells were shown to be twice as viable as adult cells in culture conditions.

Therefore, it should be borne in mind that cultures of adult tissue are not representative of prepubertal tissue.[69]

Not only has the maintenance of testicular stem cells in culture been investigated but also differentiation in vitro has been studied. Izadyar et al reported differentiation from bovine type A spermatogonia into spermatocytes and spermatids.[70] Culture at 37°C in minimal essential medium containing 2.5% fetal calf serum (FCS) provided an optimal condition for survival, proliferation and differentiation of bovine type A spermatogonia.

In-vitro tissue explants represent an alternative strategy to culture testicular cells. Bovine testicular tissue pieces were maintained in culture for 2 weeks and an increase in colony numbers indicated that testicular stem cell proliferation had taken place.[71]

Testicular tissue grafting

Testicular tissue containing stem cells can also be grafted. Attempts have been made to graft immature and adult testicular tissue in both ectopic locations and homotopic locations. In all studies of mouse-to-mouse grafts, mouse testicular tissue derived from newborn mice completed spermatogenesis. Grafting to the mouse was also successful using tissue from hamster, pig, goat, calf, rabbit and monkey. Grafting with frozen–thawed testicular tissue was also found to be efficient.[72–74] However, results obtained from adult tissue grafting were less promising. Recently published experiments show that prepubertal murine tissue can be grafted successfully, with spermatogenesis in almost all the grafts, whereas adult murine and adult human grafts are generally lost because of sclerosis or atrophy, although spermatogonia may survive.[75,76]

Cryopreservation of testicular stem cells

Cryopreservation of testicular stem cells would be a valuable tool for any clinical application. But cryopreservation could also be valuable for the conservation of the genetic material of endangered species or valuable laboratory animals.

In 1996, Avarbock and co-workers were the first to report on successful cryopreservation of testicular stem cells. Although frozen–thawed suspensions of murine testicular cells were able to colonize recipient testes and initiate spermatogenesis, the search for an optimal freezing protocol is still ongoing.[77] In 2002, a non-controlled-rate freezing protocol was described using minimal essential medium; it contained 10% FCS, 10% DMSO (dimethyl sulfoxide) and 0.07 mol/L sucrose to yield the highest number (70%) of surviving cells after freeze–thawing.[78] Interestingly, the rate of survival of stem cells was higher than that of other testicular cells, which resulted in an enrichment of stem cells in the final suspension. We were not able to confirm this. With our best freezing protocol (uncontrolled, 1.5 mol/L DMSO), we observed spermatogenesis in only 22.7% of the tubules after transplantation, whereas in fresh, unfrozen controls, spermatogenesis was obtained in 90% of the tubules, which indicated an important loss of functional stem cells after freezing.[79]

An alternative way of preserving stem cells is to freeze the whole testicular tissue. A protocol has recently been proposed using 0.7 mol/L DMSO as a cryoprotectant. The structure of the tissue was well-preserved with, especially, the spermatogonia as surviving cells.[9] However, these experiments should be validated using (xeno-)grafting as a functional assay.

Transfection of testicular stem cells

Testicular stem cells are the only stem cells in the human that can transmit parental genetic information to the offspring, making them an attractive target cell population for transgenesis. Mouse testicular stem cells have been successfully transfected with the use of a retroviral vector. Germ cells were incubated with (1) retroviral-producing cells alone; (2) an STO feeder layer and retroviral-producing cells; and (3) an STO feeder layer with periodic exposure to retroviral-particles. All methods generated stably transfected stem cells that colonized recipient testes, with the third protocol yielding the highest level of infection. In addition, co-injection of retroviral particles and germ cells into recipient testes also resulted in incorporation of the reporter gene. It is now possible to transfect both adult and immature stem cells by retroviral-mediated gene delivery in vitro[66] and in vivo[80] by using a retrovirus vector.

This method has multiple applications, such as cell therapy, the introduction of genes into certain animal species and the genetic modification of stem cells, to answer fundamental questions about the self-renewal and differentiation of stem cells.

ASSOCIATED PATHOLOGIES

Male infertility

Infertility occurs in 13–18% of the couples seeking to have children. In at least 20% of these couples, the cause of infertility is of paternal origin. Some specific male factor disorders can be treated, but, for non-specific male factor infertility, treatment is difficult. In order to understand, and eventually treat these defects, it is critical to identify the regulating mechanisms at the various stages of spermatogenesis. The culture system as well as the transplantation technique, together with transfection of testicular stem cells, may prove very useful methods in achieving more knowledge of testicular stem cells and their proliferation. Studies using these methods may not only reveal more insight into the disease. It may also help to identify markers for diagnostic purposes or serve as a model in pharmacological studies.

Contraceptive strategy

Since condoms and vasectomy are currently the only available methods for male contraception, new contraceptive strategies for the male are more than welcome. There are several approaches to male contraception, but research and development of male hormonal contraceptives is the only one under clinical investigation.

The use of testicular stem cell culture systems might provide better insights into factors regulating spermatogenesis and may eventually lead to alternative methods of male contraception.

Testicular germinal cancers

Testicular cancers are the most frequent tumor affecting the young adult (20–35 years old). Although most of these cancers can be cured, testicular cancer still represents a significant public health problem. The current understanding is that tumors progress from a carcinoma in situ, which are malignant cells derived from gonocytes.[81] Because there is still no animal model representing the characteristics of the human germinal tumors, studies carried out on testicular stem cells in culture or in an animal host will be of great significance.

Preservation of fertility for oncological patients

Oncological diseases such as leukemia and Hodgkin's disease occur with an incidence of about 1 in 600 children before the age of 15 years. In recent years, remarkable progress has been made in the treatment of childhood cancers, and up to 75% of the patients can now be cured. At present, 1 in 1000 adults in the age group of 20–30 years is a childhood cancer survivor.[82] From these figures, it is evident that the prevention of sterility in childhood cancer survivors will become a major challenge in reproductive medicine. When an adult man undergoes a sterilizing cytotoxic treatment, sperm can be frozen in order to circumvent sterility after his treatment. However, no such prevention is possible before puberty, since no active spermatogenesis is present. The introduction of the testicular stem cell transplantation technique in a clinical setting would create new prospects for the preservation of fertility in prepubertal cancer patients.[52] Since current cancer treatments may destroy all dividing cells, including testicular stem cells, and since prepubertal boys do not as yet produce spermatozoa, it is not possible for them to preserve their fertility. However, testis tissue could be removed before any cancer treatment and cryopreserved. After the patient has been cured, the testicular cells could be transplanted back to the testis. Before such an application can be approved, safety needs to be evaluated. In the mouse, it was shown that sperm cells obtained after testicular stem cell transplantation were able to fertilize and produce normal embryos after assisted reproduction. It remains to be shown whether this technique is clinically efficient as well, especially when frozen–thawed cells are to be transplanted.

An important part of the treatment is the storage of the testicular tissue. Cryopreservation of testicular tissue or cell suspensions is one option. Another possibility is the long-term organ or cell culture, and a third option may be the transplantation of the cells or grafting of the tissue into host animals.

It is obvious that the reintroduction of malignant cells into a cured patient must be omitted. A selection of spermatogonia or an elimination of cancer cells before transplantation should be carried out. Elimination of cancer cells can be achieved by decontaminating the testis sample or by grafting a tissue piece onto a host. The first approach makes use of

MACS or FACS to select out cancer cells and/or positively select spermatogonia on the basis of certain membrane molecules (e.g. cancer cells:HLA^+; spermatogonia:HLA^-). This approach, used by Fujita et al, was found to overcome malignant contamination by depleting the cell suspension from leukemic cells by FACS prior to transplantation.[83] However, in our experiments, MACS and FACS were found not efficient enough to deplete testicular cell suspensions from malignant cells.[84] The second way avoiding the reinjection of cancer cells into the remaining testis is by grafting a testicular tissue piece on the back of a host mouse. When spermatogenesis has established, mature spermatozoa might be retrieved and cryopreserved for later use.

Although all the aforementioned methods may have clinical potential, the technique of testicular stem cell transplantation is considered to be the most promising tool for fertility preservation. Also, compared with xenografting, autologous testicular stem cell transplantation may be ethically more acceptable.

Acknowledgment

We would like to thank Michael Whitburn for proofreading the manuscript.

REFERENCES

1. Lawson KA, Pederson RA. Clonal analysis of cell fate during gastrulation and early neurulation in the mouse. In: Post Implantation Development in the Mouse. CIBA Foundation Symposium 165. New York: John Wiley and Sons, 1992: 3–26.
2. Tam P, Snow MH. Proliferation and migration of primordial germ cells during compensatory growth in the mouse embryo. J Embryol Exp Morphol 1981; 64: 133–47.
3. Fleischman RA. From white spots to stem cells: the role of Kit receptor in mammalian development. Trends Genet 1993; 9: 285–90.
4. Sapsford CS. Changes in the cells of the sex cords and the seminiferous tubules during development of the testis of the rat and the mouse. Austr J Zool 1962; 10: 178–92.
5. Huckins C, Clermont Y. Evolution of gonocytes in the rat testis during late embryonic and early post-natal life. Arch Anat Histol Embryol 1968; 51: 343–54.
6. Vergouwen RP, Jacobs SG, Huiskamp R, Davids JA, de Rooij DG. Proliferative activity of interstitial cells, Sertoli cells and gonocytes during testicular development in the mouse. J Reprod Fertil 1991; 93: 233–43.
7. Manova K, Huang EJ, Angeles M et al. The expression pattern of the c-kit ligand in gonads of mice supports a role for the c-kit receptor in oocyte growth and in proliferation of spermatogonia. Dev Biol 1993; 157: 85–99.
8. Pellegrini M, Grimaldi P, Rossi P et al. Developmental expression of BMP4/ALK3/SMAD5 signaling pathway in the mouse testis: a potential role of BMP4 in spermatonia differentiation. J Cell Sci 2003; 116: 3363–72.
9. Keros V, Rosenlund B, Hultneby K et al. Optimizing cryopreservation of human testicular tissue: comparison of protocols with glycerol, propanediol and dimethylsulphoxide as cryoprotectants. Hum Reprod 2005; 20: 1676–87.
10. Schrans-Stassen BH, van de Kant HJ, de Rooij DG et al. Differential expression of c-kit in mouse undifferentiated and differentiating type A spermatogonia. Endocrinology 1999; 140: 5894–900.
11. Shinohara T, Avarbock MR, Brinster RL. β_1- and α_6-integrin are surface markers on mouse spermatogonial stem cells. Proc Natl Acad Sci USA 1999; 96: 5504–9.
12. Kanatsu-Shinohara M, Toyokuni S, Shinohara T. CD9 is a surface marker on mouse and rat male germline stem cells. Biol Reprod 2004; 70: 70–5.
13. Kubota H, Avarbock MR, Brinster RL. Growth factors essential for self-renewal and expansion of mouse spermatogonial stem cells. Proc Natl Acad Sci USA 2004; 101: 16489–94.
14. Reijo RA, Dorfman DM, Slee R et al. DAZ family proteins exist throughout male germ cell development and transit from nucleus to cytoplasm at meiosis in humans and mice. Biol Reprod 2000; 63: 1490–6.
15. Buaas FW, Kirsh AL, Sharma M et al. Plzf is required in adult male germ cells for stem cell self-renewal. Nat Genet 2004; 36: 647–52.
16. Costoya JA, Hobbs RM, Barna M et al. Essential role of Plzf in maintenance of spermatogonial stem cells. Nat Genet 2004; 36: 653–9.
17. Oulad-Abdelghani M, Bouillet P, Decimo D et al. Characterization of a premeiotic germ cell-specific cytoplasmic protein encoded by Stra8, a novel retinoic acid-responsive gene. J Cell Biol 1996; 135: 469–77.
18. Falender AE, Freiman RN, Geles KG et al. Maintenance of spermatogenesis requires TAF4b, a gonad-specific subunit of TFIID. Genes Dev 2005; 19: 794–803.
19. Kubota H, Avarbock MR, Brinster RL. Spermatogonial stem cells share some, but not all, phenotypic and

functional characteristics with other stem cells. Proc Natl Acad Sci USA 2003; 100: 6487–92.

20. Van Pelt AMM, Roepers-Gajadien HL, Gademan IS et al. Establishment of cell lines with rat spermatogonial stem cell characteristics. Endocrinology 2002; 143: 1845–50.
21. Hofmann MC, Braydich-Stolle L, Dettin L et al. Immortalization of mouse germ line stem cells. Stem Cells 2005; 23: 200–210.
22. Guan K, Nayernia K, Maier LS et al. Pluripotency of spermatogonial stem cells from adult mouse testis. Nature 2006; 440: 1199–203.
23. Kanatsu-Shinohara M, Inoue K, Lee J et al. Generation of pluripotent stem cells from neonatal mouse testis. Cell 2004; 119: 1001–12.
24. Huckins C. The spermatogonial stem cell population in adult rats. I. Their morphology, proliferation and maturation. Anat Rec 1971; 169: 533–58.
25. Oakberg EF. Spermatogonial stem-cell renewal in the mouse. Anat Rec 1971; 169: 515–32.
26. Lajtha LG. Stem cell concepts. Differentiation 1979; 14: 23–34.
27. Clermont Y, Bustos-Obregon E. Re-examination of spermatogonial renewal in the rat by means of seminiferous tubules mounted in 'toto'. Am J Anat 1968; 122: 237–48.
28. Clermont Y, Hermo L. Spermatogonial stem cells in the albino rat. Am J Anat 1975; 142: 159–76.
29. Dym M, Clermont Y. Role of spermatogonia in the repair of the seminiferous epithelium following x-irradiation of the rat testis. Am J Anat 1970; 128: 265–82.
30. Clermont Y, Hermo L. Spermatogonial stem cells and their behavior in the seminiferous epithelium of rats and monkeys. In: Cairnie AB, Lala PK, Osmond DG, eds. Stem Cells of Renewing Cell Populations. New York: Academic Press, 1976: 273–86.
31. Ehmcke J, Simorangkir DR, Schlatt S. Identification of the starting point for spermatogenesis and characterization of the testicular stem cell in adult male rhesus monkeys. Hum Reprod 2005; 20: 1185–93.
32. Dobrinski I, Avarbock MR, Brinster RL. Transplantation of germ cells from rabbits and dogs into mouse testes. Biol Reprod 1999; 61: 1331–9.
33. Brinster RL, Zimmerman JW. Spermatogenesis following male germ-cell transplantation. Proc Natl Acad Sci USA 1994; 91: 11289–302.
34. de Rooij DG, Janssen JM. Regulation of the density of spermatogonia in the seminiferous epithelium of the Chinese hamster. Anat Rec 1987; 217: 124–36.
35. van Beek ME, Meistrich ML, de Rooij DG. Probability of self-renewing divisions of spermatogonial stem cells in colonies formed after fission neutron irradiation. Cell Tissue Kinet 1990; 23: 1–16.
36. Meng X, Lindahl M, Hyvonen ME et al. Regulation of cell fate decision of undifferentiated spermatogonia by GDNF. Science 2000; 287: 1489–93.
37. Nishimune Y, Haneji T. Testicular DNA synthesis in vivo: comparison between unilaterally cryptorchid testis and contralateral intact testis in mouse. Arch Androl 1981; 6: 61–5.
38. Koshimizu U, Sawada K, Tajima Y et al. White-spotting mutations affect the regenerative differentiation of testicular germ cells: demonstration by experimental cyptorchidism and its surgical reversal. Biol Reprod 1991; 45: 642–8.
39. Tajima Y, Sakamaki K, Watanabe D et al. Steel-Dickie (Sld) mutation affects both maintenance and differentiation of testicular germ cells in mice. J Reprod Fertil 1991; 91: 441–9.
40. van Pelt AM, van Dissel-Emiliani FM, Gaemers IC et al. Characteristics of A spermatogonia and preleptotene spermatocytes in the vitamin A-deficient rat testis. Biol Reprod 1995; 53: 570–8.
41. van Pelt AM, de Rooij DG. Retinoic acid is able to reinitiate spermatogenesis in vitamin A-deficient rats and high replicate doses support the full development of spermatogenic cells. Endocrinology 1991; 128: 697–704.
42. Beamer WG, Cunliffe-Beamer TL, Shultz KL et al. Juvenile spermatogonial depletion (jsd): a genetic defect of germ cell proliferation of male mice. Biol Reprod 1988; 38: 899–908.
43. Mizunuma M, Dohmae K, Tajima Y et al. Loss of sperm in juvenile spermatogonial depletion (jsd) mutant mice is ascribed to a defect of intratubular environment to support germ cell differentiation. J Cell Physiol 1992; 150: 188–93.
44. Allard EK, Hall SJ, Boekelheide K. Stem cell kinetics in rat testis after irreversible injury induced by 2,5-hexanedione. Biol Reprod 1995; 53: 186–92.
45. Kangasniemi M, Huhtaniemi I, Meistrich ML. Failure of spermatogenesis to recover despite the presence of A spermatogonia in the irradiated LBNF1 rat. Biol Reprod 1996; 54: 1200–8.
46. Meistrich ML, Kangasniemi M. Hormone treatment after irradiation stimulates recovery of rat spermatogenesis from surviving spermatogonia. J Androl 1997; 18: 80–7.
47. Beumer TL, Roepers-Gajadien HL, van Buul PP et al. The role of the tumor suppressor gene p53 in spermatogenesis. Cell Death Differ 1998; 5: 669–77.
48. Rodriguez I, Ody C, Araki K et al. An early and massive wave of germinal cell apoptosis is required for the development of functional spermatogenesis. EMBO J 1997; 16: 2262–70.

49. Yan W, Samson M, Jegou B, Toppari J. Bcl-w forms complexes with Bax and Bak, and elevated ratios of Bax/Bcl-w and Bak/Bcl-w correspond to spermatogonial and spermatocyte apoptosis in the testis. Mol Endocrinol 2000; 14: 682–99.

50. Brinster RL, Avarbock MR. Germline transmission of donor haplotype following spermatogonial transplantation. Proc Natl Acad Sci USA 1994; 91: 11303–7.

51. Nagano M, Avarbock MR, Leonida EB et al. Culture of mouse spermatogonial stem cells. Tissue Cell 1998; 30: 389–97.

52. Tournaye H, Goossens E, Verheyen G et al. Preserving the reproductive potential of men and boys with cancer: current concepts and future prospects. Hum Reprod Update 2004; 10: 525–32.

53. Nagano M, Shinohara T, Avarbock MR et al. Retrovirus-mediated gene delivery into male germ line stem cells. FEBS Lett 2000; 475: 7–10.

54. Goossens E, Frederickx V, De Block G, Van Steirteghem AC, Tournaye H. Reproductive capacity of sperm obtained after germ cell transplantation in a mouse model. Hum Reprod 2003; 18: 1874–80.

55. Goossens E, Frederickx V, De Block G, Van Steirteghem A, Tournaye H. Blastocyst development after assisted reproduction using spermatozoa obtained after testicular stem cell transplantation in mice. Hum Reprod 2006; 21: 1759–64.

56. Goossens E, Frederickx V, De Block G, Van Steirteghem A, Tournaye H. Evaluation of in vivo conception after testicular stem cell transplantation in a mouse model shows altered post-implantation development. Hum Reprod 2006; 21: 2057–60.

57. França LR, Ogawa T, Avarbock MR et al. Germ cell genotype controls cell cycle during spermatogenesis in the rat. Biol Reprod 1998; 59: 1371–7.

58. Ogawa T, Dobrinski I, Avarbock MR et al. Xenogeneic spermatogenesis following transplantation of hamster germ cells to mouse testes. Biol Reprod 1999; 60: 515–21.

59. Nagano M, McCarrey JR, Brinster RL. Primate spermatogonial stem cells colonize mouse testes. Biol Reprod 2001; 64: 1409–16.

60. Reis MM, Tsai MC, Schlegel PN et al. Xenogeneic transplantation of human spermatogonia. Zygote 2000; 8: 97–105.

61. Nagano M, Patrizio P, Brinster RL. Long-term survival of human spermatogonial stem cells in mouse testes. Fertil Steril 2002; 78: 1225–33.

62. Shinohara T, Orwig KE, Avarbock MR et al. Spermatogonial stem cell enrichment by multiparameter selection of mouse testis cells. Proc Natl Acad Sci USA 2000; 97: 8346–51.

63. von Schonfeldt V, Krishnamurthy H, Foppiani L, Schlatt S. Magnetic cell sorting is a fast and effective method of enriching viable spermatogonia from Djungarian hamster, mouse, and marmoset monkey testes. Biol Reprod 1999; 61: 582–9.

64. Dirami G, Ravindranath N, Pursel V et al. Effects of stem cell factor and granulocyte macrophage-colony stimulating factor on survival of porcine type A spermatogonia cultures in KSOM. Biol Reprod 1999; 61: 225–30.

65. Morena A, Boitani C, Pesce M et al. Isolation of highly purified type A spermatogonia from prepubertal rat testis. J Androl 1996; 17: 708–17.

66. Nagano M, Ryu BY, Brinster CJ et al. Maintenance of mouse male germ line stem cells in vitro. Biol Reprod 2003; 68: 2207–14.

67. Kanatsu-Shinohara M, Ogonuki N, Inoue K et al. Restoration of fertility in infertile mice by transplantation of cryopreserved male germline stem cells. Hum Reprod 2003; 18: 2660–7.

68. Kanatsu-Shinohara M, Miki H, Inoue K et al. Long-term culture of mouse male germline stem cells under serum- or feeder-free conditions. Biol Reprod 2005; 72: 985–91.

69. Creemers LB, den Ouden K, van Pelt AM et al. Maintenance of adult mouse type A spermatogonia in vitro: influence of serum and growth factors and comparison with prepubertal spermatogonial cell culture. Reproduction 2002; 124: 791–9.

70. Izadyar F, den Ouden K, Creemers LB et al. Proliferation and differentiation of bovine type A spermatogonia during long-term culture. Biol Reprod 2003; 68: 272–81.

71. Oatly JM, de Avila DM, Reeves JJ et al. Testis tissue explant culture supports survival and proliferation of bovine spermatogonial stem cells. Biol Reprod 2004; 70: 625–31.

72. Honaramooz A, Snedaker A, Boiani M et al. Sperm from neonatal mammalian testis grafted in mice. Nature 2002; 418: 778–81.

73. Schlatt S, Kim S, Gosden R. Spermatogenesis and steroidogenesis in mouse, hamster and monkey testicular tissue after cryopreservation and grafting. Reproduction 2002; 124: 323–9.

74. Shinohara T, Inoue K, Ogonuki N et al. Birth of offspring following transplantation of cryopreserved immature testicular pieces and in-vitro microinsemination. Hum Reprod 2002; 17: 3039–45.

75. Schlatt S, Honaramooz A, Ehmcke J et al. Limited survival of adult human testicular tissue as ectopic xenograft. Hum Reprod 2006; 21: 384–9.

76. Geens M, De Block G, Goossens E et al. Spermatogonial survival after grafting human testicular

tissue to immunodeficient mice. Hum Reprod 2006; 21: 390–6.

77. Avarbock MR, Brinster CJ, Brinster RL. Reconstitution of spermatogenesis from frozen spermatogonial stem cells. Nat Med 1996; 2: 693–6.

78. Izadyar F, Matthijs-Rijsenbilt JJ, den Ouden K et al. Development of a cryopreservation protocol for type A spermatogonia. J Androl 2002; 23: 537–45.

79. Frederickx V, Michiels A, Goossens E et al. Recovery, survival and functional evaluation by transplantation of frozen-thawed mouse germ cells. Hum Reprod 2004; 19: 948–53.

80. Kanatsu-Shinohara M, Toyokuni S, Shinohara T. Transgenic mice produced by retroviral transduction of male germ line stem cells in vivo. Biol Reprod 2004; 71: 1202–7.

81. Jorgensen N, Muller J, Giwercman A et al. Clinical and biological significance of carcinoma in situ of the testis. Cancer Surv 1990; 9: 287–302.

82. Hawkins MM, Stevens MC. The long-term survivors. Br Med Bull 1996; 52: 898–923.

83. Fujita K, Ohta H, Tsujimura A et al. Transplantation of spermatogonial stem cells isolated from leukemic mice restores fertility without inducing leukaemia. J Clin Invest 2005; 115: 1855–61.

84. Geens M, De Block G, Goossens E et al. The efficiency of MACS and FACS in the decontamination of testicular cell suspensions in cancer patients. Hum Reprod; in Press.

CHAPTER 8

Human embryonic stem cells: a model for trophoblast differentiation and placental morphogenesis

Thaddeus G Golos and Behzad Gerami-Naini

OVERVIEW

The derivation over a decade ago of cell lines from rhesus blastocyst stage in-vivo-produced embryos with many properties of embryonic stem cells (ESCs)[1] paved the way for the derivation of similar cell lines from human in-vitro fertilization (IVF)-derived embryos.[2] Strictly speaking, these lines have not yet been shown to fulfill all criteria of ESCs as derived from mouse (e.g. contribution to in-vivo organogenesis in chimeric embryos); however, they will be referred to as human ESCs as has become the convention. While these advances have generated substantial and deserved enthusiasm regarding the therapeutic potential of human embryo-derived cells, the significance of these cells for basic research into the fundamental processes of early human development is equally compelling. It was demonstrated early on that both rhesus and human cell lines shared a novel property not readily demonstrated with mouse ESCs: namely, the spontaneous (if perhaps inefficient) differentiation to cells of the trophoblast lineage. Several diverse paradigms have been developed that amplify this property of human ESCs. In this chapter, these paradigms will be summarized, the potential phenotype of the differentiated trophoblasts will be discussed and their significance for understanding the specification of the trophoblast lineage as well as the mechanisms by which the distinct trophoblast compartments within the placenta are formed during development will be presented.

ESTABLISHMENT OF THE TROPHOBLAST LINEAGE IN EMBRYONIC DEVELOPMENT

The formation of the trophoblast lineage is initiated typically within 1 week post fertilization, with the compaction of the embryo at the morula stage of development demonstrating the differential gene expression required for the formation of the blastocyst. Intercellular junctions between blastomeres at the embryonic surface demonstrate their specialization as the first epithelium, and underlie in part their role in fluid transport to create the blastocoele cavity. Following escape of the blastocyst from the zona pellucida, subsequent embryo development and formation of the placenta varies widely among mammals in the length of time before attachment of the embryo, the nature of the mode of placentation and attendant degree of invasiveness and the characteristic organization of the maternal endometrium and fetal extra-embryonic tissues. The genetic control of this fascinating diversity of structures among mammalian species remains poorly understood in most species. Because of this diversity, in this chapter we will primarily restrict our discussion to human hemochorial placentation and placental morphogenesis. Excellent recent reviews of mouse placental development with reference to substantial strides in the 21st Century are recommended.[3,4]

IMPLANTATION AND FORMATION OF THE HUMAN PLACENTA

Following attachment of the blastocyst-stage embryo to the uterine luminal endometrium, the trophectoderm (TE) layer forms terminally differentiated syncytiotrophoblast (STB) and proliferating cytotrophoblast (CTB) elements. Placental development during these early weeks of pregnancy has been evaluated, essentially exclusively, by morphological approaches,[5] with no immunohistochemical (IHC) or molecular studies possible in the immediate human postimplantation period. Examination of the implanting embryo during the 1st week after attachment demonstrated that fetal mesenchyme begins to appear within the cords of proliferating CTB referred to as the trabeculae. As vasculogenesis is initiated, mesodermal derivatives begin to form endothelial tubes distributed through this mesenchyme, which over the 1st month of postimplantation development will ultimately coalesce with vasculogenesis within the umbilical cord and become contiguous with the fetal vasculature proper (see References 6 and 7 for excellent reviews). It is most interesting to note that in human implantation the appearance of fetal mesenchyme and vascular elements is temporally consistent with the formation of the characteristic organization of the chorionic villi, which includes the STB layer in direct contact with maternal blood pooling in the placental lacunae, an underlying proliferating layer of mononuclear CTB and cell columns forming the anchoring villi attached to the maternal decidua. From the tips of the cell columns, extravillous CTB (EVT) migrate into the decidua and are found in interstitial, perivascular and endovascular locations within the stroma and the maternal spiral arteries.[8] It is intriguing that this fetal epithelium should choose to detach and migrate from the cell–cell contacts within the cell column. Many epithelial tissues are tightly associated with (and their phenotype is regulated by) an underlying basement membrane, while other laminar epithelia form regenerating tissues from a proliferative basal layer (e.g. skin, esophagus).

Disruption of villous morphogenesis (including vascularization) or the arrested differentiation of columnar trophoblasts into the extravillous cells is associated with poor pregnancy outcomes, including pre-eclampsia and intrauterine growth restriction.[9,10] Thus, these earliest stages of development are relevant to human fertility and maternal and fetal health, and are clearly important areas for investigation. However, there are substantial gaps in our knowledge of the early formation of the placenta, owing to ethical limitations on the experimental study of human embryos, as well as the fact that implantation sites from the first weeks of pregnancy are not generally available for research. Thus, we and others have addressed the development of alternative experimental models of human embryos. While transformed immortal trophoblast cells as well as culture of primary trophoblasts isolated from human placentas are widely used for research in these areas, some areas of investigation will be extremely difficult to move forward when relying on models in which the relevant cells are already committed to the trophoblast lineage and have been 'imprinted' by the process of formation of the placenta as it already occurred in vivo.

TROPHOBLAST DIFFERENTIATION FROM HUMAN EMBRYONIC STEM CELLS

When primate ESCs were first derived from the rhesus monkey[1] and then the common marmoset[11] embryos over a decade ago, it was clear that while they exhibited the criteria of pluripotency (demonstrated by differentiation to all embryonic germ lineages with differentiation in vitro, or in vivo by the formation of teratocarcinomas in immunodeficient mice), another novel attribute was noted, in that the spontaneous differentiation to trophoblasts could consistently be detected as assayed by secretion of chorionic gonadotropin (CG), and the transcription of the genes for both the α and β CG subunits.[1,11] Thus, it was not unexpected that, similarly, human ESCs (hESCs) also initiated human chorionic gonadotropin (hCG) secretion during their differentiation upon withdrawal of conditioned medium and fibroblast growth factor 2 (FGF2),[2] the critical components of the original culture medium that sustains undifferentiated growth of hESCs.

However, while this spontaneous differentiation was sufficient to allow the formation of a small number of trophoblasts, we anticipated that it would also be possible to demonstrate the formation of trophoblasts in vivo upon teratoma formation using IHC and molecular approaches. Although we have been able to detect the low-level expression of hCG subunit mRNAs as well as several other genes associated with trophoblast differentiation (Durning and Golos, unpublished work), in general we have failed to find significant or widespread trophoblast differentiation in teratomas derived from either rhesus monkey or human ESCs injected into the hindlimb muscle of severe combined immunodeficient (scid) mice using IHC staining for the CG β subunit.[12] Recent studies from several laboratories have shown that the local environment (or cellular extracts from specific organs) can influence the differentiation decisions by undifferentiated hESCs. For example, co-culture with bone marrow stroma,[13] pancreas,[14] or nervous system[15] environments results in the expression of genes and cellular differentiation appropriate for the organotypic environment into which the cells have been introduced. Further studies will address morphologically whether trophoblast differentiation may be preferentially directed by a hormonal or growth factor environment from a different growth site.

BMPS AND EMBRYONIC STEM CELL DIFFERENTIATION

With spontaneous differentiation in-vitro, there was consistent but low trophoblast differentiation, as detected by assay for hCG.[2] Investigators have developed additional paradigms for studying trophoblast differentiation. In efforts to stimulate the formation of mesodermal tissues, Xu et al[16] treated H1, H7, H9 or H14 hESC with BMP4. Unexpectedly, a homogeneous population of cells with epithelial morphology was consistently obtained in these studies, and subsequent microarray analysis revealed that a number of genes characteristic of trophoblast differentiation were up-regulated by BMP4, or related factors (BMP2, BMP7, GDF5) in subsequent experiments.[16] We[17] and others[18] have subsequently confirmed these results with the H1 and H7 hESC lines, respectively. The significance of these observations for in-vivo trophoblast differentiation remains unclear. For example, examination of microarray data for BeWo and JEG3 cells[19] revealed expression of BMPR1A but not BMPR1B in both JEG3 and BeWo cells. In addition, BMPR2 was only detectable in one of three arrays with JEG3 cells. BMP10 was the only consistently detectable family member in these microarrays (BMPs 1–8 were consistently absent). Conversely, BMP1 and BMP7 were up-regulated in the differentiation of primary cultures of human villous CTBs to STBs.[20] Thus, the roles of BMPs and their receptors in differentiated human placental cells remains poorly understood and clearly deserving of further study. It may be that the primary role of BMPs is in the early differentiation of embryonic cells or the formation of the TE. Although studies of BMP or BMP receptor knockouts has not revealed a role for these genes in trophoblast specification or differentiation in the mouse,[21] the observation that LIF (leukemia inhibitory factor), which is essential for mouse implantation and the undifferentiated growth of mouse ESCs, has no role in maintenance of primate ESC pluripotency,[1,2] underscores the likelihood that there are additional differences between rodents and primates in the mechanisms which underlie trophoblast lineage determination and differentiation.

Interestingly, the effects of BMPs on the differentiation of HES1 cells[22] reveal differences among the existing hESC lines. The Pera laboratory has reported that BMP2 promoted differentiation to the mesodermal lineage and hematopoietic differentiation,[23] and only rarely resulted in the differentiation of small colonies of cells similar to the H1-derived trophoblasts.[16] Further experiments suggested that it was unlikely that the culture conditions, medium or surface strata used was the basis of the differential response to BMP4, but may more likely reflect an intrinsic property of the ESC lines.

OCT4 AND TROPHOBLAST DIFFERENTIATION

The homeobox transcription factor Oct4 is central to the maintenance of undifferentiated pluripotency in mouse and human ESCs.[24] The formation of the TE is associated with the loss of Oct4 expression in mouse, monkey and human blastocyst stage embryos.[24–27] Several recent studies have demonstrated that, as predicted from these observations, down-regulation of Oct4 expression in hESCs is associated with an up-regulation of the expression of genes associated with trophoblast differentiation, summarized in Table 8.1. This outcome had previously been demonstrated in mouse ESCs.[28,29] Recent studies have demonstrated at least one mechanism by which Oct4 expression controls TE determination is through a reciprocal

Table 8.1 Differentiation of human embryonic stem cells to trophoblasts

Stimulus	*Line*	*Reference*
BMP4/BMP2/GDF9	H1, H7, H9, H14	Xu et al;[16] Ezashi et al;[18] Liu et al[17]
Oct4 RNA interference	H1, H9, H7, H14	Matin et al;[48] Hay et al[49]
Nanog RNA interference	H9, H1, hES-NCL1	Zaehres et al;[50] Hyslop et al[50]
Embryoid body formation	H1, H9	Gerami-Naini et al;[32] Liu et al;[17] Harun et al[33]

interaction with cdx2 in the early development of the mouse embryo.[30] Although enlightening for mouse placental development, we wish to point out that, as of yet, there is no evidence that cdx2 plays a role in human placental development or trophoblast differentiation. Our own studies have failed to detect cdx2 mRNA in JEG3 or BeWo choriocarcinoma cells,[19] in the human or rhesus monkey placenta, in undifferentiated hESCs (Liu, Grendell and Golos, unpublished work), or in human extravillous trophoblasts (M Knofler, University of Vienna, pers comm). We suggest that additional work is needed before a judgment regarding cdx2 and human trophoblast differentiation can be made. There is further discussion of cdx2 and other factors later in this chapter, in the context of trophoblast stem cell differentiation.

TROPHOBLAST DIFFERENTIATION IN THE EMBRYOID BODY PARADIGM

When resuspended under conditions that do not provide signals to maintain pluripotency, undifferentiated mouse ESC colonies will anneal into spherical structures called embryoid bodies (EBs) and initiate differentiation and the formation of endoderm, mesoderm and ectoderm derivatives. Human and rhesus monkey EBs likewise will differentiate into components of the embryonic germ layers, and paradigms promoting mesoderm formation are well described.[31] We hypothesized that the EB paradigm, while clearly not recapitulating embryogenesis, may provide an opportunity to consolidate trophoblast differentiation revealed in ESC spontaneous differentiation. The formation of EBs from rhesus ESCs is associated with a rapid increase in hCG secretion, although this hormonal activity is relatively transient and modest in magnitude compared with differentiated human trophoblast cultures.[32] This may be related to recent observations from the Moore laboratory that there is differential activation of hCG secretion among individual hESC-derived EBs.[33] Examination of hESC-derived EBs by IHC also revealed that a consistent feature of hESC differentiation in EBs was the formation of a cytokeratin-positive superficial epithelial population which also co-expressed hCG.[32]

We reasoned that the modest secretion of hCG in suspension culture may be due to the lack of extracellular cues that would provide the external signals for trophoblast differentiation and hormone secretion characteristic of advanced differentiation at implantation. Thus, we developed an approach in which the EBs are manually introduced into 'rafts' of Matrigel prepared by sequential addition of Matrigel droplets onto a microscope cover glass (see Reference 32, and Table 8.2 for details of this procedure). Transfer of EBs to this three-dimensional (3D) Matrigel environment promoted a prolonged and consistent increase in the secretion of hCG as well as progesterone and estradiol-17β into the culture medium.[32] Intriguingly, there were two other variables which in our initial studies appear to give rise to differential secretion within these experiments. First, the level of hCG secreted per day by EBs in the 3D context was highly dependent on the frequency of medium changes: daily medium change resulted in dramatically higher hCG secretion in all experiments in which this was evaluated (Reference 32; Table 8.3). This effect is generally consistent in progesterone and estradiol-17β secretion by EBs (Figure 8.1), in that daily medium change promoted the highest level of steroid hormone secretion as well.

In addition, the number of days of suspension culture for which the EBs were maintained before transfer to the Matrigel also influenced the maximal levels of hCG produced,[32] with a consistently higher

Table 8.2 Formation of Matrigel rafts for embryoid (EB) body culture

(1) Place circular microscope cover glasses (Fisherbrand Cat. #12-546-2 25Cir-2) into a glass Petri dish layered with gauze pads and autoclave. Place sterile cover slips onto a sterile surface using forceps. A sterilized tube rack is a convenient surface as it allows for leaving a portion of the cover slip to hang over the side to so that it can be easily grasped using forceps

(2) Thaw a 100 μL Matrigel (BD Biosciences, Bedford, MA; Cat. #356231) aliquot on ice. Pipet equal amounts (about 30 μL) of Matrigel onto three separate areas of the cover slip, taking care to ensure the droplets maintain a spherical shape

(3) After approximately 5 minutes has elapsed, thaw another 100 μL Matrigel aliquot and pipet equal volumes onto each of the previous Matrigel droplets to build up a larger sphere of gelled matrix. Repeat this procedure a third time so that each droplet is 100 μL

(4) Allow the droplets to gel more completely by leaving them undisturbed for 45 minutes. Cover slips should be placed on a microscope slide in a 100 mm Petri dish, with the cover in place to prevent evaporation

(5) Using a pipettor with fine-point plastic pipet tip, pipet approximately 50–70 EBs into as small a volume as possible. Insert the pipet tip into the center of a Matrigel droplet and very slowly expel the EBs into the Matrigel. Some EBs may escape, but a majority should be left behind as you carefully and slowly withdraw the pipet tip. Repeat this for the other two droplets

(6) Using a pair of forceps and a razor blade, scrape the injected Matrigel droplets into a 35 mm dish containing 3 ml of EB culture medium. Hold the cover slip at an angle with the forceps and scrape the underside of the Matrigel droplet as it will have adhered to the cover slip

(7) Place the dish onto a rocking platform in the incubator (Thermolyne Platform Vari–Mix Rocker, Thermolyne Dubuque, IA; Cat. #M79735). Evaluate the dishes daily to make sure that the suspended Matrigel rafts have not adhered to the dish. Outgrowing trophoblasts will secrete hCG and confound comparison with non-attached dishes

Table 8.3 Effect of suspension culture on hCG secretion in three-dimensional Matrigel culture (ng/ml/day)

	Days in suspension before Matrigel placement			
Medium change	*1.5 days*	*5 days*[a]	*8 days*	*37 days*
Every 5 days	45.80	73.1	26.02	16.22
Every 3 days	117.18	191.76	–[b]	21.28
Every day	242.32	662.48	802.59	944.35

[a]3 days with ESC medium + 5 days in EB differentiation medium
[b]A 3-day group was not included in this experiment

level in experiments in which EBs were maintained in suspension for 18 or 37 days, in comparison with 8 days or 2 days (see Table 8.3); interestingly, this effect did not appear to be retained for progesterone or estrogen secretion (see Figure 8.1). We do not know if this hCG effect is due to expansion of a trophoblast progenitor population, which then results in higher hormone secretion, or if there is formation of a trophoblast population of equal numbers, which then has an enhanced differentiation potential. To directly address this question we are working to develop methods for quantitatively isolating trophoblasts

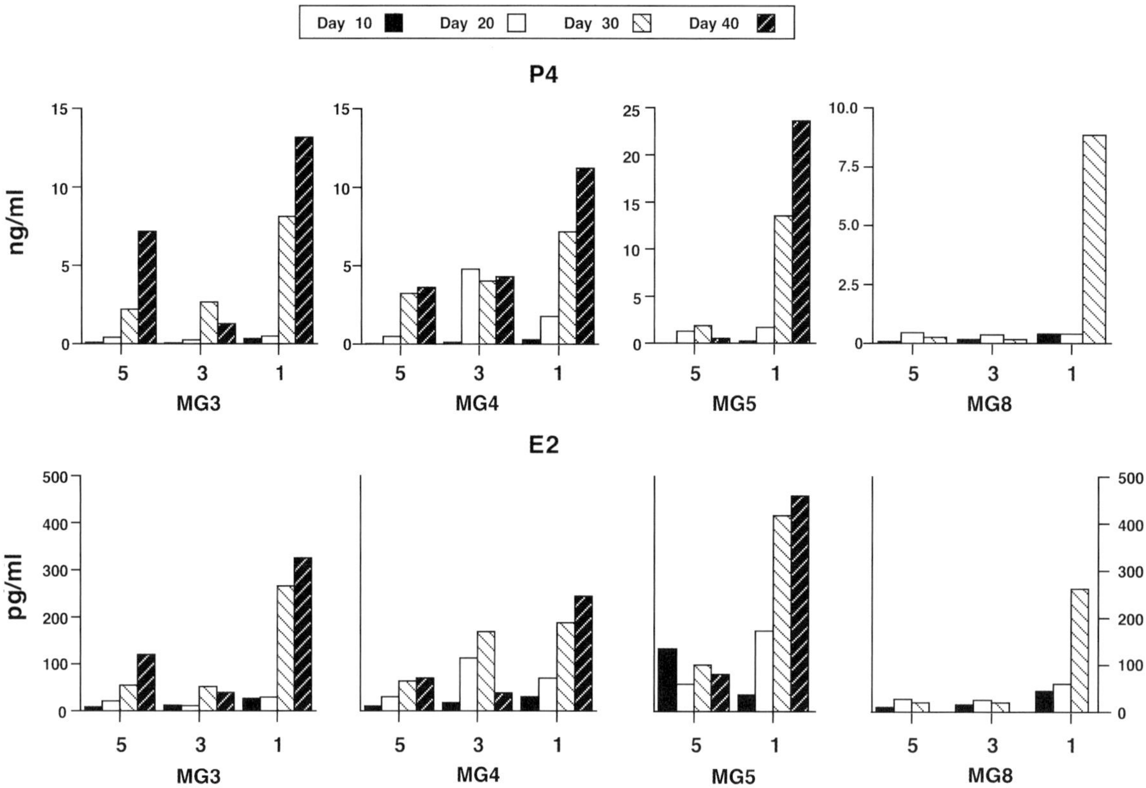

Figure 8.1 Secretion of progesterone (P4) and estradiol-17β (E2) by embryoid bodies (EBs) in three-dimensional Matrigel culture. For each experiment, bars are shown representing cells in which medium was changed every day, every 3 days or every 5 days (see *x*-axis). Four experiments are shown in which EBs were cultured in EB medium suspension for 2 (MG3), 5 (MG4), 8 (MG5) or 37 (MG8) days before placing in Matrigel. The data are normalized for ng/mL/day (P4) or pg/mL/day (E2)

from suspension cultured EBs, as well as evaluating these EBs stereologically to define the number of trophoblasts that are present both in prolonged culture and in 3D culture in Matrigel. The recovery of cells from Matrigel explants has proved to be a challenging task.

The formation and proliferation of differentiated trophoblasts is not restricted to the 3D growth paradigm. We have previously reported that if EBs are plated on Matrigel-coated culture dishes (two-dimensional or 2D) rather than the 3D explant system, there is also the formation of differentiated trophoblasts and their proliferation and outgrowth associated with the secretion of hCG[32] as well as progesterone and estradiol-17β. Interestingly, these cells will not sustain high hCG secretion, but rather hormone secretion decreases with time in culture.[32] These results could mean that (1) there is loss of the differentiated cells themselves through culture, (2) there is loss of differentiated function of the trophoblasts that nonetheless are still maintained or (3) there is the increasing expression of inhibitors of hCG secretion. Further studies will be needed to discern between these interpretations.

The question arises as to what is the trophoblast differentiation process that EB growth in a 3D Matrigel environment is modeling. There are several possibilities. The possibility which first comes to mind would be that the Matrigel environment represents the decidual matrix that the embryo encounters at implantation. In this view, the trophoblast outgrowths from the EB would be analogous to cell columns. However, given the consistent expression of hCG in these outgrowths, we are not certain that this interpretation is accurate since the STBs are the most significant hCG source in vivo, yet within the EBs mononuclear cells are clearly expressing hCG. The second possibility is that, within the in-vivo chorionic villi, a basement membrane impacts on the phenotype of the villous CTBs and their differentiation into the STBs.[8] Thus, the interaction of cells at the external surface of the EB with the Matrigel at the 'apical' surface of the EB may be interpreted as a basal extracellular matrix (ECM) of the chorionic villus. Finally, a third possibility is that soluble factors which are minor components of the Matrigel (growth factors, etc.) are the key factors promoting trophoblast differentiation, rather than ECM. This possibility seems least likely, as our preliminary studies (Gerami et al, in prep) have shown at least partial stimulation of trophoblast differentiation by purified matrix protein surfaces (e.g. collagen IV). The ability to evaluate these possibilities will require a more detailed understanding of not only the phenotype of the EB-derived trophoblasts but also the expression of integrins and 'endogenous' ECM proteins within the EBs themselves.

Integrin–ECM interactions are not only relevant simply to anchoring or movement vis-à-vis the tissue location of an individual cell but also they represent opportunities for the microenvironment to influence cellular function and direct appropriate responses via integrin signaling through focal adhesion kinase (FAK) activation. For example, interactions of integrins expressed by breast epithelial cells with collagen I convey important information regarding not only the presence of specific ECM molecules but also their flexibility to the cell, which has important effects on whether the cell will exhibit a normal differentiated phenotype (flexible collagen I environment) or a transformed proliferative phenotype (rigid collagen I environment).[34] It is possible that a similar influence of the nature of the matrix can be discerned in our EB experiments. We have conducted studies in which EBs are plated onto Matrigel-coated culture dishes in a 2D environment. A summary of the comparison of the hCG secretion between 2D and 3D is presented in Figure 8.2a. We noted that there is rapid proliferation of cells with a trophoblast-like morphology from the adherent EBs, consistent with the hCG secretion profile (Figure 8.2b). However, this secretion is comparatively transient when considered alongside the profile of secretion seen in EBs noted in 3D cultures (Figure 8.2c). We also noted that proliferation of cells from the surface of the EBs is substantially lower than that seen in culture dishes (see Figure 8.2), an observation which is remarkably consistent with the results seen with breast epithelium[34] described above. Although technical issues at this time limit quantitative recovery of the cells from the 3D Matrigel rafts and prevent strict normalization of the data, there is clearly a different pattern and achievement of endocrine secretory activity upon trophoblast differentiation, depending on the nature of the growth environment.

The EB approach has recently been adapted by Harun et al[33] for individual culture and optimization, using hCG secretion to guide the derivation of trophoblast cell lines. Using the H9 human ESC line, culture of individual EBs in microtiter plate wells allowed the identification of EBs with enhanced hCG secretion and allowed the selective isolation of trophoblast cell lines from these individual EBs. Cells were expanded and shown to express hCG, to be able to form multinuclear STBs, and to demonstrate differential proliferation influenced by cell culture conditions.[33] These cell lines are discussed further below in the context of trophoblast stem cell (TSC) isolation.

TROPHOBLAST STEM CELLS AND PLACENTAL DEVELOPMENT

The TE gives rise in mammals to a diverse population of trophoblasts within the mature placenta. The molecular control of placental development is most completely understood to date in the mouse, owing to the ease of genetic manipulation. This section will focus on the TSCs in the mouse,[35] with consideration of data from hESC studies. For more comprehensive analyses of the molecular control of mouse placental development, please refer to excellent reviews by Rossant and Cross[36] and Hemberger and Cross.[3]

Upon attachment of the mouse blastocyst to the uterine epithelium, there is differential regional pathway selection for trophoblast formation from the TE. The mural TE not adjacent to the inner cell mass rapidly undergoes differentiation to invasive primary giant cells, which initiate DNA endoreduplication. These giant cells are terminally differentiated and are the source of early placental lactogen secretion, which is important for maintenance of the corpus luteum in rodent pregnancy.[37] The TE adjacent to the inner cell mass (polar TE) will form the extraembryonic ectoderm and the ectoplacental

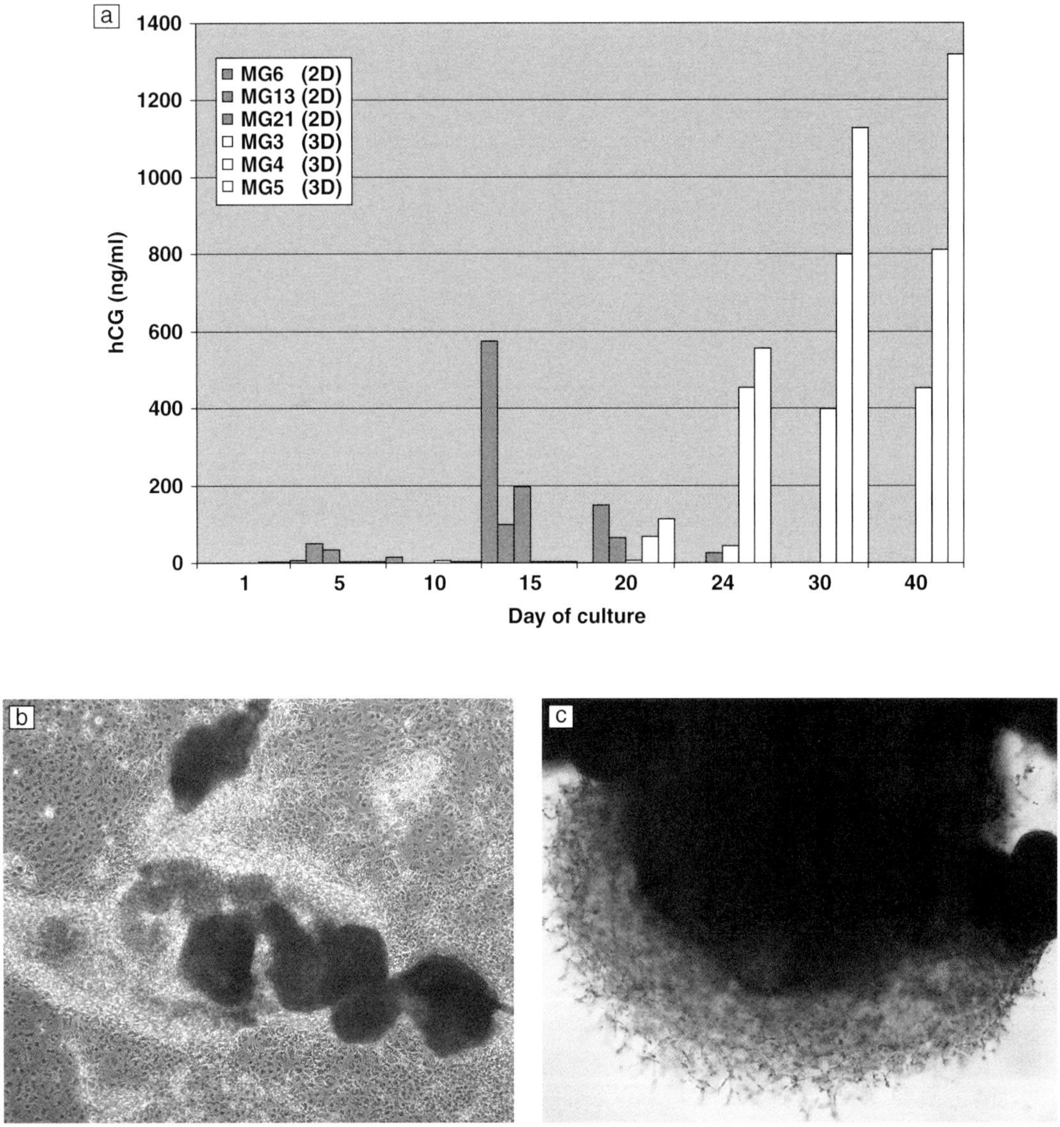

Figure 8.2 (a) Summary of hCG secretion in two-dimensional (2D) and three-dimensional (3D) embryoid body (EB) culture experiments. Culture medium was collected daily from all studies, and all determinations represent the mean of 2–3 wells per experiment. The data are not normalized for the number of EBs per well; 2D and 3D experiments included approximately 250 EBs per well. Typical appearance of proliferation from embryoid bodies in 2D (b) or 3D (c) culture. Both are shown approximately 2 weeks after placement on or in the Matrigel environment

cone, where a population of multipotent TSCs has been identified.

TSCs were first derived following the perceptive observation that FGF4 produced by the inner cell mass of the mouse blastocyst was able to sustain a proliferating population of cells with trophoblast characteristics within the extraembryonic ectoderm of the ectoplacental cone at the mouse implantation site.[38] TSCs were obtained by repeated dispersal and replating of blastocyst trophectodermal outgrowths under feeder cell conditions in the presence of FGF4 and heparin (see Quinn et al[39] for an excellent description

Table 8.4 Mouse knockout models relevant to understanding trophoblast stem cell function

Gene	*Reference*	*Phenotype*
FGF4	Feldman et al[52]	Postimplantation lethality
cdx2	Beck et al[40]	Failure to specify/maintain trophectoderm
ERRβ	Luo et al[53]	Loss of proliferating diploid trophoblasts
eomes	Russ et al[42]	Failure of trophectoderm differentiation

of the details of TSC derivation protocols). FGF4 expressed by the epiblast binds the FGFR2 and downstream ERK1/2-activated pathways at least in part sustain the TSC population within the extraembryonic ectoderm.[35] Analysis of several mouse knockout phenotypes supports the concept of the TSC as central to placental development. A summary of the relevant mutants and their molecular phenotypes is presented in Table 8.4. Briefly, FGF4 promotes the expression of critical transcription factors which maintain the TSC phenotype, including the homeobox gene cdx2, the nuclear hormone receptor superfamily member ERRβ and the T-box gene eomesodermin (eomes).[40–42] Deletion of these genes by homologous recombination results in developmental defects consistent with their support of the TSC phenotype. Subsequently, in normal placental development, TSC will support differentiation to trophoblast giant cells, as well as spongiotrophoblast, glycogen cells and STBs.

Since this original report,[38] there has been progress with the mouse TSC model in understanding the cellular and molecular requirements for TSC formation and growth. It has been reported that *Nodal* expression within the epiblast activates FGF4 expression, which in turn promotes cdx2, eomes and ERRβ expression in the extraembryonic ectoderm, and suppresses expression of mash2, which would direct ectoplacental cone differentiation to spongiotrophoblast.[43] Within the extraembryonic ectoderm, furin and PACE4 act to promote Nodal activation. Nodal also acts directly on the extraembryonic ectoderm to maintain its stem cell characteristics. Mouse TSCs are derived and expanded on mouse embryonic fibroblasts (MEFs). The active components of MEF-conditioned medium (CM) which sustain TSC growth include (but may not be limited to) TGF-β and activin, and long-term culture is possible with only FGF4 and activin added in the absence of MEF-CM.[44] Hand1, stra13 and gcm1, other transcription factors which play important roles in development of the placenta,[36] override FGF4 signaling to promote terminal differentiation of TSC,[45] and mash2 alone was not capable of promoting differentiation although it was able to sustain some proliferation in the absence of FGF4. Hand1 and stra13 promote TGC formation, whereas gcm1 promotes STB. Thus, the TSCs exist in a balance of transcriptional control, promoting multipotent proliferation and differentiation to specific terminal phenotypes.

The criteria for defining a TSC population can be adapted from the general principles of stem cell biology. First, the cells should be able to be sustained more or less indefinitely in culture. In addition, they should be multipotent in that they can give rise to all trophoblast populations in the placenta, but their differentiation capacity should be restricted to the trophoblast phenotype. These criteria have been demonstrated for FGF4-derived mouse TSCs. A number of laboratories have derived these cells routinely[43–45] and they can be propagated for prolonged periods of time, although their maximal proliferative capacity has not been defined. With in-vitro culture systems, they have been shown to have a tendency to differentiate spontaneously towards the giant cell as well as the STB phenotype, although spongiotrophoblast and glycogen cell genes are expressed during TSC differentiation in culture. The most important criterion of differentiation with TSCs is the demonstration that they exclusively contributed to the placenta in chimeric embryos, giving rise to the formation of all trophoblast lineages.[38]

DO HUMAN EMBRYONIC STEM CELL-DERIVED CELLS FULFILL CRITERIA FOR TROPHOBLAST STEM CELLS?

The question arises whether hESC-derived trophoblasts may represent human TSCs as formulated from the literature in the mouse. First, consider the evidence that BMP4-treated hESCs initiate the expression of a variety of genes associated with human trophoblast differentiation.[16] Examination of these genes indicates that, within an intact placenta, they are expressed in different trophoblast populations. For example, HLA-G is primarily expressed in extravillous trophoblasts (and more controversially, in villous trophoblasts as well[46,47]), whereas hCGβ is a major product of the STB. Thus, a clear villous or extravillous phenotype is not evident. While BMP4-treated ESCs expressed low levels of ERRβ (detectable by reverse transcription polymerase chain reaction [PCR]), the expression of other TSC markers (cdx2, eomes) was not detected by microarrays (Reference 16, Supplemental Table S6). Morphologically, under some culture conditions, such as passage into low cell density, BMP4-differentiated trophoblasts will form syncytial structures,[16] which may be consistent with giant cell formation at low-density mouse TSC culture.[39] However, it is not clear that conditions can be defined that direct extravillous or villous phenotype expression with BMP-derived cells.

Culture of hESC-derived EBs to promote trophoblast differentiation has now been reported by two groups independently, with remarkably consistent results.[32,33] The hESC-derived trophoblasts from 2D or 3D Matrigel cultures, or the trophoblasts derived from EBs cultured individually in gelatin-coated 96-well plates express hCG as a characteristic phenotypic hallmark, and are uniformly cytokeratin-positive. In addition, a subset of the cells derived from individual EBs are HLA-G-positive.[33] EB-derived cells in 3D Matrigel culture also have detectable HLA-G expression (Golos et al, in prep). These data suggest that both villous and extravillous lineages can arise from the formation of EBs by hESCs. However, at this time, the culture systems which are being used would benefit substantially from refinement such that precise conditions that promote differentiation of hESC-derived trophoblasts towards the villous or extravillous lineage can be developed. In addition, a more global analysis, including evaluation of integrin and ECM as well as transcription factor expression, will be of great significance for determining whether ESC-derived trophoblasts represent the human TSC phenotype.

Finally, with regards to the realization of the final criterion, i.e. in-vivo demonstration of the capacity of TSC to repopulate all placental trophoblast lineages, this is a study that will not be possible with human cells for obvious ethical reasons. It is possible that tests short of in-vivo function, such as differentiation and morphogenesis with co-culture in-vitro systems, may be an appropriate alternative.

FURTHER AREAS OF INVESTIGATION

The studies presented above clearly demonstrate that hESCs represent a promising model not only for novel therapeutic approaches and regenerative medicine but also for developing new paradigms to study basic aspects of early human development. Nonetheless, there are a number of areas that will benefit from further investigation and optimization:

- Determine the relative contributions of the proteins of the ECM (collagen IV, laminin, perlecan) vis-à-vis the spatial cues that they present in two and three dimensions.
- Define the coordinate specification and differentiation of additional extraembryonic lineages with the EB (or other) paradigms.
- Develop 3D scaffolding approaches to differentiate between biochemical and spatial cues, and the signaling pathways that transduce the ECM and 3D signals.
- Extend trophoblast induction paradigms to a broader array of hESC lines.
- Determine whether non-human primate ESCs share the differentiation potential for trophoblast differentiation. If so, non-human primates may provide an ultimate model for defining the in-vivo potential of primate TSC.

Acknowledgments

The authors wish to acknowledge particularly the contributions of Oksana Dovzhenko and Maureen Durning in these studies, assistance from Bob Becker in figure preparation, microarray data analysis from Rick Grendell and the WNPRC hormone assay laboratory for conducting protein and steroid hormone assays. This work was supported by March of Dimes Grant 00-041, and NIH Grants R01 HD34215 and R21 HD046919 to T.G.G., HD38843 to R.R. Magness and T.G.G., RR000167 to the WNPRC, and NCRR-supported construction grants to the WNPRC facilities. The opinions expressed in this work are solely those of the authors and do not reflect the positions of NIH or NCRR.

REFERENCES

1. Thomson JA, Kalishman J, Golos TG et al. Isolation of a primate embryonic stem cell line. Proc Natl Acad Sci USA 1995; 92: 7844–8.
2. Thomson JA, Itskovitz-Eldor J, Shapiro SS et al. Embryonic stem cell lines derived from human blastocysts. Science 1998; 282: 1145–7.
3. Hemberger M, Cross JC. Genes governing placental development. Trends Endocrinol Metabol 2001; 12: 162–8.
4. Cross JC. How to make a placenta: mechanisms of trophoblast cell differentiation in mice – a review. Placenta 2005; 26(Suppl A): S3–9.
5. Adams EC, Hertig AT, Rock J. A description of 34 human ova within the first 17 days of development. Am J Anat 1956; 98: 435–93.
6. Kaufmann P, Burton G. Anatomy and genesis of the placenta. In: Knobil E, Neill JD, eds. The Physiology of Reproduction, 2nd edn. New York: Raven Press, 1994: 441–84.
7. Kaufmann P, Mayhew TM, Charnock-Jones DS. Aspects of human fetoplacental vasculogenesis and angiogenesis. Placenta 2004; 25: 114–26.
8. Red-Horse K, Zhou Y, Genbacev O et al. Trophoblast differentiation during embryo implantation and formation of the maternal–fetal interface. J Clin Invest 2004; 114: 744–54.
9. Mayhew TM, Wijesekara J, Baker PN, Ong SS. Morphometric evidence that villous development and fetoplacental angiogenesis are compromised by intrauterine growth restriction but not by pre-eclampsia. Placenta 2004; 25: 829–33.
10. Mayhew TM, Charnock-Jones DS, Kaufmann P. Aspects of human fetoplacental vasculogenesis and angiogenesis. III. Changes in complicated pregnancies. Placenta 2004; 25: 127–39.
11. Thomson JA, Kalishman J, Golos TG et al. Pluripotent cell lines derived from common marmoset (*Callithrix jacchus*) blastocysts. Biol Reprod 1996; 55: 254–9.
12. Golos TG, Pollastrini LM, Gerami-Naini B. Human embryonic stem cells as a model for trophoblast differentiation. Semin Reprod Med 2006; in press.
13. Vodyanik MA, Bork JA, Thomson JA, Slukvin II. Human embryonic stem cell-derived CD34+ cells: efficient production in the coculture with OP9 stromal cells and analysis of lymphohematopoietic potential. Blood 2005; 105: 617–26.
14. Brolen GK, Heins N, Edsbagge J, Semb H. Signals from the embryonic mouse pancreas induce differentiation of human embryonic stem cells into insulin-producing beta-cell-like cells. Diabetes 2005; 54: 2867–74.
15. Benninger F, Beck H, Wernig M et al. Functional integration of embryonic stem cell-derived neurons in hippocampal slice cultures. J Neurosci 2003; 23: 7075–83.
16. Xu RH, Chen X, Li DS et al. BMP4 initiates human embryonic stem cell differentiation to trophoblast. Nat Biotechnol 2002; 20: 1261–4.
17. Liu YP, Dovzhenko OV, Garthwaite MA et al. Maintenance of pluripotency in human embryonic stem cells stably over-expressing enhanced green fluorescent protein. Stem Cells Dev 2004; 13: 636–45.
18. Ezashi T, Das P, Roberts RM. Low O_2 tensions and the prevention of differentiation of hES cells. Proc Natl Acad Sci USA 2005; 102: 4783–8.
19. Burleigh DW, Kendziorski CM, Choi YJ et al. Microarray analysis of BeWo and JEG3 trophoblast cell lines: identification of differentially expressed transcripts. Placenta 2006; Jun 22; [Epub ahead of print].
20. Aronow BJ, Richardson BD, Handwerger S. Microarray analysis of trophoblast differentiation: gene expression reprogramming in key gene function categories. Physiol Genomics 2001; 6: 105–16.
21. Ying Y, Zhao GQ. Detection of multiple bone morphogenetic protein messenger ribonucleic acids and their signal transducer, *Smad1*, during mouse decidualization. Biol Reprod 2000; 63: 1781–6.
22. Reubinoff BE, Pera MF, Fong CY, Trounson A, Bongso A. Embryonic stem cell lines from human blastocysts: somatic differentiation in vitro. Nat Biotechnol 2000; 18: 399–404.
23. Pera MF, Andrade J, Houssami S et al. Regulation of human embryonic stem cell differentiation by BMP-2 and its antagonist noggin. J Cell Sci 2004; 117: 1269–80.
24. Pesce M, Scholer HR. Oct-4: gatekeeper in the beginnings of mammalian development. Stem Cells 2001; 19: 271–8.
25. Mitalipov SM, Kuo HC, Hennebold JD, Wolf DP. Oct-4 expression in pluripotent cells of the rhesus monkey. Biol Reprod 2003; 69: 1785–92.
26. Hansis C, Grifo JA, Krey LC. Oct-4 expression in inner cell mass and trophectoderm of human blastocysts. Mol Hum Reprod 2000; 6: 999–1004.
27. Cauffman G, Van de Velde H, Liebaers I, Van Steirteghem A. Oct-4 mRNA and protein expression during human preimplantation development. Mol Hum Reprod 2005; 11: 173–81.
28. Velkey JM, O'Shea KS. Oct4 RNA interference induces trophectoderm differentiation in mouse embryonic stem cells. Genesis 2003; 37: 18–24.

29. Niwa H, Miyazaki J, Smith AG. Quantitative expression of Oct-3/4 defines differentiation, dedifferentiation or self-renewal of ES cells. Nat Genet 2000; 24: 372–6.

30. Niwa H, Toyooka Y, Shimosato D et al. Interaction between Oct3/4 and Cdx2 determines trophectoderm differentiation. Cell 2005; 123: 917–29.

31. Itskovitz-Eldor J, Schuldiner M, Karsenti D et al. Differentiation of human embryonic stem cells into embryoid bodies compromising the three embryonic germ layers. Mol Med 2000; 6: 88–95.

32. Gerami-Naini B, Dovzhenko OV, Durning M et al. Trophoblast differentiation in embryoid bodies derived from human embryonic stem cells. Endocrinology 2004; 145: 1517–24.

33. Harun R, Ruban L, Matin M et al. Cytotrophoblast stem cell lines derived from human embryonic stem cells and their capacity to mimic invasive implantation events. Hum Reprod 2006; 21: 1349–58.

34. Wozniak MA, Desai R, Solski PA, Der CJ, Keely PJ. ROCK-generated contractility regulates breast epithelial cell differentiation in response to the physical properties of a three-dimensional collagen matrix. J Cell Biol 2003; 163: 583–95.

35. Kunath T, Strumpf D, Rossant J. Early trophoblast determination and stem cell maintenance in the mouse – a review. Placenta 2004; 25(Suppl A): S32–8.

36. Rossant J, Cross JC. Placental development: lessons from mouse mutants. Nat Rev Genet 2001; 2: 538–48.

37. Soares MJ. The prolactin and growth hormone families: pregnancy-specific hormones/cytokines at the maternal–fetal interface. Reprod Biol Endocrinol 2004; 2: 51.

38. Tanaka S, Kunath T, Hadjantonakis AK, Nagy A, Rossant J. Promotion of trophoblast stem cell proliferation by FGF4. Science 1998; 282: 2072–5.

39. Quinn J, Kunath T, Rossant J. Mouse trophoblast stem cells. Methods Mol Med 2006; 121: 125–48.

40. Beck F, Erler T, Russell A, James R. Expression of Cdx-2 in the mouse embryo and placenta: possible role in patterning of the extra-embryonic membranes. Dev Dyn 1995; 204: 219–27.

41. Tremblay GB, Kunath T, Bergeron D et al. Diethylstilbestrol regulates trophoblast stem cell differentiation as a ligand of orphan nuclear receptor ERRβ. Genes Dev 2001; 15: 833–8.

42. Russ AP, Wattler S, Colledge WH et al. Eomesodermin is required for mouse trophoblast development and mesoderm formation. Nature 2000; 404: 95–9.

43. Guzman-Ayala M, Ben-Haim N, Beck S, Constam DB. Nodal protein processing and fibroblast growth factor 4 synergize to maintain a trophoblast stem cell microenvironment. Proc Natl Acad Sci USA 2004; 101: 15656–60.

44. Erlebacher A, Price KA, Glimcher LH. Maintenance of mouse trophoblast stem cell proliferation by TGF-β/activin. Dev Biol 2004; 275: 158–69.

45. Hughes M, Dobric N, Scott IC et al. The Hand1, Stra13 and Gcm1 transcription factors override FGF signaling to promote terminal differentiation of trophoblast stem cells. Dev Biol 2004; 271: 26–37.

46. Hunt JS, Petroff MG, Morales P et al. HLA-G in reproduction: studies on the maternal–fetal interface. Hum Immunol 2000; 61: 1113–17.

47. Sargent IL. Does “soluble” HLA-G really exist? Another twist to the tale. Mol Hum Reprod 2005; 11: 695–8.

48. Matin MM, Walsh JR, Gokhale PJ et al. Specific knockdown of Oct4 and beta2-microglobulin expression by RNA interference in human embryonic stem cells and embryonic carcinoma cells. Stem Cells 2004; 22: 659–68.

49. Hay DC, Sutherland L, Clark J, Burdon T. Oct-4 knockdown induces similar patterns of endoderm and trophoblast differentiation markers in human and mouse embryonic stem cells. Stem Cells 2004; 22: 225–35.

50. Zaehres H, Lensch MW, Daheron L et al. High-efficiency RNA interference in human embryonic stem cells. Stem Cells 2005; 23: 299–305.

51. Hyslop L, Stojkovic M, Armstrong L et al. Downregulation of NANOG induces differentiation of human embryonic stem cells to extraembryonic lineages. Stem Cells 2005; 23: 1035–43.

52. Feldman B, Poueymirou W, Papaioannou VE, DeChiara TM, Goldfarb M. Requirement of FGF-4 for postimplantation mouse development. Science 1995; 267: 246–9.

53. Luo J, Sladek R, Bader JA et al. Placental abnormalities in mouse embryos lacking the orphan nuclear receptor ERR-beta. Nature 1997; 388: 778–82.

CHAPTER 9

Adult stem cells in the human endometrium

Caroline E Gargett

INTRODUCTION

The human endometrium regenerates with each menstrual cycle, following parturition, almost complete curettage and in postmenopausal women taking estrogen replacement therapy. The concept that endometrial stem/progenitor cells are responsible for the remarkable regenerative capacity of endometrium was proposed many years ago, but attempts to isolate and characterize them has only been undertaken recently as experimental approaches to identify adult stem cells in other tissues have been developed. This latter endeavor has been fueled by enormous interest in the clinical potential of human embryonic stem cells (hESCs) as the new therapeutic agent for regenerating tissues damaged by injury and the aging process. The controversy surrounding the use of embryos to generate hESCs has encouraged exploration of other sources of stem cells from adult tissues.

This chapter reviews the evidence available to date for the existence of adult stem/progenitor cells in human endometrium and provides some basic information on adult stem cells, in particular their varying potentialities and hierarchies. Key adult stem cell concepts, including self-renewal, proliferative potential and differentiation, are explained, as are concepts relating to adult stem cell behavior in other tissues that have relevance to the endometrium, including the stem cell niche, molecular pathways involved in regulating stem cell activity and the role of adult stem cells in tissue homeostasis, repair and regeneration. Approaches used in other tissues that will inform future studies in human endometrium and have the potential to significantly increase our knowledge and understanding of adult stem/progenitor cells in endometrial regeneration are described. Application of these fundamental studies to current knowledge on the pathophysiology of common gynecological diseases associated with abnormal endometrial proliferation are also discussed. The possible use of endometrial stem/progenitor cells in tissue engineering applications relevant to urogynecology are mentioned.

ADULT STEM CELLS

Definitions and concepts

Stem cells are rare undifferentiated cells present in many adult tissues and organs. Their rarity and lack of distinguishing morphological features and specific markers make it difficult to identify their location in tissues. Rather, adult stem cells are defined by their functional properties, which include high proliferative potential, substantial self-renewal capacity and ability to differentiate along specific molecular pathways to produce large numbers of at least one type of differentiated functional progeny[1–3] (Figure 9.1). Self-renewal or the ability to produce identical daughter stem cells is necessary to maintain the stem cell pool in tissues. Asymmetric cell division is one mechanism for producing an identical daughter cell and a more differentiated daughter. However, stem cells also undergo symmetric divisions, producing two daughter stem cells or two transit amplifying (TA) progenitors. Differentiation is defined as a change in

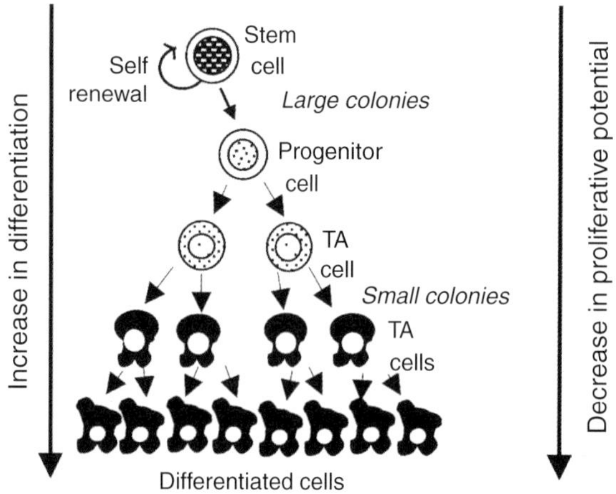

Figure 9.1 Hierarchy of stem cell differentiation. Stem cells undergo asymmetric cell divisions, which enable them to self-renew and replace themselves, or differentiate to give rise to committed progenitors. These proliferate and give rise to more differentiated transit amplifying (TA) cells, which rapidly proliferate and finally differentiate to produce a large number of terminally differentiated functional cells with no capacity for proliferation. The possible relationship of colony types initiated by human endometrial epithelial and stromal cells to the hierarchical model is shown. We postulate that the large colonies are initiated by putative stem/progenitor cells and the small colonies initiated by putative TA cells. (Reproduced with permission from Chan et al.[27])

cell phenotype due to expression of different genes usually associated with the function of the cell rather than cell division.[4] Stem cells exhibit a wide range of differentiation potential. The zygote is totipotential, producing all cell types in the embryo and extra-embryonic tissues. hESCs are pluripotential stem cells found in the inner cell mass of the blastocyst with capacity to differentiate into all cell types of the three embryonic layers: ectoderm, mesoderm and endoderm. The differentiation potential of these cells becomes increasingly restricted in lineage potential as embryonic development proceeds.[3] Arising from their progeny are the multipotential stem cells or adult stem cells that differentiate into several cell lineages and produce the component cells of the tissue in which they reside. Hematopoietic stem cells (HSCs) are an example of multipotent stem cells. Progenitor cells are derived from adult stem cells, are committed to a particular differentiation pathway and have limited ability to self-renew.[5,6] Tissue-specific stem cells may be considered progenitors. Unipotential stem cells are those with capacity to differentiate into a single, mature end-stage cell type. A classical example is the germ stem cell of the testis that produces sperm.[7] TA cells have properties intermediate between stem cells and end-stage differentiated cells, with limited proliferative potential, and inability to self-renew, but they undergo several rounds of cell division, progressively acquiring differentiation markers as part of the cellular amplification process, to produce numerous terminally differentiated cells[2,8] (see Figure 9.1).

Recent evidence suggests that the dogma of hierarchical differentiation of stem cells and their progeny is more flexible than shown in Figure 9.1. For HSCs there is a continuum of stem cell and progenitor capacity to self-renew and differentiate that is dependent on cell cycle phase and the specific microenvironment, suggesting that stem cells and progenitors are the same cell with different phenotypes under different conditions.[9] Similarly, epidermal stem cells, TA cells and differentiating keratinocytes all have capacity to regenerate a fully stratified epidermis with appropriate spatial and temporal expression of differentiation markers.[10]

The stem cell niche

In 1978 Schofield first proposed that stem cells were regulated by a specific physiological microenvironment, which he termed the niche.[11] Much of our current knowledge on the structure, function and operation of germ stem cell and adult stem cell niches has been derived from elegant studies in model organisms, in particular the *Drosophila melanogaster* ovary and testis and the *Caenorhabditis elegans* gonad, where the location of each cell is well characterized.[12] Far less is known about mammalian adult stem cell niches, which are anatomically more complex in comparison and more difficult to study. Common features between the *Drosophila* stem cell niche and those of mammalian adult stem cells include the precise location of stem cells in close relationship to one or more surrounding differentiated cells (niche cells), which, together with the extracellular matrix and various secreted molecules, provides a microenvironment to regulate key adult stem cell functions.[7,8] Signals from this niche microenvironment impinge on intrinsic adult stem cell signaling to regulate stem cell proliferation and cell fate decisions.[3]

Stem cell niches vary in their cellular composition, structure and location for adult stem cells in different tissues. They have been identified and well characterized for epidermal stem cells in the hair follicle bulge of epidermis,[8] for epithelial stem cells in the intestinal crypts,[13] the periosteum for HSCs[14] and neural stem cells in the subventricular and subgranular zones of the central nervous system.[15] Niche cells have been identified as osteoblasts lining the surface of trabecular bone in the HSC niche,[7,14] as endothelial cells in the neural stem cell niche[15] and subepithelial mesenchymal cells in the intestinal stem cell niche.[7,8] Adhesion molecules and niche cells anchor the adult stem cell in place during periods of stem cell inactivity and manage the asymmetric stem cell divisions to allow the controlled release of stem cells destined for proliferation and differentiation out of the stem cell niche.[7,8] Adhesion molecules identified as having a role in stem cell niches include cadherins mediating adhesive interactions between stem and niche cell(s), and integrins, which interact with the extracellular matrix.[14] Niche cells maintain adult stem cells in a dormant state (G_0) through signaling pathways inhibitory for growth and differentiation, often involving transforming growth factor-β (TGF-β) and bone morphogenetic protein (BMP) family members.[7]

A key function of niche cells is to sense the need for tissue replacement, and communicate proliferative and cell fate determining signals to the resident stem cell. While these mechanisms are well characterized for *Drosophila* germ stem cell niches, the signaling pathways appear to be conserved across species from fly to man and from germ stem cell to adult stem cell niches.[3] These include the Wnt/β-catenin and BMP pathways.[7,14,16] Other pathways include Notch and Hedgehog signaling, whereas growth factors such as fibroblast growth factor-2 (FGF2), insulin-like growth factor and vascular endothelial growth factor also have roles in certain niches. For example, the Notch pathway is important in regulating self-renewal of HSC, whereas Wnt/β-catenin signaling maintains HSC in an undifferentiated state,[16] promotes intestinal stem cell activation and self-renewal, and acts on bulge epidermal stem cells to regulate hair follicle development and regeneration.[8]

Adult stem cell plasticity

Of considerable controversy in the stem cell field is the concept of adult stem cell plasticity. A substantial body of literature suggests that adult stem cell fates are not restricted to the tissue in which they reside or within embryonic germ layer boundaries.[3,17,18] Transdifferentiation describes the conversion of cells of one tissue lineage into cells of a different lineage, with concomitant loss of original tissue-specific markers and function, and acquisition of markers and function of the new cell type, without an intervening cell division.[18,19] It involves nuclear reprogramming and represents a form of metaplasia or alteration of key developmental genes.[20] Plasticity, the capacity of adult stem cells to switch fate and differentiate into other lineages, results from changes in the extracellular environment, often in response to tissue damage.[9,17,19] Experiments have shown that bone marrow stem cells traffic via the bloodstream and incorporate into damaged tissues, changing into skeletal muscle cells, neurons and glia, hepatocytes, endothelial cells, myocardial cells and epithelial cells of gut, skin and lung, while neuronal cells produce blood cells and skeletal muscle cells.[17] This plasticity has been detected in tissues of gender-mismatched bone marrow transplant recipients by their co-expression of newly acquired tissue-specific antigens in Y chromosome-containing cells, or by tracking genetically tagged (e.g. green fluorescent protein [GFP]) transplanted cells. In the clinical setting, chimerism has been detected in the liver, gut and endometrium[21] of bone marrow transplant recipients and in solid organ transplantation, where circulating recipient cells have colonized donor hearts and kidneys.[22] These surprising findings suggest that adult stem cells are more ESC-like than originally thought and have major implications for therapeutics, providing hope for their eventual use in autologous cell-based therapies without histocompatability or ethical problems posed by use of hESC derivatives.[5] The concept of stem cell plasticity has been refuted, and in many studies it is a rare event.[18] There is some evidence that stem cell plasticity results from transplantation of multiple stem cell types, especially if the source is bone marrow, cell fusion, dedifferentiation after extensive in-vitro culture or the presence of truly pluripotent cells residing in the adult.[3,5] An extremely rare, multipotential adult progenitor cell (MAPC) isolated from bone marrow,[5] with properties similar to hESC, requires prolonged culture at low density, but it is not known if these cells exist in vivo. Greater rigor in demonstrating robust and persistent engraftment of stem cells in regenerating tissues and demonstration of their functional capacity has been advocated, since many studies have relied on morphology and immunostaining alone.[5,18]

Role in tissue homeostasis, repair and regeneration

Adult stem cells have a key role in tissue homeostasis, providing replacement cells in regenerating tissues and cells lost by apoptosis or injury.[7,23] Adult stem cell function is highly regulated to ensure an appropriate balance in stem cell replacement and provision of sufficient differentiated mature cells for tissue and organ function, without production of tumors. A balance between self-renewal and differentiation is imperative and is regulated by the stem cell niche.

It has become apparent that adult stem cells not only reside and function in highly regenerative tissues such as bone marrow, intestine and epidermis where they produce a steady supply of differentiated cells to maintain blood cell numbers and replace shed intestinal epithelial cells and skin cells, but also are found in tissues of low cell turnover, such as neural, liver, prostate and pancreas. In these tissues, adult stem cells function in maintaining tissue homeostasis by replenishing functional tissue cells lost by apoptosis.[24] Following injury, normally quiescent adult stem cells undergo cell division, producing TA cells that undergo rapid proliferation and expansion to eventually repair the lost tissue with functional end-stage cells. In some cases, such as liver and pancreas, fully mature cells have the capacity to revert to a proliferative phenotype to effect tissue replacement.[25] These processes are not fully understood and it is not clear if mature cells dedifferentiate into stem-like cells with a concomitant change in transcriptional profiles, or if fully mature cells have latent stem cell capacities.

IDENTIFICATION OF ADULT STEM CELLS AND STEM CELL ASSAYS

Identification and characterization of adult stem cells is a major challenge because of the paucity of these cells in tissues and the lack of defining cell surface markers that enable their isolation for study. Stem cell assays have been developed and are well characterized for identifying the hierarchies of HSCs, which are much easier to analyze than other adult stem cells due to their non-adherent growth, circulation in the bloodstream and capacity to home to bone marrow and reconstitute blood-forming tissue for each of their 8 lineages. A number of surface markers have been identified that make identification of HSCs and their differentiating progeny relatively easy to investigate. Although adaptation of these assays to assess various functions of adult stem cells in tissues with a very different architecture of adherent cells is rapidly developing, it is proving a difficult task.[26] There is a real challenge to develop predictive surrogate assays for tissue stem cell activity in cell populations removed from their natural microenvironment.[26] This is particularly the case for endometrial stem cells for which there are no phenotypic markers or, until recently, assays of their function.[27]

Adult stem cell markers

There are no specific phenotypic markers of adherent adult stem cells. A major research effort has recently been conducted to identify specific markers of epithelial stem cells from a range of adult tissues. The goal is to prospectively isolate pure populations of stem cells for further characterization, identification of stem cell location in situ and eventual use in the clinic as cell-based therapies. Many studies have simply designated a population of cells as stem cells based on marker expression, but often the same markers are also present on other mature cells: e.g. CD34 is an HSC marker and a mature endothelial cell marker, and CD90 is an HSC marker and a marker of endometrial functionalis stromal cells (Gargett and Schwab, unpublished work). Furthermore, cells alter their phenotype in culture, and marker expression of cultured stem cells may not reflect the in-vivo situation.[26] This becomes particularly important when examining plasticity of stem cells. Expression of a stem cell marker does not necessarily imply stem cell activity. Before a population of cells are designated stem cells on the basis of phenotypic marker expression, it is first necessary to validate stem cell function using at least one surrogate stem cell assay.[26] For example, fluorescence-activated cell sorting (FACS) endometrial stromal cells expressing a mesenchymal stem cell marker, Stro-1,[28] does not isolate cells with greater colony-forming efficiency (Gargett and Schwab, unpublished work).

In-vitro assays of adult stem cell activity

In-vitro assays examining the functions of adult stem cells include clonogenicity, proliferative potential, self-renewal and differentiation, whereas in-vivo assays include self-renewal and tissue regeneration.

Clonogenicity is the ability of single cells to initiate colonies of cells when seeded at extremely low seeding densities on cloning plates or by limiting dilution. These colony-forming assays have been extensively used for characterizing HSCs and their progenitors,[26,29] and provide a useful read-out assay for assessing potential stem cell markers when first characterizing candidate adult stem cells from epithelial and stromal tissues.[27,30–32] Proliferative potential is examined by determining the total number of progeny or number of cell divisions (population doublings) from a single cell or population of putative stem cells by serial passage until senescence. Depending on the adult stem cell, this may result in 10–30 population doublings with the production of many millions of cells.[20] This assay has been used as a read-out to assess the proliferative potential of human cells prospectively isolated by FACS or magnetic bead sorting for putative stem cell markers of mammary epithelial and mesenchymal stem cells.[32,33] Assays for self-renewal can be investigated both in vitro in serial cloning assays[20] and in vivo by serial transplantation methods.[34,35] In-vitro serial cloning assays rely on the ability of the initial colony-forming cell to undergo a self-renewing division during colony formation, and that the resultant cell has the same colony-initiating capacity after replating the harvested clone at limiting dilution. Ideally, adult stem cells should have capacity to self-renew multiple times and hence undergo multiple rounds of serial cloning.[20] These techniques will identify adult stem cells and progenitor cells, the difference being the extent to which they can undergo self-renewal.[20] The differentiation potential of isolated populations of candidate stem cells is evaluated after culturing the cells in specific differentiation–induction media, or by transplanting them and analyzing the tissue formed for phenotypic differentiation markers or expression of tissue-specific transcription factors. Mesenchymal stem cells isolated from bone marrow, adipose tissue and dental pulp have been characterized for their capacity to differentiate into a number of mesenchymal lineages, including adipocytic, smooth muscle, chondrocytic and osteoblastic lineages.[31,36,37]

Tissue reconstitution assays of adult stem cell activity

The gold standard assay of adult stem cell activity involves in-vivo reconstitution of the tissue from which the putative stem cell population was derived.[26,29,38] This assay requires the use of immunocompromised mice (e.g. NOD/SCID) as hosts for xenotransplantion of putative human adult stem cell populations to assess their capacity for tissue reconstitution.[39] These assays are well established for murine stem cell populations, particularly HSCs, mammary and prostate epithelial stem cells, and use sophisticated genetic approaches to distinguish the transplanted stem cell populations and their progeny from host cells.[29,35,40] For HSCs, competitive repopulation of stem cell and support cell populations enables quantitation, but resident stem cells must first be depleted by conditioning or ablation regimens in the host.[26,35] Development of analogous in-vivo tissue reconstitution assays for candidate human epithelial stem cell populations has been problematic and needs further development.[41] Inclusion of mesenchymal niche cells in the design of these assays is warranted. Putative stem cell populations are often transplanted into ectopic sites, such as the kidney capsule or subcutaneous tissue. Although these sites do not reproduce the tissue microenvironment of the stem cell niche or provide inductive cues, the kidney capsule does provide a rich vascular supply and contains the transplanted cells in a local region.[40] Supportive cells co-transplanted with stem cell populations in a matrix (e.g. collagen gels) may provide appropriate niche signals. Another important issue is the ability to track transplanted cells and identify their progeny.

Approaches include tagging cells with membrane-intercalating dyes such as PKH26, or genetic marking of putative stem cell populations with GFP. The specificity of antibodies to detect species differences can also be used. The value of these approaches is that transplanted cells and their derivatives can be identified within the architecture of the newly derived tissue. Successful reconstitution of bone and bone marrow tissue constituents has been demonstrated for candidate human mesenchymal stem cell populations xenotransplanted subcutaneously together with scaffold material.[33] In-vivo self-renewal capacity of putative stem cell populations extends the above approaches and involves harvesting the reconstituted tissue, obtaining single cell suspensions and retransplanting them back into another host to evaluate their ability for reconstituting appropriate tissue a second time. Serial tissue reconstitution indicates that the original transplanted stem cells underwent self-renewing cell divisions in vivo. Whereas this has been done for mouse adult stem cells,[29,34] it has yet to be achieved for human tissue stem cells.

A range of possibilities for endometrial reconstitution from putative stem cell populations exist. Endometrium grows ectopically as endometriosis in the peritoneal cavity and there are numerous transplantation models of endometriosis that could be adapted for assaying putative endometrial stem/progenitor cells.

EVIDENCE FOR ADULT STEM/PROGENITOR CELLS IN HUMAN ENDOMETRIUM

Indirect evidence for human endometrial stem cells

The human endometrium is a highly regenerative tissue and the concept that this regeneration is mediated by stem cells located in the basalis layer was first postulated over 35 years ago[42] and reiterated by Padykula et al in 1984.[43] Evidence from early kinetic studies of endometrial cell proliferation show zonal differences that predict an orderly replacement of functionalis endometrial epithelial and stromal cells from rarely proliferating putative stem/progenitors residing in the basalis near the endometrial–myometrial junction.[44,45] The progeny are the rapidly proliferating TA cells observed in the functionalis. More recently, a disjunction between the proliferative index of endometrial glands in the basalis and functionalis has been observed in both the proliferative and secretory stages of artificially cycled macaques using phosphorylated histone H3 as a proliferation marker.[46] Further support of this hypothesis comes from primate studies and clinical practice, where endometrium completely regenerated and supported pregnancy after surgical removal of almost all endometrial tissue by curettage.[47,48] In another clinical situation, pockets of endometrial tissue are observed to regenerate in a minority of women treated with electrosurgical ablation for menorrhagia.[49] Clinical evidence suggesting the presence of adult stem cells in human endometrium comes from observations that it has the propensity to undergo ossification, often after termination of pregnancy, and while the calcified tissue is not of fetal origin, it is usually associated with chronic inflammation and trauma,[50] conditions known to promote incorporation of mesenchymal stem cells into regenerating tissues.[29] Smooth muscle, bone and cartilage have also been found in endometrium.[51,52] Mesenchymal stem cells have the capacity to differentiate into smooth muscle, fat, bone and cartilage in vivo and in vitro[33] and, together, these observations suggest that under certain circumstances resident endometrial or bone marrow-derived multipotent mesenchymal stem cells may undergo an inappropriate differentiation.

More recent evidence indicates that endometrial glands are monoclonal in origin, suggesting that they arise from a single progenitor or stem cell. In almost half of histologically normal proliferative endometrial samples, rare glands have been observed that fail to express PTEN protein (PTEN null glands) because of a mutation and/or deletion in the *PTEN* gene.[53] These PTEN-mutant glandular clones persist in the basalis between menstrual cycles to regenerate their respective glands in the functional layer in subsequent cycles. PTEN null glands are increased in the endometrium of women in conditions of unopposed estrogen, particularly endometrial hyperplasia, a monoclonal epithelial proliferative disorder. Monoclonality was also detected in carefully dissected individual endometrial glands using a polymerase chain reaction (PCR)-based assay for non-random X chromosome inactivation of the androgen receptor gene.[54] Adjacent glands $\leq$1 mm apart shared clonality, indicating that well-circumscribed regions of endometrium were derived from the same precursor cell, which suggests that several glands share the same stem cell. This raises questions on the precise locality of candidate human epithelial stem/progenitor cells.

Recent functional studies in mouse endometrium using DNA synthesis label retention analysis has identified rare epithelial label-retaining cells (LRCs) in the luminal epithelium that do not express estrogen receptor-α (ERα), and stromal LRCs in a perivascular location near the endometrial–myometrial junction and beneath the luminal epithelium, some of which express ERα[55] supports the concept that endometrial stem/progenitor cells probably exist in human endometrium.

Evidence for human endometrial stem/progenitor cells from functional studies

Despite the likelihood that the amazing regenerative potential of human endometrium is mediated via

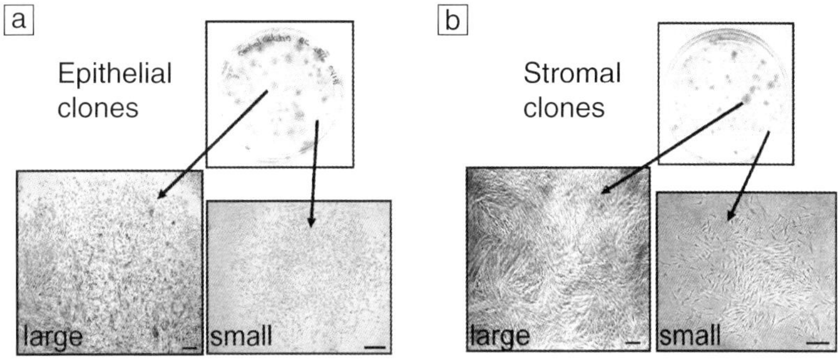

Figure 9.2 Human endometrial (a) epithelial and (b) stromal colonies formed when single-cell suspensions are seeded at cloning density and cultured for 15 days in serum-containing medium. The cells in the rare large clones were small and densely packed, with a high nuclear–cytoplasmic ratio, and the clones typically contained >4000 cells, whereas those in small clones were large, loosely arranged and contained between 50 and 3500 cells. Scale bars, 200 μm. (Adapted from Chan et al.[27])

resident stem/progenitor cells, it was only very recently that the first evidence based on functional assays was published.[27,56,57] Since a substantial stromal component supports both the glands and surface epithelium in human endometrium, it was reasoned that stromal or mesenchymal stem cells may also be found in human endometrium.[57] Using purified single-cell suspensions obtained from hysterectomy tissues, it was demonstrated that 0.22 ± 0.07% of endometrial epithelial cells and 1.25 ± 0.18% of stromal cells formed individual colonies of >50 cells/colony within 15 days when seeded at clonal density.[27] Two types of colony formed for both epithelial and stromal cells (Figure 9.2). The large colonies were rare (Table 9.1), contained >4000 cells and comprised small, densely packed cells with high nuclear-cytoplasmic ratio that were postulated to be initiated by candidate endometrial stem/progenitor cells. The more common, small colonies (see Table 9.1) were composed of large, loosely arranged cells with low nuclear–cytoplasmic ratio initiated by more mature cells, probably TA cells (see Figure 9.1) Further work has shown that the percentage of clonogenic epithelial and stromal cells in human endometrium does not vary significantly across the menstrual cycle[56] (Figure 9.3). This contrasts with a cloning study on endometrial stromal cells derived from Pipelle biopsy tissues at various stages across the menstrual cycle which demonstrated very high levels of cloning, ranging from 45% in the early proliferative stage to 27% in the late proliferative stage, using a limiting-dilution assay and plating at

Table 9.1 Cloning efficiency of human endometrial epithelial and stromal cells

	Clonogenicity (%)	
Clones	*Epithelial*	*Stromal*
Large	0.08 ± 0.03	0.02 ± 0.01[b]
Small	0.14 ± 0.04	1.23 ± 0.18[b]
Total	0.22 ± 0.07[a]	1.25 ± 0.18[a]

Data are mean ± SEM for $n=16$ epithelial and 13 stromal samples
[a]$p = 0.0001$
[b]$p = 0.0002$

0.2 cells/well.[58] However, in this study, the average size of the clones after 14 days was only 12 cells and the proliferative output of these clones bore no relationship to the original colony size. It would appear that the putative stem/progenitor cells may have been overlooked in this study, since a total of 25 000 wells would be required to isolate one large colony-initiating stromal cell. It also explains the inability to detect a relationship between proliferative potential and colony size. In another limiting-dilution cloning study, 13% of endometrial cells from a single sample that had been in continuous culture for 6 months were clonogenic.[59] The resulting clones exhibited high proliferative potential as they continued to proliferate in culture for another 24 months. It would appear that the culture conditions favored self-renewing cell divisions of

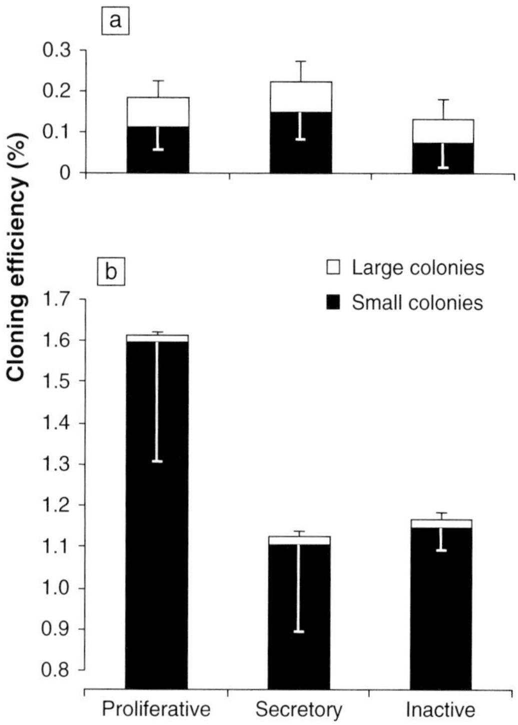

Figure 9.3 Cloning efficiency of human endometrial (a) epithelial and (b) stromal cells from proliferative, secretory and inactive endometrium cultured in serum-containing medium. Each bar consists of the cloning efficiency for small (black bars) and large (white bars) colonies, which together represent the total cloning efficiency observed. Results shown are means ± SEM of 4–7 samples. Inactive endometrium was from four samples, which included perimenopausal women and women taking oral contraceptives. (Adapted with permission from Schwab et al,[56] with permission from the American Society for Reproductive Medicine.)

putative endometrial stem/progenitor cells present in the original sample.

A number of growth factors required for human endometrial epithelial and stromal cell colony formation have been identified. In serum-free medium, clonogenic epithelial cells require either epidermal growth factor (EGF) or transforming growth factor-α (TGF-α) or platelet-derived growth factor B (PDGF-BB) and fibroblast feeder layers to establish clonal growth,[27] indicating the importance of stromal–epithelial cell interactions in the endometrial epithelial stem/progenitor cell niche. It is probable that colony-forming endometrial epithelial cells express EGF receptors, whereas PDGF-BB proliferative effects are probably mediated via PDGF receptor-β (PDGF-Rβ) on the fibroblast feeder cells. Clonogenic stromal cells also required either EGF, TGF-α or PDGF-BB, but were also clonogenic in FGF2-containing serum-free medium,[27,56] indicating that clonally derived stromal cells express EGF receptors, PDGF receptor-β and FGF receptors. Whether combinations of these growth factors further enhance growth of clonogenic endometrial cells has not been determined. Cell type-specific markers were used to characterize the cellular phenotype of the endometrial colonies.[27] Whereas small epithelial clones expressed epithelial cell adhesion molecule (Ep-CAM) and cytokeratin, the large colonies did not express Ep-CAM and weakly expressed cytokeratin. They expressed α_6-integrin subunits (CD49f), a marker expressed on the basal membrane of endometrial epithelium in tissue, but epithelial clones did not express the stromal cell marker collagen I. Both large and small stromal clones expressed CD90, a fibroblast marker. A significant proportion of stromal clones contained α-smooth muscle actin-expressing cells, indicative of myofibroblast or smooth muscle cell differentiation. Since it has been hypothesized that endometrial stem cells reside in the basalis, it is not surprising that clonally derived stromal cells have differentiated into myofibroblast or smooth muscle cell lineages as there are considerable numbers of myofibroblasts in the basalis,[60] and myometrium develops from undifferentiated müllerian duct mesenchyme.[51]

Current studies examining stem cell attributes of the rare epithelial and stromal cells initiating large colonies have demonstrated their high proliferative potential as they undergo 30–32 population doublings before senescence.[61] These clonally derived endometrial cells also undergo self-renewing cell divisions in vitro as demonstrated by their serial cloning ability. This high proliferative potential of endometrial stromal cells has been noted earlier in kinetic growth studies of serially passaged bulk cultures (as opposed to clonally derived cells) where 50% of specimens underwent more than 24 population doublings, and several between 60 and 100.[62] It is likely that a number of stromal stem/progenitor cells present in these cultures were responsible for this enormous proliferative capacity. Large secondary stromal clones also exhibit multilineage differentiation into four mesenchymal lineages – adipocytes, smooth muscle cells, chondrocytes and osteoblasts – in vitro, similar to bone marrow and adipose tissue mesenchymal stem cells.[61] In contrast, epithelial and stromal cells initiating the small colonies failed to serially clone and underwent limited proliferation up to 10 population doublings, indicating they are more differentiated endometrial cells with limited proliferative potential and self-renewal capacity.[61] These data suggest that the rare epithelial (1 in 1100 epithelial cells) and stromal (1 in 5000 stromal cells) cells initiating the large colonies (see Table 9.1) have characteristic properties of endometrial epithelial progenitor cells and mesenchymal stem cells, respectively, and are probably responsible for the remarkable, cyclical, regenerative capacity of human endometrium. These initial findings lay the groundwork for further studies to characterize stem cell properties in vivo, and for the discovery of specific endometrial stem/progenitor cell markers. A schematic showing the possible location of putative human endometrial stem/progenitor cells in the basalis is shown in Figure 9.4.

In a unique study, endometrial epithelial stem cell kinetics were investigated by examining epigenetic errors encoded in methylation patterns of individual glands in human endometrium.[64] This approach depends on endogenous DNA sequences becoming polymorphic as epigenetic variants arise during cell division, when methylation at CpG sites alters within a particular gene. In a cyclically, remodeling tissue like human endometrium, a persistent polymorphism indicates heritable epigenetic variants in the stem cells, since those variants or mutations that occur in TA or mature cells are lost during shedding. Thus, the total number of stem cell divisions may be inferred from the numbers of adult errors accumulated within individual glands.[65] Methylation sites of the *CSX* gene, which is not expressed in human endometrium, was examined to ensure that any changes in methylation patterns would have no functional consequences, and are probably due to a random process associated with aging.[64] The extent of endometrial gland methylation increased with age until menopause, after which it remained relatively constant, indicating that the number of epigenetic errors reflected the mitotic activity of endometrial stem cells.[64] Mathematical modeling of the data was more consistent with an individual gland containing a stem cell niche with an unknown number of long-lived stem cells, rather than a single immortal stem cell that always divides asymmetrically. It would appear that symmetric and asymmetric epithelial stem cell divisions occurred in a stochastic manner to maintain a constant number of stem cells in the endometrial gland niche.[64] There was no evidence for a reduction in stem cell number with aging because gland diversity remained constant after menopause, consistent with the finding of

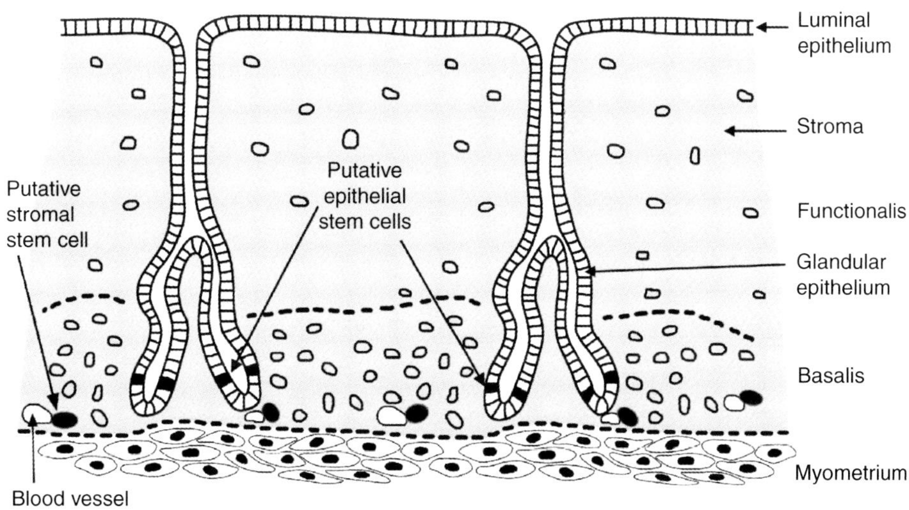

Figure 9.4 The possible location of putative endometrial stem/progenitor cells in human endometrium. It is predicted that candidate epithelial stem/progenitors will be located in the basalis in the base of the glands and stromal stem/progenitors near blood vessels. (Adapted from Gargett[63].)

clonogenic epithelial cells in inactive perimenopausal endometrium.[56] These random replication errors that accumulate in a clock-like manner provide a record of endometrial stem cell replication history that may be useful to investigate the role that putative endometrial stem/progenitor cells may have in proliferative disorders of the endometrium.

Markers of human endometrial stem/progenitor cells

Currently, there are no known single markers for endometrial epithelial stem/progenitor cells that distinguish them from their mature progeny. However, sorting endometrial stromal cells by magnetic beads or FACS and examining the sorted populations for clonogenic activity have now excluded several potential markers. These include Stro-1, a mesenchymal stem cell marker, which did not enrich for endometrial stromal cells with clonogenic activity, and CD133, an HSC marker (Gargett and Schwab, unpublished work). However, co-expression of two perivascular cell markers, CD146 and PDGF-Rβ, does give a significant 10-fold enrichment of multipotent, clonogenic stromal cells from human endometrium.[66] This rare population of candidate endometrial stromal stem/progenitor cells, postulated to reside near blood vessels in the basalis (see Figure 9.4), still needs to be tested for stem cell properties in vivo. At this stage there has been no progress made in identifying markers recognizing endometrial epithelial progenitor cells.

There have been a number of expression studies examining endometrial tissues using antibodies to stem cell markers. Bearing in mind the caveats outlined previously, these studies may assist in determining which markers might be worth examining for prospective isolation and subsequent testing in stem cell assays. Many classical stem cell markers have been examined in human endometrium for other purposes, but few have examined the basalis, making them less informative. The expression of HSC markers, CD34, c-kit/CD117 and the survival marker, bcl-2, has been examined in hysterectomy tissues. Basically, this study found immunostaining for all three markers in basalis glands and stroma, with CD34 specific for basalis stroma.[67] Flow cytometric analysis of fresh and cultured decidual stromal cells showed that some expressed Stro-1 and CD34, although their co-expression was not determined.[68] Whether any of these markers have value in identifying endometrial epithelial or stromal stem/progenitor cells has yet to be determined. Recently it was discovered that rare cells in the endometrial stroma of approximately 44% of women (11/25) immunostain for Oct-4, a pluripotency marker and transcription factor of hESC.[69] Although neither the frequency of Oct-4$^+$ endometrial stromal cells nor their location in the basalis or functionalis was reported, and their phenotype (stromal fibroblasts, vascular cells or leukocytes) was not determined, their presence suggests the possible presence of adult stem cells in human endometrium. Oct-4 cannot be used to prospectively isolate endometrial mesenchymal stem-like cells as it is not a surface marker, but its expression in human endometrial stromal clones and putative endometrial mesenchymal stem cell populations should be examined.

Source of human endometrial stem/progenitor cells

The embryonic female reproductive tract has its origins in the intermediate mesoderm which forms soon after gastrulation. As this embryonic tissue proliferates, it is thought that some cells undergo mesenchymal to epithelial transition to give rise to the coelomic epithelium that later invaginates to form the paramesonephric ducts.[70] These ducts, also known as Müllerian ducts, comprise surface epithelium and underlying urogenital ridge mesenchyme. During fetal life the glands commence development as the undifferentiated uterine surface epithelium invaginates into the underlying mesenchyme. Smooth muscle differentiation of the mesenchyme also commences to form the myometrium.[71] A small number of fetal epithelial and mesenchymal stem cells are thought to remain in adult endometrium and contribute to tissue replacement during its cyclic regeneration.[23]

Whether there is an ultimate uterine stem cell that has the capacity to replace all endometrial and myometrial cell types, including epithelial, stromal, vascular and smooth muscle, or whether there are separate epithelial and mesenchymal stem cells is unknown. The different phenotypes, growth factor dependence and frequency of clonogenic endometrial epithelial and stromal cells suggest that there are at least two types of endometrial progenitor cell. However, this does not exclude the possibility of the existence of an unidentified, more primitive precursor in human endometrium. Sophisticated studies examining the relative reconstitution capacity of endometrial cells separated using lineage-specific and differentiation stage markers that have yet to be elucidated are required to distinguish these possibilities. Another possible source of endometrial stem cells is the bone marrow. Increasingly, it is being recognized that bone marrow stem cells circulate, albeit in low numbers, and populate various organs.[17] Furthermore, a significant level of chimerism, ranging from 0.2% to 52% was detected in the endometrial glands and stroma of several women who received single antigen HLA-mismatched bone marrow transplants, suggesting that bone marrow stem cells contributed to endometrial regeneration in a setting of cellular turnover and inflammatory stimuli (Chapter 10).[21] This observation, together with the similar percentage of donor-derived epithelial and stromal cells in each patient, suggests that there may be a single endometrial stem cell responsible for production of both glands and stroma. These interesting observations rely solely on marker expression, but they raise a number of questions requiring further research to determine whether transdifferentation of bone marrow stem cells into functional endometrial cells occurs. Bone marrow contains at least three different stem cells – HSCs, mesenchymal stem cells and endothelial progenitors – and all circulate. Just which bone marrow stem cells or even myeloid cells contribute to endometrial regeneration needs to be determined. Whether bone marrow-derived cells regularly engraft the endometrium with each menstrual cycle or at the time of the bone marrow transplant, or subsequently on the resumption of endometrial cycling, is not known. Does this engraftment of endometrium with bone marrow stem cells occur under normal physiological conditions? Certainly, large numbers of mature bone marrow-derived cells traverse the endometrium on a regular basis. Whether the local tissue damage associated with menstruation is sufficient to attract bone marrow stem cells into the endometrium for permanent residence remains to be determined. Where do bone marrow-derived stem cells incorporate into endometrial tissue: the basalis, functionalis or both? The studies required to answer some of these questions are not possible in the human and will rely on animal studies using transgenic reporter mice (Chapter 10).

HUMAN ENDOMETRIAL STEM/PROGENITOR CELLS – CLINICAL PERSPECTIVE

Gynecological disease

A number of gynecological conditions are associated with abnormal endometrial proliferation, and it is possible that putative endometrial stem/progenitor cells may play a role in the pathophysiology of diseases such as endometrial hyperplasia, endometrial cancer, endometriosis and adenomyosis.[57] Alterations in the number, function, regulation and location of epithelial and/or stromal endometrial stem/progenitor cells may be responsible for any one of these endometrial disorders. Furthermore, clonogenic epithelial and stromal cells are present in noncycling and peri-menopausal endometrium[56] and may be responsible for regenerating endometrium in women given estrogen replacement therapy.

There is increasing interest amongst researchers and oncologists in the concept that cancers contain small numbers of cells with stem cell properties that are responsible for their growth and spread.[72,73] There is considerable similarity in the properties of adult stem cells in normal tissues and cancer stem cells. Cancer stem cells have a long life span, enormous proliferative potential and self-renewal capacity enabling them to maintain and expand the cancer cell population, although they themselves are quiescent and rarely proliferate. They also produce abnormally differentiated cancer cell progeny with limited proliferative potential that form the bulk of the cancer.[74] Many features of carcinoma can be explained by the stem cell concept, including clonal origin and heterogeneity of tumors, some associated with TA cells or progenitors, the mesenchymal influence on cancer behavior, the local formation of precancerous lesions and the plasticity of tumor cells.[73] Only a small proportion of the tumor actually comprises cancer stem cells, ~0.02–1%. Thus, cancer stem cells act as precursor cells that produce the proliferating, more differentiated cancer cells killed by chemotherapy or radiation. Cancer stem cells differ from normal tissue stem cells in that their proliferation is no longer controlled by the neighboring cells of the stem cell niche.[72] It is likely that cancer stem cells arise from adult stem cells that have accumulated multiple genetic and epigenetic changes over a period of time, giving them selective proliferative advantage and allowing their clonal expansion and succession in the stem cell niche.[73] Thus, cancer stem cells are likely to be the key tumor cells involved in the initiation, progression, metastasis and recurrence of tumors after treatment. A key role of cancer stem cells has been established in acute myeloid leukemia, breast cancer and glioblastoma.[72] Key genes involved in the self-renewal pathways that regulate adult stem cells, such as Wnt/β-catenin, sonic hedgehog and PTEN tumor suppressor gene, are associated with a range of cancers. Microsatellite instability or mutations in the *PTEN* gene are known to be involved in endometrial hyperplasia and endometrioid endometrial carcinoma, but whether endometrial cancer stem cells are involved is not currently known. Furthermore, the Wnt/β-catenin signaling pathway is involved in endometrial carcinoma and endometrial stromal sarcomas.[75,76] Endometrial carcinoma is the commonest female genital tract malignancy and the incidence of new cases is increasing. Based on epidemiological data, there are two distinct types of endometrial carcinoma.[77] Type 1 accounts for about 80% of all endometrial cancers and occurs in younger and perimenopausal women in a setting of estrogenic stimulation and endometrial hyperplasia. Type 2 tumors include high-grade, poorly differentiated endometrioid endometrial carcinoma and aggressive serous and clear cell carcinomas that occur in older postmenopausal women and are not associated with estrogen.[77] It is currently unknown whether cancer stem cells have a role in endometrial cancers, or in endometrial hyperplasia, but this is an area open for future research. Surgery is the main treatment for endometrial cancer;[77] however, possible future therapies targeting cancer stem cells, perhaps blocking molecules regulating asymmetric cell division, may improve the prospects for those women with advanced or type 2 tumors.

Endometriosis, defined as the growth of endometrium outside the uterine cavity, is a common gynecological disorder affecting 6–10% of women. It is a major clinical problem, causing inflammation, pain and infertility. Despite its common occurrence, little is known about its pathogenesis. The most commonly held theory on the etiology of endometriosis is that viable endometrial cells reach the peritoneal cavity through retrograde menstruation.[78] However, it is well known that menstrual debris is present in the peritoneal cavity of 90% of menstruating women, suggesting that only some endometrial cells from some women are capable of establishing endometriotic implants. Several theories have been suggested, including abnormal endometrium, genetic factors, altered peritoneal environment, reduced immune surveillance and increased angiogenic capacity.[78] It is possible that in 6–10% of women who develop endometriosis, endometrial stem/progenitor cells are inappropriately shed during menstruation and reach the peritoneal cavity, where they adhere and establish endometriotic implants.[57] Whereas long-term endometriotic lesions may develop from endometrial stem/progenitor cells, those lesions that resolve may have been established by more mature TA cells. The monoclonality of some endometriotic lesions and the increasing evidence that endometriosis can develop into ovarian clear cell and endometrioid carcinomas[79] are consistent with the concept that endometriosis could have a stem cell origin. This is further supported by the demonstration of clonogenic cells in a long-term culture derived from a sample of endometriosis tissue.[59] If bone marrow stem cells have the capacity to seed the endometrium and transdifferentiate into functional endometrial cells, it is possible that they may have the capacity to behave similarly outside the endometrial environment, particularly in sites other than the peritoneal cavity.[21] Alternatively, it has been postulated that some forms of endometriosis may arise from remnant fetal Müllerian cells, which have characteristic stem cell properties of high proliferative potential, multipotency and self-renewal.

Adenomyosis, a condition affecting 1% of women, results from basal endometrium undergoing extensive invasion of the myometrium and is associated with smooth muscle hyperplasia; it is also considered to arise from fetal Müllerian cells.[80] It is possible that endometrial stem/progenitor cells or their niche cells demonstrate abnormal behavior in adenomyosis, and these putative stem cells have an abnormally orientated niche such that their differentiating progeny move toward the myometrium rather than functionalis, producing pockets of endometrial tissue deep within the myometrium. Alterations in the putative endometrial stem cell niche, particularly in the niche cells regulating stem cell fate decisions, may result in excessive smooth muscle differentiation of putative endometrial stem/progenitor cells, producing the observed myometrial hyperplasia. Much research is required to establish a role for endometrial progenitors or bone marrow stem cells in the pathogenesis of endometriosis or adenomyosis.

Tissue engineering applications

There is great interest in the use of both embryonic and adult stem cells in tissue engineering applications for restoring function to aging or diseased tissues and organs. Medical advances have ensured increasing longevity, and the aging population has many tissues in need of repair.[81] The failure of artificial implants to last longer than 10–15 years and the problems associated with non-degradable synthetic materials make cell-based therapies for tissue replacement attractive.[82] There is now a focus on using a combination of temporary biological scaffold materials to provide initial support and stem cells to promote appropriate tissue genesis and regeneration of functional tissue.[82] This is particularly important for the provision of supportive tissues and could be adapted for tissue engineering support of the female reproductive tract. Pelvic floor prolapse is a major problem, resulting in 10% of women requiring surgery with approximately 30% of these requiring repeat surgery.[83] The use of artificial and biological scaffolds for pelvic floor prolapse surgery has improved outcomes to a limited degree. Thus, the use of tissue constructs comprising scaffolds and autologous endometrial mesenchymal stem/progenitor cells may provide a possible solution for treatment of pelvic floor prolapse in the future.

CONCLUSIONS AND FUTURE DIRECTIONS FOR HUMAN ENDOMETRIAL STEM/PROGENITOR CELL RESEARCH

Human endometrial stem cell research is in its infancy, but major advances have already been made that have identified rare populations of epithelial and stromal cells with progenitor activity in human endometrium that are probably responsible for its remarkable regenerative capacity. Whether there is a single more primitive endometrial stem cell that produces all endometrial cell types is yet unknown and whether the endometrial stromal progenitor has full mesenchymal stem cell activity in vivo is yet to be determined. Much still needs to be done to fully identify and characterize endometrial epithelial and mesenchymal stem/progenitor cells. There is a need to identify specific markers of both cell types to allow their prospective isolation for molecular characterization and determination of their precise location in the endometrium. Animal xenotransplantation models are needed to examine key stem cell properties of self-renewal and tissue reconstitution in vivo. Whether the bone marrow is a source of endometrial stem/progenitor cells as a major or minor contributor needs to be determined under physiological conditions. The putative endometrial stem cell niches for epithelial and stromal stem/progenitors need characterization once they can be localized with single markers. How estrogen and progesterone interact with endometrial stem/progenitor cells or their neighboring niche cells needs to be explored. The signaling pathways that regulate endometrial stem/progenitor cell activity have yet to be investigated and candidate pathways involving the Wnt, hedgehog, BMP pathways and the *HOX* genes should be investigated, as these molecules or pathways have already been detected in endometrium or have important roles during endometrial development or decidualization when stromal cells undergo terminal differentiation.

As endometrial stem/progenitors cells become characterized, their role in gynecological disorders associated with abnormal endometrial proliferation can be assessed. This not only increases understanding of the pathogenesis of endometrial hyperplasia, endometrial cancer, endometriosis and adenomyosis but also has the potential to change the way these diseases may be treated in the future, particularly as therapeutic agents that target key stem cell functions are developed.

Acknowledgments

The author thanks the National Health and Medical Research Council (ID 284344), the Royal Australian and New Zealand College of Obstetricians and Gynaecologists, the Australian and New Zealand Charitable Trusts, the CASS Foundation and the Helen MacPherson Smith Trust for financial support, Rachel Chan, Kjiana Schwab and Rachel Zillwood for their major contributions to these studies; and Nancy Taylor and Nicki Sam for collection of human tissues.

REFERENCES

1. Weissman IL. Stem cells – scientific, medical, and political issues. N Engl J Med 2002; 346: 1576–9.
2. Potten CS, Loeffler M. Stem cells: attributes, cycles, spirals, pitfalls and uncertainties. Lessons for and from the crypt. Development 1990; 110: 1001–20.
3. Eckfeldt CE, Mendenhall EM, Verfaillie CM. The molecular repertoire of the 'almighty' stem cell. Nat Rev Mol Cell Biol 2005; 6: 726–37.

4. Bach SP, Renehan AG, Potten CS. Stem cells: the intestinal stem cell as a paradigm. Carcinogenesis 2000; 21: 469–76.
5. Lakshmipathy U, Verfaillie C. Stem cell plasticity. Blood Rev 2005; 19: 29–38.
6. McCulloch EA, Till JE. Perspectives on the properties of stem cells. Nat Med 2005; 11: 1026–8.
7. Li L, Xie T. Stem cell niche: structure and function. Annu Rev Cell Dev Biol 2005; 21: 605–31.
8. Fuchs E, Tumbar T, Guasch G. Socializing with the neighbors: stem cells and their niche. Cell 2004; 116: 769–78.
9. Quesenberry PJ, Dooner G, Colvin G, Abedi M. Stem cell biology and the plasticity polemic. Exp Hematol 2005; 33: 389–94.
10. Li A, Pouliot N, Redvers R, Kaur P. Extensive tissue-regenerative capacity of neonatal human keratinocyte stem cells and their progeny. J Clin Invest 2004; 113: 390–400.
11. Schofield R. The relationship between the spleen colony-forming cell and the haemopoietic stem cell. Blood Cells 1978; 4: 7–25.
12. Ohlstein B, Kai T, Decotto E et al. The stem cell niche: theme and variations. Curr Opin Cell Biol 2004; 16: 693–9.
13. Booth C, Potten CS. Gut instincts: thoughts on intestinal epithelial stem cells. J Clin Invest 2000; 105: 1493–9.
14. Wilson A, Trumpp A. Bone-marrow haematopoietic-stem-cell niches. Nat Rev Immunol 2006; 6: 93–106.
15. Doetsch F. A niche for adult neural stem cells. Curr Opin Genet Dev 2003; 13: 543–50.
16. Reya T, Duncan AW, Ailles L et al. A role for Wnt signalling in self-renewal of haematopoietic stem cells. Nature 2003; 423: 409–14.
17. Blau HM, Brazelton TR, Weimann JM. The evolving concept of a stem cell: entity or function? Cell 2001; 105: 829–41.
18. Wagers AJ, Weissman IL. Plasticity of adult stem cells. Cell 2004; 116: 639–48.
19. Tosh D, Slack JM. How cells change their phenotype. Nat Rev Mol Cell Biol 2002; 3: 187–94.
20. Reynolds BA, Rietze RL. Neural stem cells and neurospheres – re-evaluating the relationship. Nat Methods 2005; 2: 333–6.
21. Taylor HS. Endometrial cells derived from donor stem cells in bone marrow transplant recipients. JAMA 2004; 292: 81–5.
22. Korbling M, Estrov Z. Adult stem cells for tissue repair – a new therapeutic concept? N Engl J Med 2003; 349: 570–82.
23. Snyder EY, Loring JF. A role for stem cell biology in the physiological and pathological aspects of aging. J Am Geriatr Soc 2005; 53: S287–S291.
24. Clarke RB, Smith GH. Stem cells and tissue homeostasis in mammary glands. J Mammary Gland Biol Neoplasia 2005; 10: 1–3.
25. Dor Y, Brown J, Martinez OI et al. Adult pancreatic beta-cells are formed by self-duplication rather than stem-cell differentiation. Nature 2004; 429: 41–6.
26. Kaur P, Li A, Redvers R, Bertoncello I et al. Keratinocyte stem cell assays: an evolving science. J Investig Dermatol Symp Proc 2004; 9: 238–47.
27. Chan RW, Schwab KE, Gargett CE. Clonogenicity of human endometrial epithelial and stromal cells. Biol Reprod 2004; 70: 1738–50.
28. Simmons PJ, Torok-Storb B. Identification of stromal cell precursors in human bone marrow by a novel monoclonal antibody, STRO-1. Blood 1991; 78: 55–62.
29. van Os R, Kamminga LM, de Haan G. Stem cell assays: something old, something new, something borrowed. Stem Cells 2004; 22: 1181–90.
30. Pellegrini G, Golisano O, Paterna P et al. Location and clonal analysis of stem cells and their differentiated progeny in the human ocular surface. J Cell Biol 1999; 145: 769–82.
31. Gronthos S, Mankani M, Brahim J et al. Postnatal human dental pulp stem cells (DPSCs) in vitro and in vivo. Proc Natl Acad Sci USA 2000; 97: 13625–30.
32. Stingl J, Eaves CJ, Zandieh I, Emerman JT. Characterization of bipotent mammary epithelial progenitor cells in normal adult human breast tissue. Breast Cancer Res Treat 2001; 67: 93–109.
33. Gronthos S, Zannettino ACW, Hay SJ et al. Molecular and cellular characterisation of highly purified stromal stem cells derived from human bone marrow. J Cell Sci 2003; 116: 1827–35.
34. Kordon EC, Smith GH. An entire functional mammary gland may comprise the progeny from a single cell. Development 1998; 125: 1921–30.
35. Shackleton M, Vaillant F, Simpson KJ et al. Generation of a functional mammary gland from a single stem cell. Nature 2006; 439: 84–8.
36. Pittenger MF, Mackay AM, Beck SC et al. Multilineage potential of adult human mesenchymal stem cells. Science 1999; 284: 143–7.
37. Zuk PA, Zhu M, Ashjian P et al. Human adipose tissue is a source of multipotent stem cells. Mol Biol Cell 2002; 13: 4279–95.
38. Joseph NM, Morrison SJ. Toward an understanding of the physiological function of mammalian stem cells. Dev Cell 2005; 9: 173–83.
39. Greiner DL, Hesselton RA, Shultz LD. SCID mouse models of human stem cell engraftment. Stem Cells 1998; 16: 166–77.
40. Xin L, Lawson DA, Witte ON. The Sca-1 cell surface marker enriches for a prostate-regenerating cell subpopulation that can initiate prostate tumorigenesis. Proc Natl Acad Sci USA 2005; 102: 6942–7.

41. Stingl J, Raouf A, Emerman JT et al. Epithelial progenitors in the normal human mammary gland. J Mammary Gland Biol Neoplasia 2005; 10: 49–59.

42. Prianishnikov VA. On the concept of stem cell and a model of functional-morphological structure of the endometrium. Contraception 1978; 18: 213–23.

43. Padykula HA, Coles LG, McCracken JA et al. A zonal pattern of cell proliferation and differentiation in the rhesus endometrium during the estrogen surge. Biol Reprod 1984; 31: 1103–18.

44. Ferenczy A, Bertrand G, Gelfand MM. Proliferation kinetics of human endometrium during the normal menstrual cycle. Am J Obstet Gynecol 1979; 133: 859–67.

45. Padykula HA, Coles LG, Okulicz WC et al. The basalis of the primate endometrium: a bifunctional germinal compartment. Biol Reprod 1989; 40: 681–90.

46. Brenner RM, Slayden OD, Rodgers WH et al. Immunocytochemical assessment of mitotic activity with an antibody to phosphorylated histone H3 in the macaque and human endometrium. Hum Reprod 2003; 18: 1185–93.

47. Hartman C. Regeneration of monkey uterus after surgical removal of endometrium and accidental endometriosis. W J Surg Obstet Gynecol 1944; 52: 87–102.

48. Wood C, Rogers PAW. Pregnancy after planned partial endometrial resection. Aust NZ J Obstet Gynaecol 1993; 33: 316–18.

49. Tresserra F, Grases P, Ubeda A et al. Morphological changes in hysterectomies after endometrial ablation. Hum Reprod 1999; 14: 1473–7.

50. Biervliet FP, Maguiness SD, Robinson J et al. A successful cycle of IVF-ET after treatment of endometrial ossification; case report and review. J Obstet Gynaecol 2004; 24: 472–3.

51. Bird CC, Willis RA. The production of smooth muscle by the endometrial stroma of the adult human uterus. J Pathol Bacteriol 1965; 90: 75–81.

52. Roth E, Taylor HB. Heterotopic cartilage in the uterus. Obstet Gynecol 1966; 27: 838–44.

53. Mutter GL, Lin MC, Fitzgerald JT et al. Changes in endometrial PTEN expression throughout the human menstrual cycle. J Clin Endocrinol Metab 2000; 85: 2334–8.

54. Tanaka M, Kyo S, Kanaya T et al. Evidence of the monoclonal composition of human endometrial epithelial glands and mosaic pattern of clonal distribution in luminal epithelium. Am J Pathol 2003; 163: 295–301.

55. Chan RWS, Gargett CE. Identification of label-retaining cells in mouse endometrium. Stem Cells 2006; 24: 1529–38.

56. Schwab KE, Chan RW, Gargett CE. Putative stem cell activity of human endometrial epithelial and stromal cells during the menstrual cycle. Fertil Steril 2005; 84: 1124–30.

57. Gargett CE. Stem cells in gynaecology. Aust NZ J Obstet Gynaecol 2004; 44: 380–6.

58. Loughney AD, Redfern CP. Menstrual cycle related differences in the proliferative responses of cultured human endometrial stromal cells to retinoic acid. J Reprod Fertil 1995; 105: 153–9.

59. Tanaka T, Nakajima S, Umesaki N. Cellular heterogeneity in long-term surviving cells isolated from eutopic endometrial, ovarian endometrioma and adenomyosis tissues. Oncol Rep 2003; 10: 1155–60.

60. Fujii S, Konishi I, Mori T. Smooth muscle differentiation at the endometrio–myometrial junction. Virchows Arch A Pathol Anat Histopathol 1989; 414: 105–12.

61. Gargett CE, Zillwood R, Schwab KE. Characterising the stem cell activity of human endometrial cells. Hum Reprod 2005; 20(Suppl 1): i95.

62. Holinka CF, Gurpide E. Proliferative potential and polymorphism of human endometrial stromal cells. Gynecol Endocrinol 1987; 1: 71–81.

63. Gargett CE. Endometrial stem cells. In Alpin JD, Fazleabas AT, Gassnel SR, Giudice LC, eds. The endometrium: molecular, cellular and clinical perspectives. 2nd edn. London: Informa Healthcare 2007 (in press).

64. Kim JY, Tavare S, Shibata D. Counting human somatic cell replications: methylation mirrors endometrial stem cell divisions. Proc Natl Acad Sci USA 2005; 17739–44.

65. Ro S, Rannala B. Methylation patterns and mathematical models reveal dynamics of stem cell turnover in the human colon. Proc Natl Acad Sci USA 2001; 98: 10519–21.

66. Schwab KE, Gargett CE. Prospective isolation of putative human endometrial mesenchymal stem cells using CD146 and plalelet-derived growth factor receptor-β. J Soc Gynecol Invest 2006; 13(Suppl): 186A – Abstract 370.

67. Cho NH, Park YK, Kim YT et al. Lifetime expression of stem cell markers in the uterine endometrium. Fertil Steril 2004; 81: 403–7.

68. Garcia-Pacheco JM, Oliver C, Kimatrai M et al. Human decidual stromal cells express CD34 and STRO-1 and are related to bone marrow stromal precursors. Mol Hum Reprod 2001; 7: 1151–7.

69. Matthai C, Horvat R, Noe M et al. Oct-4 expression in human endometrium. Mol Hum Reprod 2006; 12: 7–10.

70. Kobayashi A, Behringer RR. Developmental genetics of the female reproductive tract in mammals. Nat Rev Genet 2003; 4: 969–80.

71. Spencer TE, Hayashi K, Hu J et al. Comparative developmental biology of the mammalian uterus. Curr Top Dev Biol 2005; 68: 85–122.

72. Pardal R, Clarke MF, Morrison SJ. Applying the principles of stem-cell biology to cancer. Nat Rev Cancer 2003; 3: 895–902.

73. Miller SJ, Lavker RM, Sun TT. Interpreting epithelial cancer biology in the context of stem cells: tumor properties and therapeutic implications. Biochim Biophys Acta 2005; 1756: 25–52.

74. Reya T, Morrison SJ, Clarke MF et al. Stem cells, cancer, and cancer stem cells. Nature 2001; 414: 105–11.

75. Latta E, Chapman WB. PTEN mutations and evolving concepts in endometrial neoplasia. Curr Opin Obstet Gynecol 2002; 14: 59–65.

76. Moreno-Bueno G, Hardisson D, Sanchez C et al. Abnormalities of the APC/beta-catenin pathway in endometrial cancer. Oncogene 2002; 21: 7981–90.

77. Amant F, Moerman P, Neven P et al. Endometrial cancer. Lancet 2005; 366: 491–505.

78. Giudice LC, Kao LC. Endometriosis. Lancet 2004; 364: 1789–99.

79. Van Gorp T, Amant F, Neven P, Vergote I, Moerman P. Endometriosis and the development of malignant tumours of the pelvis. A review of literature. Best Pract Res Clin Obstet Gynaecol 2004; 18: 349–71.

80. Ferenczy A. Pathophysiology of adenomyosis. Hum Reprod Update 1998; 4: 312–22.

81. Vats A, Bielby RC, Tolley NS et al. Stem cells. Lancet 2005; 366: 592–602.

82. Rahaman MN, Mao JJ. Stem cell-based composite tissue constructs for regenerative medicine. Biotechnol Bioeng 2005; 91: 261–84.

83. Delancey JO. The hidden epidemic of pelvic floor dysfunction: achievable goals for improved prevention and treatment. Am J Obstet Gynecol 2005; 192: 1488–95.

CHAPTER 10

Bone marrow-derived stem cells in the human endometrium

Ivan Araujo Penna and Hugh S Taylor

INTRODUCTION

The human endometrium is one of the most dynamic structures in the human body. The remarkable tissue remodeling that occurs in the endometrium is unparallelled in any other organ. Under the influence of the ovarian steroids hormones – estrogen and progesterone – the uterus undergoes dramatic changes in order to prepare for embryo implantation every 28 days. These modifications occur in multiple cells types, including the epithelium, the underlying stroma and the vasculature. The molecular and cellular modifications that occur during the period of these structural changes result in a functional window of receptivity for a human embryo to attach to the endometrium.[1]

The chance of conception in any menstrual cycle for many healthy fertile couples is proximally 25%.[2] Embryo quality and development of a receptive endometrium are determining factors in the establishment of gestation. If implantation does not occur, other characteristic tissue changes proceed in a similarly dynamic process, and a menses occurs about 6 days later. The re-epithelization begins simultaneously with the endometrial tissue destruction; this is followed by the regeneration of stromal components and the beginning of a new proliferative phase. The cellular basis for this dramatic remodeling is still incompletely understood; however, it probably involves stem cells.

ENDOMETRIUM IN THE MENSTRUAL CYCLE

In order to appreciate the dramatic growth, remodeling, differentiation and cell turnover that occurs in the endometrium, we will briefly describe the events of the endometrial cycle. The endometrial functional layer is regulated by the ovarian steroids estradiol and progesterone in well-characterized monthly cycles. There are three distinct phases of the menstrual cycle: the proliferative phase, the secretory phase and menstruation.

The proliferative phase is characterized by rapid regeneration of the endometrium. Development of the endometrium during the proliferative phase is driven by the action of estradiol. During the early portion of this phase, the glands are lined by a columnar epithelium; the luminal diameter is small and the glands are circular in shape. During this phase glandular mitoses are frequent. Under the control of increasing levels of estradiol during the middle of the proliferative phase, the endometrial functional layer grows and the tubular glands become more tortuous, acquiring a longitudinal shape. The mitotic index of both epithelial and stromal cells increases and, in particular, the rate of glandular mitosis is higher in this part of the proliferative phase than any other. In the late proliferative phase, the glands show increased numbers of ribosomes and endoplasmatic reticulum. The glands are more tortuous and the epithelial cells are tall and columnar, and the mitosis rate is reduced. In contrast, during the late proliferative phase, the stromal cells show an increase in mitotic index until ovulation, when mitosis peaks. Pseudostratification of the epithelial cells increases during the late proliferative phase, reaching a maximum between 4 days before and 2 days after the luteinizing hormone (LH) level peaks.[3]

The formation of the corpus luteum, leading to increased progesterone concentration in the plasma, marks the onset of the secretory phase. In the early part of the secretory phase, the level of progesterone produced by the corpus luteum rises abruptly and structural modifications in the endometrium rapidly follow. Stromal mitoses peak on the day of ovulation and within 5 days of the ovulation no further mitoses occur in the endometrial glands. The histological changes in the glands in response to the ovulatory stimulus are remarkable; by the 2nd day after the ovulation, the glands already represent 20% of the functional layer. During the first 3 days following ovulation, the glandular cell subnuclear vacuoles increase dramatically and contain newly produced glycoproteins and mucopolysaccharides. By day 5 after ovulation the intracellular accumulation is a maximum. During day 6 the glands actively secrete this material into the luminal space and their shape changes, becoming more tortuous. At this time the glands represents 25% of the endometrium. Alterations also occur in the stroma, the most evident being edema. In the second part of luteal phase, the structural transformations are slower and mostly affect the stroma and vessels. The glands involute, the epithelial cells decrease in height and nuclei appear shrunken. Infiltration of lymphocytes begins at the luminal epithelial surface. In particular, the reduction of stromal edema, on day 10 after the ovulation, increases the proportion of glands to one-third of the endometrium.[4]

The last phase of the menstrual cycle is menstruation. Menstruation is triggered by withdrawal of estradiol and progesterone, and is characterized by the loss of the functional layer with menstrual bleeding. The first event leading to menstruation occurs by day 28 of the menstrual cycle and consists of small lesions in the luminal epithelium. After that, a rapid and incomplete degeneration of all functional layers occurs, exposing blood vessels and leading to bleeding.[5] The rapid and complete loss of this tissue is followed again by rapid regeneration. The massive turnover of multiple cell types suggests the need for a source of stem cells to regenerate the endometrium.

ENDOMETRIAL ANGIOGENESIS

The blood vessels also regenerate in the endometrium, in particular during the secretory phase. The endometrial vessels and capillary networks become more extensive and apparent. Both angiogenesis and arteriogenesis are involved in this generation of abundant new vascular smooth muscle cells and endothelium which vary with the menstrual cycle and have their origin in local endothelial cells. In addition, they can originate from bone marrow precursors such as mesenchymal stem cells.[6]

Endometrial white blood cells

In addition to the endometrial epithelium and the vasculature, there are other periodically renewed cells within the endometrium. There is an enormous flux of leukocytes through the endometrium. During the first trimester of pregnancy, up to 40% of cells in the decidua are leukocytes. Neutrophils, the most common leukocyte in the human circulation, have been identified in the endometrium; they have been defined as $CD11b^{bright}$, $CD66B^{+}$ and $CD16^{+}$.[7] During the early menstrual cycle, neutrophils are almost undetectable in the normal endometrium, but in the perimenstrual period their numbers increase by 6–15%.[7] They function in conjunction with other leukocytes in menstruation by helping to remove menstrual debris. Eosinophils, another leukocyte present in the endometrium, become more prevalent prior to menstruation. Eosinophils function in late-type inflammatory reactions. Monocytes from the circulation enter the endometrium and differentiate to macrophages. Macrophages ($CD68^{+}$) have been detected in the endometrium, with increasing numbers from the proliferative through to the menstrual phase. Macrophages are also linked with chronic inflammation. Mast cells have also been demonstrated in the endometrium throughout the menstrual cycle. These cells secret nociceptive, vasoactive and proinflammatory molecules in mast cell degranulation. This process increases vascular permeability and attracts other leukocytes. B and T lymphocytes are found in basal lymphoid aggregates, scattered throughout the stroma and in intraepithelial sites of endometrium.[7] The ratio of CD8+ to CD4+ in the endometrium (2:1) is the inverse of that found in the blood; in addition, the CD3+ T cells are present in the endometrium and increase during menstruation. Natural killer cells are present in large numbers in non-pregnant endometrium (CD56+, CD2+/−, CD38+, CD16− and CD3−).[7] All these hematopoietic cells are derived from bone marrow stem cells and are found throughout the endometrium. Their function is thought to be cytotoxic during the late part of the proliferative phase. The factors that regulate the flux of leukocytes in endometrium is not fully known; however, there is an increase in both in-situ proliferation and migration from the peripheral circulation (indirectly from bone marrow) in the late luteal phase. This demonstrates an important contribution of traditional bone marrow-derived cells in the process of endometrial remodeling; it is therefore not difficult to assume that bone marrow-derived stem cells would have access to this tissue.

Without implantation, the functional layer of the endometrium is lost during menstruation, and a regeneration of all cell types occurs from multipotent and unipotent stem cells in the remaining basal layer[8] and (as described below) from bone marrow.[9] Therefore, in the endometrium, this capacity is in keeping with the function of the stem cells: to repair and regenerate tissue in specific sites.[10]

STEM CELLS

The definition of a stem cell includes two classical principles: self-renewal and totipotency or multipotency.[11] Totipotency is the capacity of a stem cell to generate all types of cells, including the germinative tissue. Multipotency is the characteristic of being able to differentiate into more than one mature cell type. Self-renewal is the capacity of a stem cell to divide without differentiation and hence generate a lasting supply of stem cells.[12] Stem cells are further subclassified based on their spatial or tissue of origin and capacity to differentiate into other specific types of cells.[13] In general, there are two origins of stem cells: embryonic (embryonic stem cells) and adult tissue (somatic stem cells). Adult stem cells or mesenchymal stem cells (MSCs) can differentiate into specific tissue in which they reside and self-renew for long periods of time within a specific niche, but, for a limited time in culture. Embryonic stem cells, however, have a different potential and are capable of self-renewing for long periods of time in culture,[14] owing to their totipotency or pluripotency; this can produce a teratoma if they are transferred into a host without a previous subtype-specific cell differentiation.[15] Embryonic stem cells are currently an active area of research, but the attainment of these cells is complicated – ethically and technically. However, MSCs are easier to study, because of the lack ethical constraints and technically due to the ease of access and the lack of concerns over immunological cross-match.[16]

Within various tissues, there are also multipotent and unipotent stem cells; the first have the potential to produce a limited number of mature cell lineages and the second have the capability of differentiating in only one lineage. Well-known examples include hematopoietic stem cells and epidermal stem cells, respectively.[17] In the adult, a fairy well-characterized source of multipotent stem cells is the bone marrow. The degree of differentiation of each type of stem cell varies with its origin.

All adult tissues have stem cells that usually constitute a small minority of the total tissue mass, with the capacity to renew and regenerate the mature tissue. However, this is a simple idea and does not express the complexity of the degree of stem cell differentiation. The tissue location where stem cells are isolated is called the 'niche'. Twenty years ago, Schofield first introduced the concept of a niche for hematopoietic stem cells.[19] The niche has the specific microenvironment to contain the stem cells and maintain them in an undifferentiated state in vivo. The microenvironment of the niche regulates access to messengers and to oxygen tension, temperature, chemical gradients and mechanical forces to provide a sheltering environment that protects the stem cells from signals triggering differentiation, apoptosis and other stimuli that reduce cell reserve.[20,21] The niche is composed of both stem cells and neighboring differentiated cell types that communicate by both negative and positive signaling, including molecular signals such as Bmp/Wnt, cell–cell contact and anatomical organization.[20] The stem cell in the niche can undergo cell division with minimal gene expression. However, some genes are expressed in the undifferentiated state of stem cells; these include vimentin, connective tissue growth factor, collagen type I α1 and eukaryotic translation elongation factor I α1.[22] The activation of this reserve of stem cells is tied to a change in the environment or with consecutive cell divisions, causing the cell to physically lose connection with the niche.[23] The environmental equilibrium can be changed by reducing oxygen, heat, chemical reagents and even changes in diet.[21] The niche can have a different location in each type of tissue, e.g. the satellite cell, and is attached to the basal lamina in muscle.[23] In the nervous system, the niche has been identified in four different locations: subventricular zone, lateral ventricles, dentate gyrus and subcortical white matter.[24,25] Schwab et al[26] and Simon have reported the presence of stem cells in the basal lamina of the endometrium and Körbling et al[27] showed donor-derived cells located in the deep Malpighian layer (skin).

Not only is the ability of the niche to retain the stem cells important but also its capacity to recruit new stem cells from other organs (bone marrow) is probably necessary. The process is called 'homing' and is known to occur after tissue damage. The molecular mechanisms mediating this process are still not characterized; however, this homing phenomenon was shown by Kai and Spraiding[28] in *Drosophila* germinative stem cell (GSC) niches. They reported that when the GSC niches are significantly decreased, the niche cells signal mesenchymal stem tissue to migrate and to repopulate the niche.

Bone marrow stem cells

The bone marrow has a well-characterized population of stem cells, the hematopoietic stem cells. Those cells were the first know somatic stem cells and represent more than 99% of bone marrow.[29] The hematopoietic stem cells are self-renewing and produce progenitors that differentiate into all of the circulating mature blood cell, such as granulocytes, erythrocytes, lymphocytes and megakaryocytes.[10] As described above, MCSs migrate into the endometrium during several periods of the menstrual cycle. The concentration and types of blood cell vary during the menstrual cycle, but all are derived from hematopoietic stem cells.

Bone marrow mesenchymal stem cells

Mesenchymal stem cells were described in 1966 by Friedenstein et al who isolated a progenitor cell from rat bone marrow.[30] While MSCs may exist in all tissue, they have only been identified in a minimal number of tissues, including liver, fetal blood, cord blood, nervous system, amniotic fluid, heart and placenta.[24,26,31] Human MSCs are extracted from marrow in the posterior iliac crest or the tibial and femoral compartment, and selected by their adherence capacity to plastic in the specific culture medium.[32] The study of these cells has two obstacles: the rarity of MSCs in the marrow aspirate and the lack of a primary single phenotype.[33] The MSCs produce neither hematopoietic (CD34, CD45, CD14) nor endothelial cell markers (CD34, CD31, VWF),[34] but they express adhesion molecules (CD44, CD29, CD90), stromal cell markers (SH-2, SH-3, SH-4) and cytokine receptors (interleukin-1 receptor [IL-1R] and tumor neurosis factor-α receptor [TNF-αR]). In an attempt to differentiate hematopoietic stem cells from MSCs in culture and tissue, Baddoo et al[35] used antibodies against CD45, CD34 and CD11b, and isolated them using negative selection. This is currently the most effective procedure used to isolate these cells. The MSCs have different degrees of multipotency and few cells are capable of multipotent differentiation, but most cells are bipotent or unipotent.[32] This characteristic varies between the tissues and MSCs analyzed. In-vitro differentiation of these cells is possible. Dexamethasone, for example, drives the MSCs into the osteogenic cell type, transforming growth factor-β (TGF-β) drives the MSCs into chondrogenic differentiation and isobutylmethylxanthine into adpocogenic differentiation.[33] The multipotentiality of mesenchymal cells has also been confirmed in vivo. MCSs contribute to regeneration in multiple tissues, including liver, neurons, heart, skin, kidney, cornea, gastrointestinal epithelium, skeletal muscle and endometrium. In the liver, the MSCs engraft as hepatocytes. Using male-to-female bone marrow transplantation in rats, mice and humans, it was first demonstrated to occur in response to liver damage.[36] Mesenchymal stem cells have been used to reverse models of degenerative central nervous system diseases, such as the Niemann–Pick disease. In a mouse model, the neurological defects and death were delayed after direct injection of mesenchymal cells, cultured and differentiated, into the nervous system.[37] In humans, after orthopedic transplantation of female hearts into males, up to 15% of the cardiac myocytes are donor derived.[38] In mice and humans, Y+ cytokeratin-positive cells are present in the skin of female recipients after bone marrow transplantation.[39]

Plasticity

A unique function of stem cells is the plasticity to become another type of cell.[40] Controversy about plasticity remains, in part, because of the inconsistent reproducibility of the models and results.[41] There are five different types of mechanism that can explain the plasticity – transdifferentiation, dedifferentiation, multiple stem cells, pluripotent stem cells and cell fusion – but only three are widely accepted: transdifferentiation, cell fusion and dedifferentiation.[17] Cell transdifferentiation is defined as the ability of one committed cell type to change its identity to that of a completely different cell type. It can be classified in two types – direct and indirect;[42] the first is transdifferentiation followed by maturation down an alternative pathway, and the second is a direct transition. Another type of plasticity mechanism, dedifferentiation, occurs when a unipotent stem cell changes to become a multipotent stem cell and subsequently differentiates into a specific tissue; however, this is an indirect transdifferentiation. Direct transdifferentiation has never been definitely established, despite the study of Bjornson et al[43] who reported a transdifferentiation of neural stem cells into hematopoietic mature cells.

A second mechanism by which a stem cell changes the cell type is cell fusion. The cell fusion theory suggests that the stem cell fuses with a somatic cell, resulting in the formation of another lineage cell.[40] The cell fusion phenomenon is known to occur in humans during many physiological processes such as fertilization, placentation, granulomatous tissue formation and monocytes/macrophage cell lineage generation. In support of this mechanism, mice with a fatal liver disease could be cured by infusion of purified stem cells; the mechanism reported to repair this tissue was cell fusion.[40] In humans, cell fusion has been reported to underlie the contributions of transplanted bone marrow stem cells to liver hepatocytes and cardiac myocytes. However, the low frequency with which such a phenomenon has been observed – around 1% in cardiomyocytes and less than 0.1% in hepatocytes – implies that it may contribute little to total tissue regeneration.[17]

The explanation that is the most widely accepted is direct differentiation. Differentiation is the capacity of stem cells to become a specific cell type in a specific environment; this is a multistep and unidirectional process in which a specific cell type is formed.[33] It is a result of activation and repression events affecting transcription factors and genes that are implicated in differentiation and self-renewal in stem cells. Portmann-Lanz et al[31] reported chondrogenic, osteogenic, adipogenic, myogenic and neurogenic differentiation of MSCs from amnion, chorion and villous stroma. LaBarge and Blau reported the differentiation of bone marrow cells into muscle stem cells, and then to mature muscle cells.[44] Similarly, Lagase et al[36] reported the differentiation of purified hematopoietic stem cells into hepatocytes.

The trigger for activation of plasticity may be damage or stress. Different types of damage models produce varying numbers of stem cell in the repaired tissue. The range of the tissue conversion after specific kinds of damage is 0.07–50% in liver, 0.2–12.5% in skeletal muscle and 1–35% in lung.[40]

For plasticity to take place, it is necessary that stem cells migrate and home to the site of tissue damage. During the prenatal period, stem cells migrate or home to all tissues. One classic example is the migration of stem cells from the fetal liver to the bone marrow.[36] However, the homing of these cells in the postnatal period is a key part of plasticity and maintains a stem cell reserve in niches in different tissues.[34] It is well characterized that bone marrow can be recolonized after stem cell injection into the circulation, but the directed migration of stem cells into damaged tissue is a relatively new concept.[36] During the process of tissue damage, some mesenchymal chemoattractants are up-regulated. Several molecules that are expressed at higher levels during this process are stromal-derived factor-1 (SDF-1), vascular endothelial growth factor (VEGF), hepatocyte growth factor/scatter factor (HGF/SF), leukemia inhibitory factor (LIF), hypoxia-regulated/induced transcription factor (HIF-1) and CXC chemokine receptor 4^+ (CXCR4). SDF-1 was first identified in osteoblasts and its blinding with CXCR4 is essential to seed stem cells from the damaged tissue. SDF-1 has the capacity to pass endothelial barriers to recruit stem cells in the bone marrow.[45] The complex SDF-1/CXCR4 is regulated for HIF-1. HIF-1 is express in the endothelial cells within bone marrow, liver, heart and brain during stress, in particular during partial hypoxia.[46] Therefore, damage and stress are implicated in regenerative potential (plasticity) of mobilized circulating stem cells. However, homing mechanisms, both in the absence or presence of tissue damage, are poorly understood.

Endogenous stem cells in endometrium

During the last 2 years, several groups have suggested that the deep basal layer of the endometrium may have a pool of stem cells, similar to a classic niche as described above. Chan et al[47] showed evidence of putative endometrial epithelial and stromal stem cells. Schwab et al[26] first demonstrated that human endometrium has both stromal and epithelial clonogenic cells. Later, they demonstrated that human epithelial and stromal cell clonogenic activity is not different between the proliferative and secretory phases of the menstrual cycle; the inactive human endometrium also contains clonogenic epithelial and stromal cells. These authors also demonstrated that several chemokines are linked to the microenvironment of stem cells in the endometrial niche; these include epidermal growth factor (EGF), transforming growth factor-α (TGF-α) and platelet-derived growth factor BB (PDGF-BB) for stromal and epithelial cells, and basic fibroblast growth factor (bFGF), insulin-like growth factor 1 (IGF-1), LIF, HGF and stem cell factor (SCF). More recently, the Simon group has demonstrated a region of BrdU (bromodeoxyuridine)-retaining cells in endometrium that also expresses stem cell markers.

Endometrial stem cells from bone marrow

While the presence of endometrial stem cells in specialized endometrial niches is not surprising, given the remarkable turnover in this tissue, more intriguing is the demonstration of bone marrow donor stem cells in the endometrium of women who had undergone bone marrow transplant. Endometrial biopsies were obtained from four female allogeneic bone marrow transplant recipients who received marrow from a single antigen-mismatched related donor; these women therefore had a human leukocyte antigen (HLA) type that allowed determination of the origin of any cell. Only female donors were used to eliminate the possibility that men may not harbor female reproductive stem cells. To reduce variability induced by the type of damage, we used only subjects that received bone marrow transplant for leukemia treatment and who had undergone similar treatment; all patients had total body radiotherapy and chemotherapy, and all were of reproductive age. The donor cells were identified using a reverse transcription polymerase chain reaction (RT-PCR) and immunohistochemistry (IHC). Monoclonal antibodies against HLA antigens (A11, A3 and B7) identified donor-derived cells. To reduce the interobserver and intraobserver errors, >200 high-power fields were counted for each subject by three observers. The RT-PCR was performed for each patient's RNA sample using primers for the mismatched HLA antigen.

We showed that donor-derived endometrial cells were present in the endometrial samples of bone marrow recipients. Although the mismatched HLA antigen was detected by RT-PCR, the RNA may have been derived from leukocytes of bone marrow donor origin. The transient leukocyte infiltrations

Table 10.1 Bone marrow transplant recipients

				Positive cells/Total No. of cells (%)	
Patient	*Age (years)*	*Regimen*	*Time from transplantation to biopsy (months)*	*Donor-derived epithelial cells*	*Donor-derived stromal cells*
1	43	TBI, cyclophosphamide, cytarabine	157	4950/10,400 (48)	96,704/187,000 (52)
2	25	Cyclophosphamide, busulfan	129	1203/12,300 (10)	20,941/193,600 (11)
3	32	TBI, cyclophosphamide	35	684/17,300 (4)	6832/156,200 (4)
4	28	TBI, cyclophosphamide	24	45/19,500 (0.2)	675/210,000 (0.3)

TBI, total body irradiation

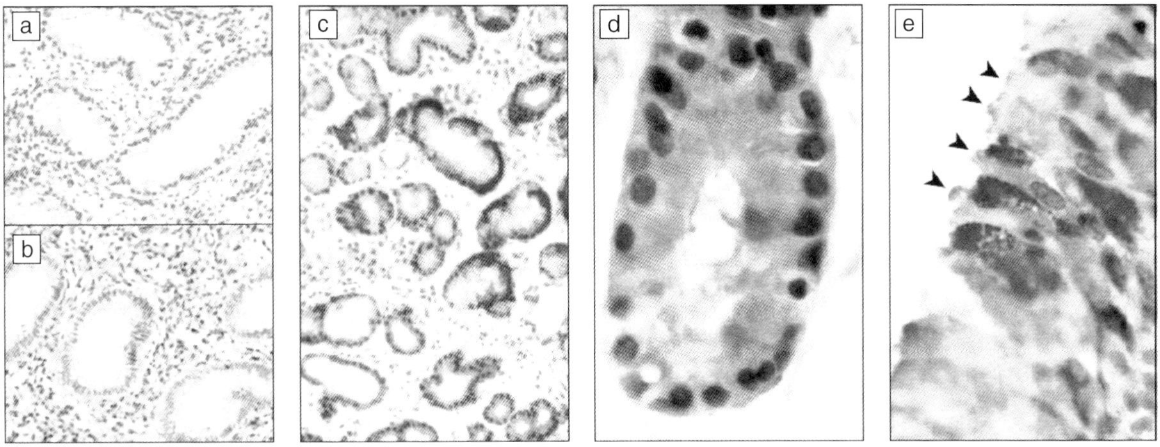

Figure 10.1 Donor-derived cells in the endometrium of an HLA-A11-mismatched bone marrow transplant recipient (patient 1). Immunohistochemistry using anti-HLA-A11 monoclonal antibody, biotin peroxidase detection system, diaminobenzidine as the chromogen (brown), and hematoxylin counterstain. (a) HLA-A11-negative control (original magnification ×200). (b) HLA-A11 immunopositivity (brown) in an HLA-A11-positive control (original magnification ×200). (c) HLA-A11 immunopositivity (brown) in patient 1. More than 50% of the cells were of donor origin (original magnification ×100). (d) Endometrial glands partially derived from cells of donor origin (brown; original magnification ×400). (e) Rare cells of donor origin (brown) in an endometrial gland. Functional differentiation is noted by characteristic cilia. Arrowheads identify the ciliated epithelial surface (original magnification ×600). (See also color plate)

were distinguished from donor-derived endometrial cell by CD45 immune staining. However, the IHC revealed differentiated epithelial and stromal cells of donor origin (Figure 10.1). These cells expressed the donor HLA antigen and no markers of differentiated white blood cells. The rates of bone marrow-derived stem cells were greater in the stroma than in the glandular epithelium. The donor-derived cells were found to constitute a small fraction of the total tissue.

Although some endometrial glands appeared to be completely composed of donor-derived cells, other glands had only a fraction of these cells, implying that not all glands are clonal in origin. The predominance of donor-derived stromal cells in relation to glandular epithelial cells demonstrates differential cell type-specific rates of transdifferentiation as well as variation in the percentage of cells of donor origin, which depends of the cell type and length of the time from treatment to biopsy. Some samples showed endometrial epithelial cells with functional cilia and calcitonin expression, indicating full differentiation. There was no double-intensity DNA signal detected, demonstrating a low-likelihood cell fusion (Figure 10.2). As expected, there were a large number of mature leukocytes of donor origin.

CLINICAL IMPLICATIONS

These results lead to several novel ways of looking at common medical problems that affect the uterus and pregnancy. We examine several of these in the following sections.

Endometrial ablation

The idea of an exogenous source of stem cells may explain why endometrial ablation is not highly effective. Current ablative techniques can destroy between 3 and 5 mm of uterine wall; theoretically, this depth should be enough to destroy the basalis layer of endometrium and lead to amenorrhea. Ablation leads to a 90% reduction in the uterine blood flow, but only half completely stops menstruating and, over time, these rates continue to drop.[48] Stem cells can be a mechanism of repair. The repair may begin within a niche or from a circulating pool of stem cells. Even if

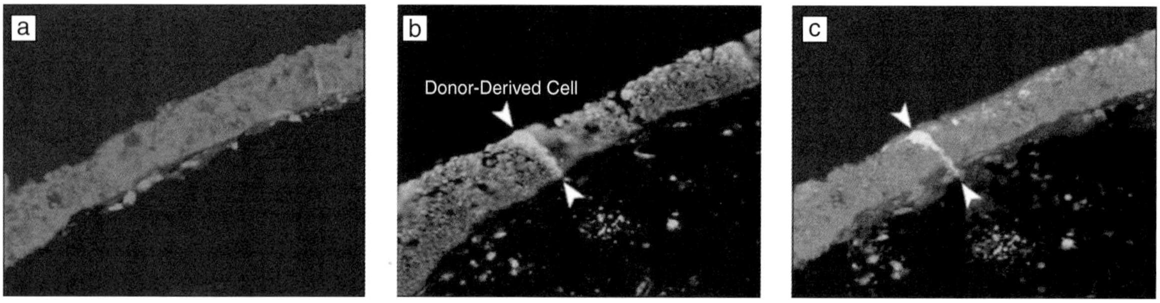

Figure 10.2 Differentiation shown by immunofluorescence in donor-derived cell in endometrial epithelial layer. Immunofluorescence using tetrarhodamine isothiocyanate for calcitonin expression (red) and fluorescein isothiocyanate for donor-derived cells (green) in endometrial epithelial cells of HLA-A11-negative transplant recipient (patient 1) who received bone marrow from an HLA-A11-positive donor. (a) Calcitonin expression in endometrial epithelium indicative of receptivity to blastocyst implantation. (b) Mismatched HLA-A11-positive endometrial epithelial cell of donor origin (arrowheads). (c) Merge demonstrating HLA-mismatched cell expressing calcitonin as a marker of functional differentiation (original magnification ×100). (See also color plate)

all endometrial cells, including endogenous stem cells are destroyed, perhaps endometrium can regenerate from circulating stem cells.

Endometriosis

The role of MSCs in the re-epithelization of endometrium can be used to understand endometriosis. Endometriosis is a disorder defined by the presence of endometrial glands and stroma outside the uterus. There are three classical theories that purport to explain its etiology: retrograde menstruation, hematological and lymphatic dissemination and coelomic metaplasia. Retrograde menstruation is widely accepted, but 70–90% of the patients have the retrograde menstruation and don't develop endometriosis.[49] The dissemination theory tries to explain the existence of endometriosis outside the pelvis through the export of cells via the lymphatic system and blood. Coelomic metaplasia is based on the presence of undifferentiated cells in the coelomic pelvis. However, the data described here lead to a novel theory for the origin of endometriosis: circulating mesenchymal stem cells can differentiate into endometrial cells in ectopic locations. Perhaps this differentiation could be mediated by inflammatory factors. This may result in endometriosis far from the uterus, in areas that are not in communication with the peritoneal cavity and are not typically areas receiving pelvic lymphatic or venous drainage. Future research will strive to identify mediators of endometrial stem cell differentiation. A better understanding of this process may lead to a mechanism to control or modify its progress and potentially to treating endometriosis.

Infertility and pregnancy

Assisted reproduction has improved in the last 20 years. New techniques, such as intracytoplasmatic sperm injection (ICSI), and new culture media have increased the success of infertility treatments. However, none of these technologies have increased implantation or endometrial receptivity.[50] Multiple embryos are transferred to obtain a reasonable clinic pregnancy rate. One of the possible areas for improvement is the implantation process, in particular endometrial receptivity during the implantation window. Whereas the full spectrum of endometrial alterations are unknown, some conditions, including uterine adhesion, endometriosis, hydrosalpinges and fibroids, are linked to poor implantation and diminished endometrial receptivity.

Women with endometriosis have increased level of cytokines, growth factors and active macrophages as a result of an immune response to ectopic tissue. These inflammatory factors probably have a deleterious effect on the endometrium, sperm and embryo, and decrease the success rates of attempts at spontaneous and assisted conception.[51] Specifically, in the endometrium, women with endometriosis show aberrant expression of several gene products, including aromatase, endometrial bleeding factor, HGF, 17β-hydroxysteroid dehydrogenase, HOXA10, HOXA11, LIF, integrins, matrix metalloproteinases 7 and 11 and progesterone receptors, all important for embryo implantation.[51,52]

The presence of hydrosalpinges reduces implantation after in-vitro fertilization (IVF)–embryo transfer. The intermittent bathing of endometrium with toxic fluid from the hydrosalpinges results in aberrant expression of HOXA10, integrins and LIF.[53]

The importance of uterine fibroids as a cause of infertility is controversial; however, the presence of fibroid distorting in the uterine cavity is an established cause of reduced implantation. The explanation is linked to the impairment of blood supply, reduction of gamete transport and reduced expression of implantation factors, as described above.[54]

In the future, stem cells may play an important role in the treatment or several of these conditions and serve as sources of new stromal, glandular epithelial cells.

These cells may also be modified to restore expression of molecular essential to the implantation process.[55]

Endometrial damage and Asherman's syndrome

Adhesions within the uterine cavity are typically caused by endometrial damage, such as infections, chemical irritation and surgery. The adhesion may obstruct the tubal ostia or reduce the amount and quality of receptive endometrium available for the embryo. The current treatment is hysteroscopic adhesiolysis, and the success rates vary from 71 to 90%.[56] Perhaps one source of cells that regenerate the endometrium once the cavity is made patent are circulating stem cells. Treatment by additional bone marrow MSCs may be a means of improving success rates after the hysteroscopic adhesiolysis.

FUTURE TREATMENTS

The goal of regenerative medicine is to restore cells, tissue and organs that are lost or damaged. Current approaches are influenced by the knowledge of embryonic development, tissue turnover and stem cell biology.[57] Stem cell plasticity opens a new field of regenerative medicine and has brought hope for the treatment of a variety of degenerative and age-related diseases. MSCs, being easy to obtain and culture, bring new promise to the field of tissue engineering.[41] MSCs have several advantages over embryonic stem cells. Embryonic stem cells are pluripotent and cannot be transplanted directly into the target tissue without previous differentiation in culture. The risk of teratoma development still needs to be addressed.[58] Another advantage to using MSCs is the possibility of reducing immunological rejection with autologous engraftments. Five different potential uses of MSCs have been explored:

- local implantation for localized diseases
- systematic transplantation of MSCs
- ex-vivo gene therapy in stem cells
- tissue engineering
- homing induction.[59]

Local implantation

Several animal models have demonstrated the efficacy of using MSCs in the treatment of bone defects.[60] In humans, local autologous MSC injection has been successfully used to treat large bone defects after fracture, vascular ischemia secondary to peripheral arterial diseases, coronary disease and non-healing chronic skin wounds.[60,61] The local injection of MSCs is a real possibility for the treatment of endometrial disease. In Asherman's syndrome, the injection can be given locally by hysteroscopy after resection of uterine adhesion in an attempt to regenerate the endometrium.

Systemic transplantation

The transplantation of hematopoietic stem cells for the treatment of hematological diseases is well characterized. Many investigators have tried similar protocols, using MSCs to treat diffuse diseases such as osteogenesis imperfecta.[62] This method could be used as a second way of delivering MSCs to the endometrium, through the uterine circulation to the basalis layer.

Ex-vivo gene therapy in stem cells

The genetic modification of stem cells is an interesting target, because they have unique characteristics such as high proliferative capacity and long-term survival.[59] Allay et al[63] demonstrated that genetically modified MSCs can express exogenous proteins such as factor VIII and interleukin-3 (IL-3) for extended periods of time and maintain this ability after transplantation.[63] Another strategy is the use of genetically modified MSCs to deliver chemotherapeutics to malignant cells in cancer patients.[33] It has been demonstrated that MSCs engineered to secrete interferon-β (IFN-β) have the ability to suppress the growth of metastases in a xenogeneic mouse model.[64] Genetically modified MSCs could be implanted in endometriosis sites with the intention of producing apoptosis or MSCs genetically modified to express high levels of HOXA10 could be transplanted into the uterus of infertility patients or those with recurrent pregnancy loss in an attempt to improve success rates. In the same way, genetically modified MSCs could be useful for the treatment of endometrial cancer, delivering chemotherapy to malignant cells.

Specific tissue engineering

Tissue engineering involves the use of three-dimensional bioscaffolds seeded with mature stem cells. These cells are cultivated in specific media to drive them to form differentiated tissue and organs such as liver, heart, cartilage or kidney.[65] There are several animal experiments that utilize this approach, e.g. the treatment of large bone defects.[66] Using tissue engineering, stem cells could be used to generate endometrial or myometrial tissue for transplanting into the uterus for treatment of Asherman's syndrome or uterine perforation.

Homing induction

Stimulating the proliferation and differentiation of endogenous stem cells is, potentially, another way of repairing endometrial damage. The advantage of this method is that it does not need an ex-vivo step; however, the exact stimuli that will induce 'homing' of stem cells to each tissue still needs to be determined.[41] Carlen et al[67] presented evidence that the new olfactory granule cells could integrate into the neural circuitry by trans-synaptical transport of virus and respond to odorant stimulation by up-regulation of phosphorylated c-fos.[67] In the endometrium, homing induction could be used for Asherman's syndrome and endometrial abnormalities linked to infertility. Alternatively these factors could be blocked to stop the homing of MSCs to endometriosis.

CONCLUSIONS

The identification of stem cells from multiple sources has tremendous implications for medicine. The regenerative potential of these cells allows us for the first time to consider autologous tissue repair and modification.

The ability of stem cells from bone marrow to contribute to endometrial regeneration has particular importance for reproductive biology and medicine. We now have the potential for a novel etiology of diseases. Endometriosis may be caused by ectopic stem cell differentiation. Stem cell biology brings new possibilities for the treatment of endometrial disorders such as Asherman's syndrome and implantation defects.

These findings may also allow ex-vivo modification of these cells to improve reproductive potential. We can expect to see rapid improvement in medical care deriving from stem cell technology.

SUMMARY

The endometrium is among the most dynamic tissues in the adult. Each month this tissue is remodeled under the influence of the ovarian steroids. The modifications that occur during the renewal process affect the entire endometrium, including the epithelium, stroma and vasculature. The primary portion of the endometrium that drives this functional regeneration is the basalis layer. This tissue is capable of producing cells for re-epithelization. Many of these cells that contribute to endometrial regeneration and the vascular system are derived from endogenous stem cells. These are a subset of endometrial cells, have high proliferative potential and can promote the remodelation of the endometrium.

While endogenous endometrial stem cells are still poorly defined, they are likely to be unipotent or multipotent, giving rise to endometrial epithelial, stromal and vascular cells. The origin of the most totipotent and pluripotent cells is the embryo. Embryonic stem cells are currently an active area of research, with vast potential. However, the bone marrow is also a rich source of stem cells. Hematopoietic stem cells have been well characterized and have the potential to give rise to all of the circulating bone marrow-derived cell types. Recently, bone marrow mesenchymal stem cells have been shown to have a remarkable capacity for transdifferentiation. The stem cells of bone marrow can differentiate into multiple non-hematopoietic cell lineages; recent reports have documented differentiation of bone marrow mesenchymal stem cells into hepatocytes, neurons, cardiomyocytes, skin, kidney, cornea, gastrointestinal epithelium and endometrium. The transdifferentiation of stem cells in these tissues is linked to regeneration and accelerated after tissue damage.

We have identified two sources of stem cells in the uterus: endogenous cells in the basalis layer of the endometrium and the bone marrow. The theory that the endometrium can be remodeled using non-hematopoietic stem cells from bone marrow was established with the demonstration of differentiated endometrial cells of bone marrow donor origin in the endometrium of bone marrow transplant recipients. The percentage of bone marrow-derived cells is greater in the stroma than glandular epithelium and was localized in focal areas. Although some endometrial glands appeared to be completely composed of donor-derived cells, others contained only a small number of individual cells of donor origin. These cells were distinct from the large number of mature leukocytes of donor origin and were capable of full differentiation to secretory endometrium. The transdifferentiation of these stem cells is probably increased by tissue damage. Chemotherapy, radiation, graft-vs-host disease, where damage to the tissue is very significant, leads to repair incorporating a greater percentage of donor cells.

The capacity of stem cells to differentiate into endometrial cells can be helpful in understanding the pathophysiology of endometrium and endometriosis. Endometrial regeneration by recruitment of bone marrow-derived stem cells may be important in endometrial receptivity and the establishment of pregnancy. Endometrial regeneration may explain failure of endometrial ablative procedures. A non-endometrial circulation of stem cells that can differentiate in the endometrium in ectopic locations is an alternative explanation for some forms of endometriosis. Finally, bone marrow-derived mesenchymal stem cells may have a use in the treatment of some endometrial diseases such as Asherman's syndrome and infertility related to defective endometrial receptivity.

REFERENCES

1. Dockery P, Khalid J, Sarani SA et al. Changes in basement membrane thickness in the human endometrium during the luteal phase of the menstrual cycle. Hum Reprod Update 1998; 5: 486–95.
2. Shahine LK, Cedars MI. Preimplantation genetic diagnosis does not increase pregnancy rates in patients at risk for aneuploidy. Fertil Steril 2006; 85: 51–6.
3. Smith SK. The menstrual cycle. In: Glasser SR, Aplin JD, Giunce LC, Tabibzadeh S, eds. The Endometrium. New York: Taylor & Francis, 2002: 73–86.
4. Dockery P. The fine structure of mature human endometrium. In Glasser SR, Aplin JD, Giunce LC, Tabibzadeh S, eds. The Endometrium. New York: Taylor & Francis, 2002: 21–39.
5. Salamonsen LA. Tissue injury and repair in the female human reproductive tract. Reproduction 2003; 125: 301–11.
6. Rogers PAW, Abberton KM. Endometrial arteriogenesis: vascular smooth muscle cell proliferation and differentiation during the menstrual cycle and changes associated with endometrial bleeding disorders. Microsc Res Techn 2003; 60: 412–19.
7. Trundley A, Moffet, A. Human uterine leukocytes and pregnancy. Tissue Antigens 2004; 63: 1–12.
8. Jabbour HN, Kelly RW, Fraser HM, Critchley HO. Endocrine regulation of menstruation. Endocr Rev 2006; 27: 17–46.
9. Taylor HS. Endometrial cells derived from donor stem cells in bone marrow transplant recipients. JAMA 2004; 292: 81–5.
10. Grove JE, Bruscia E, Krause DS. Plasticity of bone marrow-derived stem cells. Stem Cells 2004; 22: 487–500.
11. Spangrude GJ. When is a stem cell really a stem cell? Bone Marrow Transplant 2003; 32 s7–11.
12. Smith A. The battlefield of pluripotency. Cell 2005; 123: 757–60.
13. Herzog EL, Chai L, Krause DS. Plasticity of marrow-derived stem cells. Blood 2003; 102: 3483–93.
14. Ding S, Schultz PG. A role for chemistry in the stem cell biology. Nature 2004; 22: 833–40.
15. Jiang Y, Jahagirdar BN, Reinhardt RL et al. Pluripotency of mesenchymal stem cells derived from adult marrow. Nature 2002; 427: 41–9.
16. Fortier LA. Stem cells: classifications, controversies, and clinical applications. Veter Surg 2006; 34: 415–23.
17. Wagers AJ, Weissman IL. Plasticity of adult stem cells. Cell 2004; 116: 639–48.
18. Hwang WS, Ryu YJ, Park JH et al. Evidence of a pluripotent human embryonic stem cell line derived from a cloned blastocyst. Science 2004; 303: 1660–74.

19. Schofield R. The relationship between the spleen colony-forming cell and the haemopoietic stem cell. Blood Cells 1978; 4: 7–25.
20. Moorre KA, Lemischka IR. Stem cells and their niches. Science 2006; 311: 1880–5.
21. Salim A, Giaccia AJ, Longaker MT. Stem cell differentiation. Nature 2004, 22: 804–5.
22. Song L, Webb NE, Song Y, Tuan RS. Identification and functional analysis of candidate genes regulating mesenchymal stem cell self-renewal and multipotency. Stem Cell 2006; 24: 1707–18.
23. Fuchs E, Tumbar T, Guasch G. Socializing with the neighbors: stem cells and their niche. Cell 2004; 116: 769–78.
24. Sanai N, Tramontin AD, Quinones-Hinojosa A et al. Unique astrocyte ribbon in adult human brain contains neural stem cells but lacks chain migration. Nature 2004: 427: 740–4.
25. Nunes MC, Roy NS, Keyoung HM et al. Identification and isolation of multipotential neural progenitor cells from the subcortical white matter of the adult human brain. Nat Med 2003; 9: 439–47.
26. Schwab KE, Chan RW, Gargett CE. Putative stem cell activity of human endometrial epithelial and stromal cells during the menstrual cycle. Fertil Steril 2005; 84(Supp 2): 1124–30.
27. Körbling M, Katz RL, Khanna A et al. Hepatocytes and epithelial cells of donor origin in recipients of peripheral-blood stem cells. N Engl J Med 2002; 346: 738–46.
28. Kai T, Spradling A. An empty Drosophila stem cell niche reactivates the proliferation of ectopic cells. Proc Natl Acad Sci USA 2003; 100: 4633–8.
29. Fukuda K. Progress in myocardial regeneration and cell translatation. Circ J 2005; 9: 1431–46.
30. Friedenstein AJ, Piatetzky-Shapiro II, Petrakova KV. Osteogenesis in transplants of bone marrow cells. J Embryol Exp Morphol 1966; 16: 381–90.
31. Portmann-Lanz CB, Schoeberlein A, Huber A et al. Placental mesenchymal stem cells as potential autologous graft for pre- and perinatal neurogeneration. Am J Obstet Gynecol 2006; 194: 664–73.
32. Digirolamo CM, Stokes D, Colter D et al. Propagation and senescence of human marrow stromal cells in culture: a simple colony-forming assay identifies samples with the greatest potential to propagate and differentiate. Br J Haematol 1999; 107: 275–81.
33. Kemp CK, Hows J, Donaldson C. Bone marrow-derived mesenchymal stem cells. Leuk Lymph 2005; 46: 1531–44.
34. Kucia M, Reca R, Jala VR et al. Bone marrow as a home of heterogeneous population of nonhematopoietic stem cell. Leukemia 2005; 199: 1118–27.
35. Baddoo M, Hill K, Wilkison R et al. Characterization of mesenchymal stem cells isolated from murine bone marrow by negative selection. J Cell Biochem 2003; 89: 1235–49.
36. Lagase E, Connors H, Al-Dahalimy M et al. Purified hematopoietic stem cells can differentiate into hepatocytes in vivo. Nat Med 2000; 6: 1229–34.
37. Jin HK, Carter JE, Huntley GW et al. Intracerebral transplantation of mesenchymal stem cells into acid sphingomyelinase-deficient mice delays the onset of neurological abnormalities and extends their life span. J Clin Invest 2002; 109: 1183–91.
38. Quiani F, Urbanek K, Beltrami AP et al. Chimerism of the transplanted heart. N Engl J Med 2002; 346: 5–15.
39. Krause DS, Theise ND, Collector MI et al. Multi-organ, multi-lineage engraftment by a single bone marrow-derived stem cell. Cell 2001; 105: 369–77.
40. Quesenberry PJ, Dooner G, Colvin G, Abedi M. Stem cell biology and the plasticity polemic. Exp Hematol 2005; 33: 389–94.
41. Tsai RY, Kittappa R, McKay RD. Plasticity, niches, and the use of stem cells. Dev Cell 2002; 2: 707–12.
42. Choi JB, Uchino H, Azuma K et al. Little evidence of transdifferentiation of bone marrow-derived cells into pancreatic beta cells. Diabetologia 2003; 46: 1366–74.
43. Bjornson CR, Rietze RL, Reynolds BA et al. Turning brain into blood: a hematopoietic fate adopted by adult neural stem cells in vivo. Science 1999; 283: 534–7.
44. LaBarge MA, Blau HM. Biological progression from adult bone marrow to monucleate muscle stem cell to multinucleate muscle fiber in response to injury. Cell 2002; 111: 589–601.
45. Ceradini DJ, Kulkarni AR, Callaghan MJ et al. Progenitor cell trafficking is regulated by hypoxic gradients through HIF-1 induction of SDF-1. Nat Med 2004; 10: 858–64.
46. Lapidot T, Dar A, Kollet O. How the stem cells find their way home? Blood 2005; 106: 1901–10.
47. Chan RWS, Schwab KE, Gargett CE. Clonogenicity of human endometrial epithelial and stromal cells. Biol Reprod 2004; 70: 1738–50.
48. Banu NS, Manyonda IT. Alternative medical and surgical options to hysterectomy. Best Pract Res Clin Obstet Gynecol 2005; 19: 431–49.
49. D'Hooghe TM, Kyama C, Debrock S, Meuleman C, Mwenda JM. Future directions in endometriosis research. Ann NY Acad Sci 2004; 1034: 316–25.
50. Trokoudes KM, Minbattiwalla MB, Kalogirou L et al. Controlled natural cycle IVF with antagonist use and blastocyst transfer. Reprod Biomed Online 2005; 11: 685–9.
51. Giudice LC, Telles TL, Lobo S et al. The molecular basis for implantation failure in endometriosis: on

the road to discovery. Ann NY Acad Sci 2002; 955: 252–64.

52. Taylor HS, Bagot C, Kardana A et al. HOX gene expression is altered in the endometrium of women with endometriosis. Hum Reprod 1999; 5: 1328–31.

53. Seli E, Kayisli UA, Cakmak H et al. Removal of hydrosalpinges increases endometrial leukaemia inhibitory factor (LIF) expression at the time of the implantation window. Hum Reprod 2005; 20: 3012–17.

54. Benecke C, Kruger TF, Siebert TI et al. Effect of fibroids on fertility in patients undergoing assisted reproduction. A structured literature review. Gynecol Obstet Invest 2005; 59: 225–30.

55. Anker PS, Scherjon SA, Keur CK et al. Isolation of mesenchymal stem cells of fetal or maternal origin from human placenta. Stem Cells 2004; 22: 1338–45.

56. Diamond MP, Freeman ML. Clinical implications of postsurgical adhesions. Hum Reprod Update 2001; 7: 567–76.

57. Brockes JP, Kumar A. Appendage regeneration in adult vertebrates and implications for regenerative medicine. Science 2005; 310: 1919–23.

58. Odorico JS, Kaufman DS, Thomson JA. Multilineage differentiation from human embryonic stem cells lines. Stem Cell 2001; 19: 193–204.

59. Kassem M. Mesenchymal stem cells: biological characteristics and potential clinical applications. Cloning Stem Cell 2004; 6: 369–74.

60. Bruder SP, Fink DJ, Caplan AI. Mesenchymal stem cells in bone development, bone repair, and skeletal regeneration therapy. J Cell Biochem 1994; 56: 283–94.

61. Wollert KC, Meyer GP, Lotz J. Intracoronary autologous bone-marrow cell transfer after myocardial infarction: the BOOST randomized controlled trial. Lancet 2004; 364: 141–8.

62. Horwitz EM, Gordon PL, Koo WK. Isolated allogeneic bone marrow-derived mesenchymal cells engraft and stimulate growth in children with osteogenesis imperfecta. Implications for cell therapy of bone. Proc Natl Acad Sci USA 2002; 99: 8932–7.

63. Allay JA, Dennis JE, Haynesworth SE. Lacz and interleukin-3 expression in vivo after retroviral transduction of marrow-derived human osteogenic mesenchymal progenitor. Hum Gene Ther 1997; 8: 1417–27.

64. Studeny M, Marini FC, Champlin RE et al. Bone marrow-derived mesenchymal stem cells are vehicles for interferon-beta delivery into tumors. Cancer Res 2002; 62: 3603–8.

65. Stock UA, Vacanti JP. Tissue engineering: current state and prospects. Annu Rev Med 2001; 52: 443–51.

66. Kon E, Muraglia A, Corsi A et al. Autologous bone marrow stromal cells loaded onto porous hydroxyapatite ceramic accelerate bone repair in critical-size defects of sheep long bones. J Biomed Mater Res 2000; 49: 328–37.

67. Carlen M, Cassidy RM, Brismar H et al. Functional integration of adult-born neurons. Curr Biol 2002; 12: 606–8.

CHAPTER 11

Selection of embryos for stem cell derivation: can we optimize the process?

Anna Veiga, Maria Vicenta Camarasa, Begoña Aran, Angel Raya and Juan Carlos Izpisua Belmonte

INTRODUCTION

Human embryonic stem cells (hESCs) represent a great potential source of cells for therapeutic uses, including cell therapy, and for required prior research, basic or translational. Parkinson's disease, spinal cord injury, heart failure and bone marrow failure are examples of pathological conditions amenable to being corrected by means of stem cell transplantation.[1,2] However, the regenerative medicine applications of ESCs are only one aspect of hESC research potential. They are an invaluable research tool to study human development, and can serve as a platform to develop and test new drugs and treatment protocols.[3]

Since the first report of derivation from a human blastocyst in 1998,[4] most stem cell lines derived have been obtained from surplus embryos from in-vitro fertilization (IVF) programs, donated by couples not willing to use them for their own transfer or for donation to other couples. Some regulatory policies allow the use for research of embryos generated for reproductive purposes but lacking parental project, including the derivation of ESC lines. Many reports have been published on the availability of embryos for research and different patient's attitudes have been described.[5–8] Ethics committees from scientific societies have made recommendations on this topic and the European Society for Human Reproduction and Embryology (ESHRE) Task Force on Ethics and Law and the Ethics Committee of the American Society for Reproductive Medicine have established guidelines for the donation of oocytes and embryos for research, including stem cell derivation.[9,10]

Derivation methodology is still today highly empirical, and various protocols are used in the different steps of the process, including feeder cell preparation (if feeder cells are used), inner cell mass (ICM) isolation and initial steps of derivation. It is worth mentioning that the final goal in derivation attempts is to achieve derivation and hESC culture in feeder[11,12] and animal-free conditions,[13] and in chemically defined culture conditions.[14,15] Such conditions, as well as derivation in Good Manufacturing Practice (GMP) environment, are necessary for the safe clinical use of ESCs in human therapy. It is also important to note that hESCs, when considered for therapy in the European Union (EU), will have to follow the EU Tissues and Cells Directives (2004/23; 2006/17),[16,17] which regulates the use of any cells in humans.

In the present chapter, we focus on ESC derivation, especially relating to embryo origin, stage and quality as well as the first steps of hESC derivation. As described and reviewed in Tables 11.1 and 11.2, where the cell lines published to date are reported, many different protocols have been used and the efficiencies published are also very variable. We review embryo culture techniques, ICM isolation methods and alternatives, technical aspects of initial splitting from the ICM outgrowth and, finally, derivations from preblastocysts and from abnormal embryos.

Table 11.1 Reported hESC derivations: author, year, center, number of embryos, number of inner cell mass (ICM), number or names of derived cell lines, derivation efficiency per ICM

First author	*Year*	*Laboratory*	*No. of embryos*	*ICM (n)*	*Cell lines*	*Efficiency (%)*[a]
Thomson[4]	1998	WiCell, USA	36	14	H1, H7, H9, H13, H14	36
Reubinoff[31]	2000	Monash Inst, Australia/Singapore	N/A	2	HES-1, HES2	–
Lanzendorf[29]	2001	Jones Inst for Reprod Med, USA	110	18	ES-76, ES-78-1, ES-78-2	17
Amit[40]	2002	Rambam Med, Center, Israel	5	5	I-3, I-4, I-6	60
Richards[52]	2002	Dept Obstet Gynecol NU Singapore	1	1	1	–
Hovatta[32]	2003	Karolinska Inst, Sweden	5	2	HS181, HS207	40
Mitalipova[26]	2003	BresaGen, USA	19	8	BG01, BG02, BG03, BG04	50
Park J[53]	2003	MizMedi Hosp, Seoul, Korea	N/A	30	3	10
Pickering[38]	2003	Guy's, King's & St Thomas Med, UK	58	24	3	13
Baharvand[27]	2004	Royan Inst, Iran	N/A	1	Royan H11	–
Heins[54]	2004	Cellartis AB, Sweden	N/A	N/A	SA002, FC018, AS034, AS038, SA121 SA181(abn)	N/A
Cowan[33]	2004	Howard Hughes Medical Inst, USA	286 clev.+ 58 blasts	97	HUES1-17	18
Park S[55]	2004	Maria Infertility, Hosp, Korea	20 blastos 20 Pron.	11 3	MB01-07 MB08-09	64 67
Sjögren[20]	2004	Goteborg Univ, Sweden	748	114	22	19
Stojkovic[24]	2004	Univ Newcastle, UK	11 day – 2 embryos	7	HES-NCL1	14
Strelchenko[43]	2004	Reprod Genetic Inst, Chicago, USA	46 morula 39 blast 32 ICM	11 12 5	8 7 5	17 18 16
Suss-Toby[34]	2004	Rambam Med Center, Israel	60	6	19	17

(*Continued*)

Table 11.1 *(Continued)*

Chen[25]	2005	Tongji Hospital, People's Republic of China	130	10	2	20
Findikli[21]	2005	Istanbul Mem Hosp, Turkey	31	N/A	7	N/A
Genbacev[13]	2005	UCSF, USA	192 321	14 10	UCSF-2 UCSF-1	7 10
Inzunza[42]	2005	Karolinska Inst, Sweden	10	N/A	HS293, HS206	N/A
Kim HS[39]	2005	Seoul Nat Univ, Korea	47	13	N/A	N/A
Kim SJ[56]	2005	MizMedi Hosp, Korea	N/A	16	Miz-Hes 4–8, 10–13	47
Klimanskaya[12]	2005	ACT, USA	N/A	5	ACT-14	20
Lee[57]	2005	MRC MizMedi Hosp, Korea	8 PN-stage	7	Miz-endol, -2, -3	43
Li[58]	2005	Hosp Sun Yat-sen Univ, China	N/A	4	CHES-1	25
van de Stolpe[37]	2005	Hubrecht Lab, The Nederlands	22	N/A	NL-HESC1	N/A
Oh[60]	2005	MRC, Seoul Nat Univ, Korea	73	10	SNUhES1-3	30
Pickering[46]	2005	Guy's, King's & St Thomas Med, UK	N/A	N/A	CF1 abn	N/A
Simon[36]	2005	Centro de Investigación Principe Felipe, Valencia	40	16	VAL-1, VAL-2	13
Verlinsky[35]	2005	RGI Chicago, USA	72	N/A	18 abn	N/A
Wang[61]	2005	Xiinhua Hosp, China	N/A	N/A	SH1, SH2, SH7	N/A
Baharvand[48]	2006	Royan Inst, Iran	N/A	N/A	Royan H2-3-4-5-6 (abn)	N/A
Hampl[b]	2006	Acad Sci Czech Republic	98	14	CCTL8, 9, 6, 10, 12, 14	42
Ludwig[15]	2006	WiCell	N/A	N/A	WA15, WA16	N/A
Lysdahl[59]	2006	Aalborg Univ, Denmark	198	23	CLS1, CLS2, CLS3, CLS4	17

(Continued)

Table 11.1 (*Continued*)

First author	*Year*	*Laboratory*	*No. of embryos*	*ICM (B)*	*Cell lines*	*Efficiency (%)*[a]
Mandal[62]	2006	Reliance Life Sciences, India	N/A	N/A	ReliCell®hES1	N/A
Mateizel[47]	2006	Res C Reprod Genetics, Belgium	69	52	VUB 1, 2, 3, 4, 5 (abn)	10

[a]Derivation efficiency, per ICM
[b]Unpublished results. Source: www.isscr.org/science/documents/reportdvorak.pdf

Table 11.2 Reported hESC derivation parameters: fresh/frozen embryos, choice of feeders, ICM isolation, initial split conditions

First author	*Embryo source*	*Feeders*[a]	*ICM isolation*[b]	*Culture (days) before ICM isolation*[c]	*Initial split*[d]
Thomson[4]	Fresh/ frozen	Irrad MEF	IS	N/A	M/D/9–15
Reubinoff[31]	Frozen	MitoC MEF	IS	6	MD
Lanzendorf[29]	Fresh	Irrad MEF	IS	6	M4-11
Amit[40]	Frozen	MEF	IS/M	N/A	M
Richards[52]	Frozen	MitoC HF (FetMusl)	IS	N/A	MD 10
Hovatta[32]	Fresh	Irrad postnatHFF	IS	6	D9–19
Mitalipova[26]	Frozen	Irrad MEF	IS	6–7	M7–10
Park J[53]	Frozen	MitoC MEF	IS	N/A	8
Pickering[38]	Fresh/frozen	MitoC MEF	IS	5/6	M2–15
Baharvand[27]	N/A	MitoC MEF	M	6	MD10
Heins[54]	Fresh/frozen	MitoC MEF	IS/W	6–7	M7–14
Cowan[33]	Frozen	MitoC MEF	IS	N/A	M
Park S[55]	Frozen	MitoC STO	IS	N/A	M5–8
Sjögren[20]	Fresh/frozen	MEF	IS/W	6–7	N/A
Stojkovic[24]	Fresh	Irrad MEF	IS	8	M17
Strelchenko[43]	Fresh/frozen	MitoC MEF or BRL	IS/W	N/A	N/A
Suss-Toby[34]	Fresh	Inact MEF	W	N/A	M

(*Continued*)

Table 11.2 *(Continued)*

Chen[25]	Fresh	MitoC MEF	Immuno	5–8	M5–8
Findikli[21]	Fresh	MitoC MEF	IS/W	5–7	7–10
Genbacev[13]	Frozen/fresh	Human placental fibroblasts	W	6–7	M14–35
Inzunza[42]	3 frozen, 7 fresh	Irrad HFF	IS	6	M12
Kim HS[39]	Frozen	MitoC STO	IS/M/W	5–7	M7
Kim SJ[56]	Frozen	MitoC MEF	IS	N/A	M7
Klimanskaya[12]	Frozen	MitoC lysed MEFs	IS	N/A	N/A
Lee[57]	Frozen	MitoC human endometrial	IS	N/A	M6–8
Li[58]	Frozen	Irrad MEF	IS	N/A	–
var de Stolpe[37]	Fresh	MitoC MEF	IS	N/A	MD8
Oh[60]	Frozen	MitoC STO	IS/W	5–7	M7–8
Pickering[46]	Fresh PGD	N/A	N/A	N/A	M17
Simon[36]	Frozen	Human placental	No immuno	N/A	M15 M21
Wang[61]	N/A	Irrad MEF 55Gy EDF	IS	N/A	M/C 10–14
Verlinsky[35]	Fresh PGD	MitoC MEF or BRL	–	–	ED8–14
Baharvand[48]	N/A	MitoC MEF	IS	5–5	MD 10
Hampl[e]	Frozen	MEF	IS	N/A	4–12
Ludwig[15]	Frozen	–	IS	>7	M14–21
Lysdahl[59]	Fresh	Irrad HFF	IS	N/A	M10–15
Mandal[62]	–	–	–	–	–
Mateizel[47]	Frozen/fresh	Irrad/MitoC MEF	IS	N/A	N/A

[a]MitoC, inactivation by mitomycin; Irrad, inactivation by irradiation
[b]IS, Immunosurgery; M, mechanical isolation; W, whole blastocyst seeding
[c]Days of development at the time of ICM isolation
[d]Method of first split (M = mechanical; D = dispase; C = collagenase) and days after initial seeding
[e]Hampl – unpubhshed results. Source: www.isscr.org/science/documents/reportdvorat.pdf
MEF, mouse embryonic fibroblasts; STO, commercial name. Feeder cells, mouse. HFF, human foreskin fibroblasts; BRL, buffalo rat liver; PGD, preimplantation genetic diagnosis

As the hESC research field is progressing rather quickly, established guidelines and protocols are needed to standardize the methodologies involved to increase the efficiency in derivation.

EMBRYO CULTURE

Embryos donated for stem cell derivation are, most of the times, surplus embryos in excess after embryo transfer, in which the best embryos are replaced in the uterus. As a result, they are frequently frozen embryos not intended for further pregnancy attempts, even though fresh ones have been used for derivation, either from conventional IVF or from preimplantation genetic diagnosis (PGD) programs (see Table 11.2).

Embryos frozen at different developmental stages and cryopreserved for variable periods of times have been made available for hESC derivation. Embryos at the pronuclear or early cleavage stages or blastocysts can be considered as a source of hESC lines, when donated by the couples for research. An aspect to be considered is the fact that zygotes (frozen at the pronuclear stage) and early embryos (day 2 – 4 cell, day 3 – 6–8 cell) have to be cultured to achieve blastocyst development, and are typically used for hESC derivation. Also, the quality of such embryos and, as a result, the survival rate after thawing, are essential factors to be considered when attempting to improve the efficiency of derivation. Freezing protocols and the selection criteria of the embryos to be frozen have changed in recent years and it is presumed that embryos frozen a number of years ago could have reduced survival rates and, as a consequence, reduced blastocyst rates would be achieved with such material. Thus, both the survival rate of the frozen embryos and the blastocyst rate achieved with zygotes and early-cleavage embryos are important parameters to control in hESC derivation attempts.

The experience acquired in embryo culture techniques in IVF laboratories has been essential when attempting hESC derivation.[18] Embryo quality (day 2, day 4, blastocyst) is strictly correlated with the implantation potential attained in IVF programs.[19] It would seem that embryo quality is also a key factor for derivation success.

Culture of embryos to the blastocyst stage for stem cell derivation follows the same guidelines and protocols used in IVF laboratories. Thus, an important step in the establishment of an hESC line is to culture the human embryo until it forms a good-quality blastocyst.

It has been described that hESC lines are more efficiently obtained from frozen blastocysts than from frozen cleavage-stage embryos, since the poor quality of many of the latter after thawing prevents their further development.[20,21] As previously mentioned, high rates of survival after cryopreservation of good-quality embryos result in higher blastocyst rates after culture. Therefore, securing high-quality embryos and optimizing embryo culture conditions are important to increase the efficiency in the establishment of hESC lines.

Currently, culture systems in assisted reproduction involve the use of sequential media for embryo development and culture to the blastocyst stage. It has to be reminded that years ago, in the 1990s, this was achieved through the use of feeder cell support, such as primate Vero, human granulosa or endometrial cells.[22] Some of these systems are still in use in certain laboratories. An important factor to achieving good embryo quality is good overall practice in embryo manipulation and handling: quality control in IVF laboratories as well as standardization of methodologies and technological improvements help to maintain embryos in controlled and optimal conditions at all stages. Risk minimization by regular equipment control and limited workflow are very important to keep intrinsic embryo developmental potential to a maximum.

Sequential culture is routinely used from fertilization to fully expanded blastocyst stage in IVF laboratories using homemade or commercial media. The composition of the different media used tries to fulfil the requirements of the embryos at different stages of development.[23]

Recently, a culture system with three-step sequential media was described.[24] The embryos are cultured in conventional sequential media (two steps) up to day 6, followed by culture in a third medium up to day 8 (DMEM supplemented with Glasgow medium, conditioned by buffalo rat liver cell lines). The addition of leukemia inhibiting factor (LIF) improves the blastocyst rate. According to the reported results, the increase in the number of ICM cells achieved through culture to day 8 would be beneficial for improvement in derivation efficiency.

EMBRYO QUALITY: RELATIONSHIP WITH HUMAN EMBRYONIC STEM CELL DERIVATION

Embryo quality is assessed according to morphological parameters that have been clearly determined and described.

Morphological assessment that considers pronuclear patterns, number and symmetry of the cells and percentage of fragmentation is routinely used in IVF laboratories to assess proper development characteristics. The time of the first cleavage and the presence of mononucleated cells have also been proposed as predictive factors of embryo viability. Scoring systems for zygotes, early cleavage embryos and blastocysts have been described.

Regarding blastocyst quality, parameters such as the degree of expansion and the hatching status, as well as the ICM and trophectoderm (TE) development, are considered for classification (Figures 11.1 and 11.2). Different authors use different nomenclature systems for blastocyst grading, but parameters subjected to evaluation are common, as follows:

Developmental stage, expansion degree (related to the size of the blastocoelic cavity), ICM grading (morphology, size and compaction of ICM cells), trophectoderm grading (morphology of the trophectodermal epithelium).

The scoring system proposed by Gardner et al[19] classifies blastocysts as:

1 early blastocyst
2 young blastocyst
3 full blastocyst
4 expanded blastocyst
5 hatching blastocyst
6 hatched blastocyst

ICM:

A: tightly packed, many cells
B: loosely grouped, several cells
C: very few cells

TE:

A: many cells forming a cohesive epithelium
B: few cells forming a loose epithelium
C: very few large cells

The efficiency of derivation has been correlated with blastocyst developmental stage and it would seem that day 7 blastocysts achieve a higher derivation rate than earlier blastocyst stages,[20] probably owing to the larger number of ICM cells.

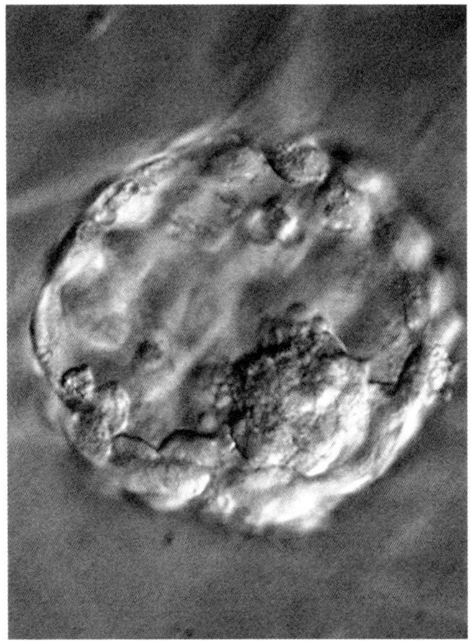

Figure 11.1 High morphological score blastocyst after zona pellucida removal

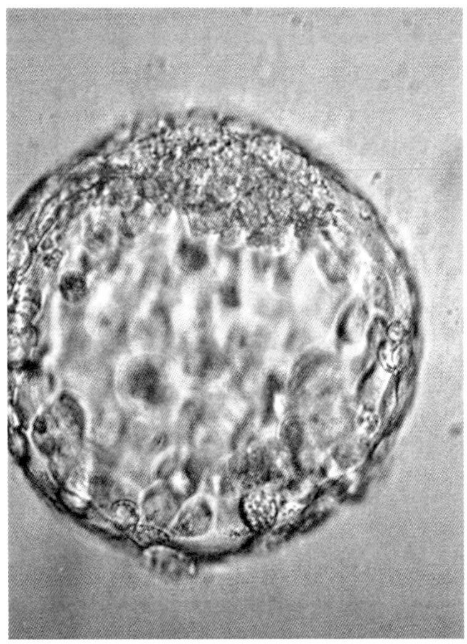

Figure 11.2 Low morphological score blastocyst

The use of poor-quality embryos, discarded after IVF procedures, is frequent in protocols of stem cell derivation. It has to be pointed out that such embryos achieve low blastocyst rates and, as a result, would achieve low efficiency in the derivation. For research purposes, these poor-quality (low morphological score) human embryos have proven useful, even with low success rates, for stem cell line derivation.

When trying to find a correlation between blastocyst quality and derivation efficiency, it has been reported that higher efficiency rates are attained with good-quality blastocysts, even though hESC lines have been obtained with low-score blastocysts.[21,25–27]

Regarding ICM morphology and size, clumps with higher numbers of cells have more chances of attaching and proliferating, although this cannot be taken as a predictive parameter isolated from the developmental history of the blastocyst. As mentioned before, prolonged culture periods favor greater cell numbers in the ICM in day 8 blastocysts and this would allow more efficient derivation of hESCs with respect to 'younger' ones.[24]

Blastocyst quality and developmental stage and parameters such as ICM size and shape have to be assessed when attempting stem cell derivation. Most probably there is a critical ICM size under which further growth towards the establishment of hESC colonies is not achievable. This threshold has yet to be established.

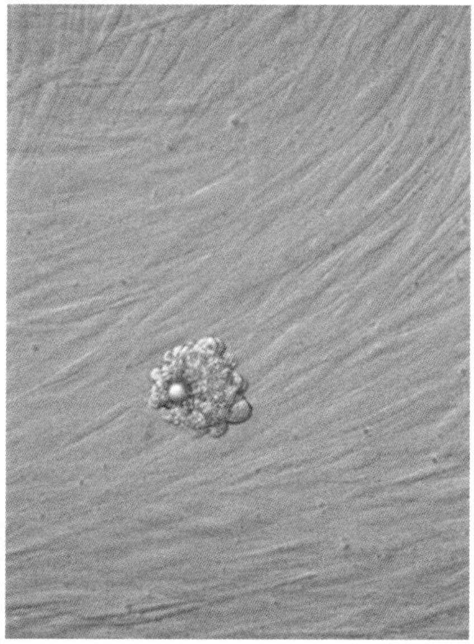

Figure 11.3 ICM isolated by immunosurgery

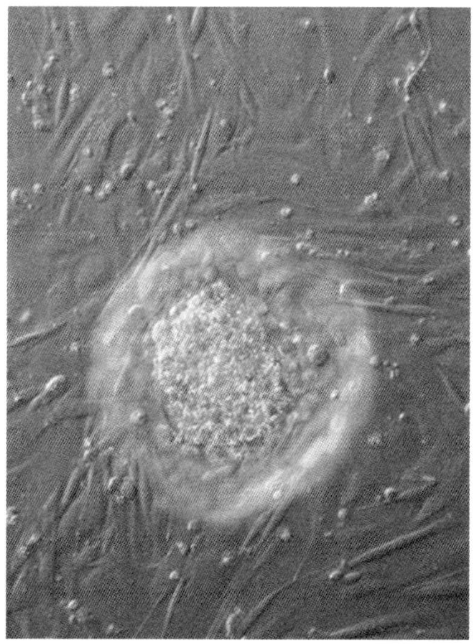

Figure 11.4 Whole blastocyst seeding

DERIVATION METHODOLOGIES

Inner cell mass isolation and seeding

The first report of the successful separation of human ICM cells and their culture in vitro was published in 1994 by Bongso and co-workers.[28] The ICM lump was separated mechanically from TE cells and produced cells with stem cell-like morphology that were cultured for at least two passages.

The mechanical isolation of the ICM was substituted by the removal of TE cells by immunosurgery (IS) using specific antibodies.[4,29] Immunosurgery was first described in mouse blastocysts by Solter and Knowles[30] and is currently the most widely used method of ICM isolation for hESC derivation (Figure 11.3).

Trophectoderm elimination and ICM isolation by immunosurgery have been used by most groups conducting hESC derivation from surplus embryos from IVF programs. Other methods of ICM isolation have been described, including total or partial mechanical isolation or no isolation, as in the case of whole embryo seeding[24,31–38] (Figure 11.4).

From the review of the literature (see Table 11.2), it is not clear whether certain hESC lines have emerged from immunosurgical or mechanical protocols, so a comparison in efficiency for both methods is not always possible. It would seem that the methodology preferred is related to the morphology and quality of the blastocyst and ICM and to the experience and skills of the group. When the comparison of results from the different techniques is possible, the use of IS shows higher derivation rates than the other methods proposed. The importance of eliminating all the TE cells prior to the seeding of the ICM seems to be relative, as some authors have derived hESC lines with partial mechanical ICM isolation or with direct culture of whole blastocyst. Trophectoderm residuals in early passages are not absolutely deleterious for ICM development and culture, although it is a common belief that TE growth can impair ICM development and the establishment of the initial colony of hESCs.

A recent publication[39] describes different derivation methodologies according to blastocyst quality, especially with respect to the morphology of the TE and the ICM. Thus, in cases when the latter is graded the best quality, a mechanical or immunosurgical protocol is preferred to isolate the ICM in order to seed as few residual trophectoderms as possible. Also, a pulled glass pipette, with a diameter slightly larger than the ICM to be isolated, is frequently used to help TE elimination by gentle pipetting after immunosurgery. Needles (27G) have been also used to remove TE cells.[40] In cases in which the ICM is small but distinguishable, and TE is not formed by many tight cells, partial biopsy by mechanical means is preferred to diminish the TE bulk in the initial seeding. A finely drawn glass pipette or a needle is used to excise the trophectoderm, separating the ICM. To isolate the ICM, minimizing cell loss, or in cases in which no ICM is distinguishable in the blastocyst, it has been reported that whole-embryo culture can be performed. After successive splitting of outgrowths and elimination of expanding TE cells, some cell lines have been derived using this approach.[39] These derivations are the most challenging, as the expansion of the TE cells can impair stem cell growth, owing to their difference in size and their overexpansion during culture.

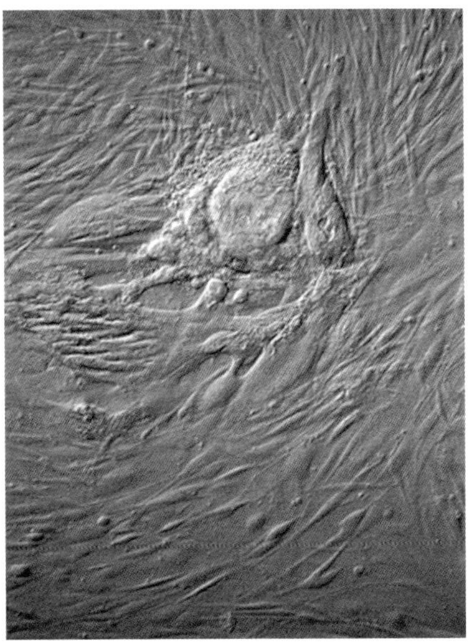

Figure 11.5 ICM outgrowth over human foreskin fibroblasts feeder layer

As stem cell research is evolving and xenobiotic-free stem cell lines derivation is pursued, the avoidance of animal antisera used for immunosurgery is a requirement so that mechanical isolation of the ICM will be the method of choice. The use of lasers, already described for blastocyst biopsy in PGD,[41] may also be a useful alternative method.

Following the ICM initial growth (Figure 11.5) up to the first distinguishable hESC colony is perhaps the most critical step during stem cell derivation. The morphology and the growth rate of the initial ICM proliferation are variable and the first structure observed is usually composed of flat, irregular cells. The first ICM outgrowth is a small, compact or tightly packed group of round cells with prominent nucleoli, organized in an individual cell colony, forming a distinct ball of cells growing on top of the rest of the outgrowth. Experience helps in differentiating adequate initial outgrowths from differentiating ones, and clearly from TE cells, which are always more flat and grow as a monolayer. The success of the derivation may be in the timing of the first split, passaging this clump of ESCs adequately. Individual follow-up of each derivation procedure is mandatory for protocol adaptation.

Nevertheless, when the whole-embryo culture method is used, and taking into account that these cases correspond to unclear and/or undistinguishable ICM, following the growth of a putative colony is more difficult. In those cases, the isolation of hESC-like outgrowth from TE and differentiated cells requires a great deal of care and caution, as well as good cell-handling skills.

Mechanical splitting of the first ICM outgrowth is performed by fine technical procedures with pulled glass pipettes or metal needles, to isolate and split the structure of packed cells that is observed on top of the feeder layer forming a 'dome', 4–14 days after ICM seeding (passage 0). To help cell line establishment,

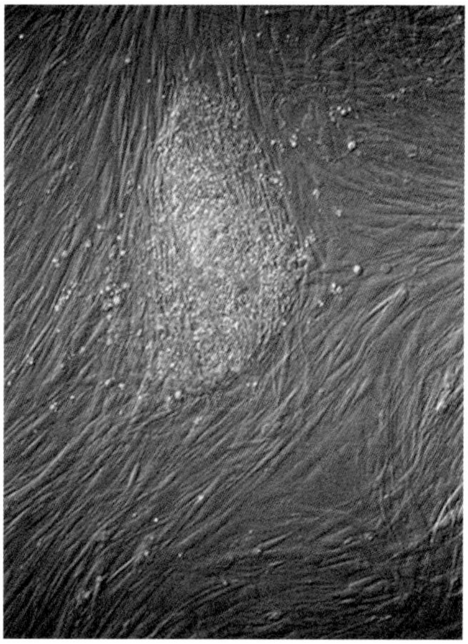

Figure 11.6 Putative stem cell colony, 1st passage

additives such as LIF, Plasmanate, insulin–transferrin–selenium (ITS) complex and/or serum can be added, which can be omitted from the culture medium after cell growth has been established.[42]

The failure to isolate the hESC initial outgrowth can be the result of suboptimal manipulation or may be due to intrinsic poor quality of the blastocysts used for derivation. Until an hESC colony with typical morphology is formed, several splits are required to effectively establish a new stem cell line, and initial outgrowths are regarded as 'progenic' hESC lines[20] (Figure 11.6).

Derivation from preblastocyst stage embryos

It is known that ESCs are pluripotent only during a narrow window during development. No embryonic stem cell lines have ever been derived from post-implantation blastocysts, but there are reports of the derivation of new hESC lines from human morula and from preblastocyst mouse embryos,[43,44] and, in the mouse and in the human, from single blastomeres.[45–46]

In hESC derivation from morulae, hESC lines are obtained after the injection of the naked morula under the feeder layer with the use of a micromanipulator. The efficiency achieved in the derivation of hESC lines from human morula is similar to that obtained with blastocysts and there are differences in morphology or in the patterns of expression markers in the hESC lines obtained with either method.[43]

A high efficiency is also reported in the derivation of mouse embryonic stem cells (mESCs) from morula and early-cleavage stages. mESC lines derived from morula or early-cleavage embryos might originate before the cells are allocated to ICM or TE. The potential of such lines has yet to be established, but it is conceivable that they may have a wider differentiation potential than the ones derived from blastocysts. It has been suggested that the stage of development from which ESCs are originated may be an important factor to take into account for their use in cell differentiation research.[44]

Cell lines from abnormal embryos: disease models

After the first proposal of PGD in the 1960s as an alternative to prenatal diagnosis in couples with known genetic disorders, embryos were first clinically sexed for selection against an X-linked disorder in 1990,[45] and, since then, the PGD field has been expanding by the addition of new diagnostic protocols for different disorders. After the establishment of diagnosis, the affected embryos are obviously not suitable for replacement, and can be used for research (e.g. stem cell derivation) if donated by the couples after informed consent.

Derivation of hESC lines has been achieved with embryos affected by genetic disorders.[35,46,47] Thalassemia, Fanconi's anemia, myotonic dystrophy, Huntington's disease, neurofibromatosis, Marfan syndrome, adrenoleukodystrophy, muscular dystrophies (Duchenne's and Becker's dystrophies), fragile site mental retardation syndrome and cystic fibrosis have been modeled now on hESC lines which are available for the research community as valuable tools for the study of the pathological mechanisms of such diseases. As a model of disease progression, naturally occurring mutations in hESCs represent a bona-fide system for elucidating the path of physiological mechanisms that underlie genetic disorders, as the mutant phenotype is expressed in its normal physiological context and proteins retain their natural expression patterns. The possibilities of having different lines with different mutations that cause the same disease in cases of complex genetic pathologies, such as muscular dystrophies, allow comparative physiopathological studies to be performed. Last but not least, pluripotential stem cells can be differentiated into many different cell types, and thus screenings for therapeutic compounds can be applied to many cell types using only one cell line.

Two triploid lines have also been derived recently. The first line was derived from a three-pronuclear embryo and the resulting cell line confirmed the triploid constitution. A mosaic triploid cell line was obtained from an apparently normally fertilized embryo.[48] The use of blastocysts resulting from abnormal fertilization patterns has been described with the derivation of a diploid cell line from a monopronuclear zygote.[34]

The possibility of self-correction of chromosomally abnormal embryos in culture by anaphase lag, non-disjunction or chromosome demolition has recently been demonstrated and thus abnormal embryos could be considered an extra source of chromosomally normal hESC.[49]

CONCLUSION

After reviewing the literature describing hESC line derivation (see Tables 11.1 and 11.2) up to August 2006, the reported details on derivations are not sufficient to identify an optimized methodology for efficient derivation. There is a wide range of efficiency rates among published studies and it is difficult to compare the data, as many different methodologies have been applied. In some of the reports, no data for analysis and comparison are available.

Embryo quality should be, as in IVF procedures, an important factor to consider for the success of hESC derivation, but there are a number of publications describing the use of poor-quality embryos and blastocysts for hESC derivation with adequate derivation rates.

Culture conditions play a major role in the first steps in derivation, and although the literature describes different methodological details and many variations in the originally reported protocol, it is clear that adequate supportive culture conditions, either with the use of feeders or with chemically defined culture media, are needed to allow initial growth of the hESCs.

Differences exist between individual hESC lines with respect to culture and passaging methods as well as to differentiation potential and it is probable that such differences may be related to the methodology used for derivation. There is a need for a standardization of the protocols used for hESC derivation in order to obtain cell lines with similar established characteristics, useful for research. Safe, proven protocols and GMP derivation are needed to envisage human therapy.

REFERENCES

1. Hoffman DI, Zellman GL, Fair CC et al. Cryopreserved embryos in the United States and their availability for research. Fertil Steril 2003; 79(5): 1063–9.
2. Trounson A. Derivation characteristics and perspectives for mammalian pluripotential stem cells. Reprod Fertil Dev 2005; 17(1–2): 135–41.
3. Pera MF, Trounson AO. Human embryonic stem cells: prospects for development. Development 2004; 131: 5515–25.
4. Thomson JA, Itskovitz-Eldor J, Shapiro SS et al. Embryonic stem cell lines derived from human blastocysts. Science 1998; 282: 1145–7.
5. Oghoetuoma JO, McKeating C, Horne G et al. Use of in-vitro fertilisation embryos cryopreserved for 5 years or more. Lancet 2000; 355: 1336.
6. Hoffman DI, Zellman GL, Fair CC et al. Society for Assisted Reproduction Technology (SART) and RAND. Cryopreserved embryos in the United States and their availability for research. Fertil Steril 2003; 79: 1063–9.
7. Bjuresten K, Hovatta O. Donation of embryos for stem cell research – how many couples consent? Hum Reprod 2003; 18: 1353–5.
8. Bangsboll S, Pinborg A, Yding Andersen C et al. Patients' attitudes towards donation of surplus cryopreserved embryos for treatment or research. Hum Reprod 2004; 19: 2415–9.
9. Ethics Committee of the American Society for Reproductive Medicine. Donating spare embryos for embryonic stem-cell research. Fertil Steril 2004; 82(Suppl 1): S224–S227.
10. ESHRE Taskforce on Ethics and Law. IV. Stem cells. Hum Reprod 2002; 17: 1409–10.
11. Amit M, Shariki C, Margulets V et al. Feeder layer- and serum-free culture of human embryonic stem cells. Biol Reprod 2004; 70: 837–45.
12. Klimanskaya I, Chung Y, Meisner L et al. Human embryonic stem cells derived without feeder cells. Lancet 2005; 365: 1636–41.
13. Genbacev O, Krtolica A, Zdravkovic T et al. Serum-free derivation of human embryonic stem cell lines on human placental fibroblast feeders. Fertil Steril 2005; 83: 1517–29.

14. Lu J, Hou R, Booth CJ et al. Defined culture conditions of human embryonic stem cells. Proc Natl Acad Sci USA 2006; 103: 5688–93.

15. Ludwig TE, Levenstein ME, Jones JM et al. Derivation of human embryonic stem cells in defined conditions. Nat Biotechnol 2006; 24: 185–7.

16. Directive 2004/23 of the European Parliament and the Council of 31 March 2004 on setting standards of quality and safety for the donation, procurement, testing, processing, preservation, storage and distribution of human tissues and cells.

17. Commission Directive 2006/17/EC of 8 February 2006 implementing Directive 2004/23 of the European Parliament and of the Council as regards certain technical requirements for the donation, procurement and testing of human tissues and cells.

18. Menezo Y, Veiga A, Benkhalifa M. Improved methods for blastocyst formation and culture. Hum Reprod 1998; 13(Suppl 4): 256–65.

19. Gardner DK, Lane M, Stevens J et al. Blastocyst score affects implantation and pregnancy outcome: towards a single blastocyst transfer. Fertil Steril 2000; 73: 1155–8.

20. Sjögren A, Hardarson T, Andersson K et al. Human blastocysts for the development of embryonic stem cells. Reprod Biomed Online 2004; 9: 326–9.

21. Findikli N, Kahraman S, Akcin O, Sertyel S, Candan Z. Establishment and characterization of new human embryonic stem cell lines. Reprod Biomed Online 2005; 10: 617–27.

22. Veiga A, Torello MJ, Menezo Y et al. Use of co-culture of human embryos on Vero cells to improve clinical implantation rate. Hum Reprod 1999; 14(Suppl 2): 112–20.

23. Gardner DK. Changes in requirements and utilization of nutrients during mammalian preimplantation embryo development and their significance in embryo culture. Theriogenology 1998; 49: 83–102.

24. Stojkovic M, Lako M, Stojkovic P et al. Derivation of human embryonic stem cells from day-8 blastocysts recovered after three-step in vitro culture. Stem Cells 2004; 22: 790–7.

25. Chen H, Qian K, Hu J et al. The derivation of two additional human embryonic stem cell lines from day 3 embryos with low morphological scores. Hum Reprod 2005; 20: 2201–06.

26. Mitalipova M, Calhoun J, Shin S et al. Human embryonic stem cell lines derived from discarded embryos. Stem Cells 2003; 21: 521–6.

27. Baharvand H, Ashtiani SK, Valojerdi MR et al. Establishment and in vitro differentiation of a new embryonic stem cell line from human blastocyst. Differentiation 2004; 72: 224–9.

28. Bongso A, Fong CY, Ng SC et al. Isolation and culture of inner cell mass cells from human blastocysts. Hum Reprod 1994; 9: 2110–17.

29. Lanzendorf SE, Boyd CA, Wright DL et al. Use of human gametes obtained from anonymous donors for the production of human embryonic stem cell lines. Fertil Steril 2001; 76: 132–7.

30. Solter D, Knowles BB. Immunosurgery of mouse blastocyst. Proc Natl Acad Sci USA 1975; 72: 5099–102.

31. Reubinoff BE, Pera MF, Fong CY et al. Embryonic stem cell lines from human blastocysts: somatic differentiation in vitro. Nat Biotechnol 2000; 18: 399–404.

32. Hovatta O, Mikkola M, Gertow K et al. A culture system using human foreskin fibroblasts as feeder cells allows production of human embryonic stem cells. Hum Reprod 2003; 18: 1404–09.

33. Cowan CA, Klimanskaya I, McMahon J et al. Derivation of embryonic stem-cell lines from human blastocysts. N Engl J Med 2004; 350: 1353–6.

34. Suss-Toby E, Gerecht-Nir S, Amit M et al. Derivation of a diploid human embryonic stem cell line from a mononuclear zygote. Hum Reprod 2004; 19: 670–5.

35. Verlinsky Y, Strelchenko N, Kukharenko V et al. Human embryonic stem cell lines with genetic disorders. Reprod Biomed Online 2005; 10: 105–10.

36. Simon C, Escobedo C, Valbuena D et al. First derivation in Spain of human embryonic stem cell lines: use of long-term cryopreserved embryos and animal-free conditions. Fertil Steril 2005; 83: 246–9.

37. van de Stolpe A, van den Brink S, van Rooijen M et al. Human embryonic stem cells: towards therapies for cardiac disease. Derivation of a Dutch human embryonic stem cell line. Reprod Biomed Online 2005; 11: 476–85.

38. Pickering SJ, Braude PR, Patel M et al. Preimplantation genetic diagnosis as a novel source of embryos for stem cell research. Reprod Biomed Online 2003; 7: 353–64.

39. Kim HS, Oh SK, Park YB et al. Methods for derivation of human embryonic stem cells. Stem Cells 2005; 23: 1228–33.

40. Amit M, Itskovitz-Eldor J. Derivation and spontaneous differentiation of human embryonic stem cells. J Anat 2002; 200(Pt 3): 225–232.

41. Veiga A, Sandalinas M, Benkhalifa M et al. Laser blastocyst biopsy for preimplantation diagnosis in the human. Zygote 1997; 5: 351–4.

42. Inzunza J, Gertow K, Stromberg MA et al. Derivation of human embryonic stem cell lines in serum replacement medium using postnatal human fibroblasts as feeder cells. Stem Cells 2005; 23: 544–9.

43. Strelchenko N, Verlinsky O, Kukharenko V et al. Morula-derived human embryonic stem cells. Reprod Biomed Online 2004; 9(6): 623–9.

44. Tesar PJ. Derivation of germ-line-competent embryonic stem cell lines from preblastocyst mouse embryos. Proc Natl Acad Sci USA 2005; 102(23): 8239–44.

45. Chung Y, Klimanskaya I, Becker S et al. Embryonic and extraembryonic stem cell lines derived from single mouse blastomeres. Nature 2006; 439(7073): 216–19.

46. Klimanskaya I, Chung Y, Becker S et al. Human embryonic stem cell lines derived from single blastomeres. Nature: advance online publication; 23 August 2006.

47. Handyside AH, Kontogianni EH, Hardy K, Winston RM. Pregnancies from biopsied human preimplantation embryos sexed by Y-specific DNA amplification. Nature 1990; 344: 768–70.

48. Pickering SJ, Minger SL, Patel M et al. Generation of a human embryonic stem cell line encoding the cystic fibrosis mutation deltaF508, using preimplantation genetic diagnosis. Reprod Biomed Online 2005; 10: 390–7.

49. Mateizel I, De Temmerman N, Ullmann U et al. Derivation of human embryonic stem cell lines from embryos obtained after IVF and after PGD for monogenic disorders. Hum Reprod 2006; 21: 503–11.

50. Baharvand H, Ashtiani SK, Taee A et al. Generation of new human embryonic stem cell lines with diploid and triploid karyotypes. Dev Growth Differ 2006; 48(2): 117–28.

51. Munne S, Velilla E, Colls P et al. Self-correction of chromosomally abnormal embryos in culture and implications for stem cell production. Fertil Steril 2005; 84: 1328–34.

52. Richards M, Fong CY, Chan WK et al. Human feeders support prolonged undifferentiated growth of human inner cell masses and embryonic stem cells. Nat Biotechnol 2002; 20: 933–6.

53. Park JH, Kim SJ, Oh EJ et al. Establishment and maintenance of human embryonic stem cells on STO, a permanently growing cell line. Biol Reprod 2003; 69: 2007–14.

54. Heins N, Englund MC, Sjoblom C et al. Derivation, characterization, and differentiation of human embryonic stem cells. Stem Cells 2004; 22(3): 367–76.

55. Park SP, Lee YJ, Lee KS et al. Establishment of human embryonic stem cell lines from frozen-thawed blastocysts using STO cell feeder layers. Hum Reprod 2004; 19(3): 676–84.

56. Kim SJ, Lee JE, Park JH et al. Efficient derivation of new human embryonic stem cell lines. Mol Cells 2005; 19(1): 46–53.

57. Lee JB, Lee JE, Park JH et al. Establishment and maintenance of human embryonic stem cell lines on human feeder cells derived from uterine endometrium under serum-free condition. Biol Reprod 2005; 72(1): 42–9.

58. Li T, Zhou CQ, Mai QY et al. Establishment of human embryonic stem cell line from gamete donors. Chin Med J (Engl) 2005; 118(2): 116–22.

59. Lysdahl H, Gabrielsen A, Minger SL et al. Derivation and characterization of four new human embryonic stem cell lines: the Danish experience. Reprod Biomed Online 2006; 12(1): 119–26.

60. Oh SK, Kim HS, Ahn HJ et al. Derivation and characterization of new human embryonic stem cell lines: SNUhES1, SNUhES2, and SNUhES3. Stem Cells 2005; 23(2): 211–19.

61. Wang Q, Fang ZF, Jin F et al. Derivation and growing human embryonic stem cells on feeders derived from themselves. Stem Cells 2005; 23(9): 1221–7.

62. Mandal A, Tipnis S, Pal R et al. Characterization and in vitro differentiation potential of a new human embryonic stem cell line, ReliCellhES1. Differentiation 2006; 74: 81–90.

CHAPTER 12

Harvesting of embryonic stem cells aimed at embryo conservation

Takumi Takeuchi, Noriko Tanaka, Queenie V Neri and Gianpiero D Palermo

INTRODUCTION

Because of their pluripotency – i.e. their ability to give rise to most tissue cell types – human embryonic stem cells (hESCs) could be used to treat debilitating or fatal conditions. For example, it appears that hESCs can be used to grow nerve cells that may help to repair spinal injuries and restore function to paralyzed limbs,[1,2] to grow heart muscle cells that can replace scar tissue after a heart attack,[3] to make neurons that would secrete dopamine and control Parkinson's disease[4] or cells producing insulin to cure diabetes.[5] It has also been proposed that hESCs may be able to regenerate bone marrow damaged by disease or radiation, to make blood cells genetically altered to resist specific infections such as human immunodeficiency virus (HIV) or simply replace diseased blood cells.[6] Because of these implications, much interest is being directed towards ESCs. On the other hand, hESC research is still controversial and some countries such as Germany, Austria, Norway and Switzerland have legislated against research that would create embryos for the sake of harvesting ESCs. Ireland, Hungary and Poland implicitly prohibit such research, stating that the right to life of the 'unborn child' must be respected and protected. In the USA, the Federal financing of such research is prohibited, but the authorization to conduct this is left to the discretion of each State, nine of which have so far prohibited such research.

ESCs are pluripotent stem cells derived from the inner cell mass (ICM) of blastocysts.[7] They can self-renew indefinitely under specific in-vitro culture conditions, resulting in daughter cells that maintain their potential for multilineage differentiation.[8,9] Techniques to obtain ESCs require the isolation of ICM cells devoid of trophoblastic and/or endodermal cells, after physically disrupting intact blastocysts[7,10] or from ICMs isolated by immunosurgical techniques.[11,12] In the human case, after demolishing an entire embryo, only up to 40% of ESC lines can be derived, even under optimal conditions,[13–17] and obviously this renders them useless for uterine transfer. Particularly in the case of hESCs, this embryo destruction has been one of the main ethical stumbling blocks to research. For many, the method in which an embryo is destroyed to obtain ESCs is unacceptable.[18]

In light of the reactions by many pro-life supporters or 'embryoists' to the present harvesting of hESCs, a number of people, including members of the US President's Council on Bioethics, have looked into other ways of obtaining hESCs: one is parthenogenesis,[19] whereas another involves the collection of hESCs from defective embryos[20] or by combining faulty embryos.[21,22]

Another method of generating ESCs, 'altered nuclear transfer' (ANT), has been proposed as a way of easing such ethical concerns.[23] ANT creates a pseudo-embryo which lacks the essential elements for continued development yet is still capable of generating ESCs. By inactivating a gene such as *Cdx2*, in a somatic donor cell, crucial for trophectoderm development, ANT will generate a pseudo-embryo that is unable to stimulate the formation of a placenta but retains the ability to differentiate an ICM lineage. In fact, it has been recently shown, at least in the mouse, that this strategy provided proof of principle for the creation of pseudo-embryos capable of generating ESCs.[24]

Finally, another approach involves the collection of stem cells from embryos after 'embryo death'. This is defined as the point when there is irreversible arrest of cell division in the embryo – measured by determinants of growth and differentiation such as the time elapsing after the cells stop dividing or by the disappearance of Oct-4.[20]

There is a compulsory need to identify feasible methods to isolate ESC precursors to limit or even avoid embryo wastage.[25] It is known that clonal propagation of single pluripotent cells can lead to the establishment of ESC lines.[26] In addition, single blastomeres isolated from 8-cell stage mouse embryos gave rise to ESCs.[25,27,28] Although with this method the efficiency of harvesting ESCs is only 3.2% per embryo, much lower than the conventional methods (20–40%), the biopsied embryos maintained their postimplantation development.[28]

Therefore, harvesting ESCs while sustaining the embryo viability would be more attractive.[25,28] This can be accomplished by propagating pluripotent precursor cells isolated through biopsy of either cleaving-stage or blastocyst-stage embryos.

It has been demonstrated that the harvesting rate per blastomere is compromised, but the utilization of the entire embryo as the denominator raised the harvesting rate to a comparable value to the conventional method.[25,28] We have also shown that isolation of single ICM cells from blastocysts yielded a higher ESC harvesting rate than plating the intact blastocyst, probably a result of less endodermal cell contamination.[29]

Another proposed method, suited to meet embryoists' objections, is called the blastocyst transfer method where a part of the ICM is extracted and cultured for ESC derivation. This approach aims to leave the biopsied embryo viable. The procedure, if the biopsied embryos achieve full-term postimplantation development, would prove crucial in pursuing embryo conservation.[18]

In this study, we have tested the possibility that individual cells, collected from cleaving-stage embryos and blastocysts without preventing their ability to develop and implant normally, can provide a source for ESCs of comparable quality to those derived by destroying blastocysts. The ESC lines so derived were comprehensively tested for their pluripotency status, and for their differentiation capability in vitro and in vivo, while the viability of the biopsied embryos was evaluated by their ability to generate healthy offspring.

MATERIALS AND METHODS

Embryos

B_6D_2-F_1 females (7–11 weeks) were superovulated with 10 IU of pregnant mare's serum gonadotrophin (Sigma, St Louis, MO, USA), then 10 IU of human chorionic gonadotropin (hCG) (Sigma), 48 hours apart, as previously described,[30] following which they were placed with males of the same strain. Mating was confirmed by the presence of a vaginal plug the following morning. Zygotes collected approximately 20 hours after hCG (embryonic day 0; d0) were cultured up to the 8-cell or the blastocyst stage in $KSOM^{AA}$ medium (Specialty Media, Phillipsburg, NJ, USA) at 37°C with 6% CO_2 in humidified air.

Embryonic cell isolation

Single blastomeres were taken from 8-cell-stage embryos by micromanipulation. Briefly, an 8-cell-stage embryo was secured by a holding pipette while the zona pellucida was penetrated by a glass microneedle pressed tangentially into the perivitelline space against the holding pipette. A single blastomere was removed in a micropipette of 20 μm inner diameter (Figure 12.1).

Alternatively, ICM cells were obtained by microdissection.[29] For this, an intact day 3 blastocyst was secured by a holding pipette, with the ICM at 9 o'clock. A biopsy pipette of 15 μm inner diameter, loaded with trypsin–EDTA solution (PBS containing 250 U/ml trypsin and 1 mmol/L EDTA), was inserted by a few piezo pulses into the blastocoele at 3 o'clock and advanced towards the ICM, and the trypsin–EDTA solution was gently expelled. Approximately 5 disaggregated ICM cells were then aspirated into the pipette (Figure 12.2).

Subsequently, blastomeres and ICM cells were seeded individually on mouse embryonic fibroblasts (MEFs) and cultured in Knockout DMEM (Ko-M, Invitrogen, Carlsbad, CA, USA) supplemented with 15% Knockout serum replacement (Ko-S, Invitrogen) in the presence of leukemia inhibiting factor (LIF).[31] Some intact fully expanded or hatching blastocysts were also plated as controls.

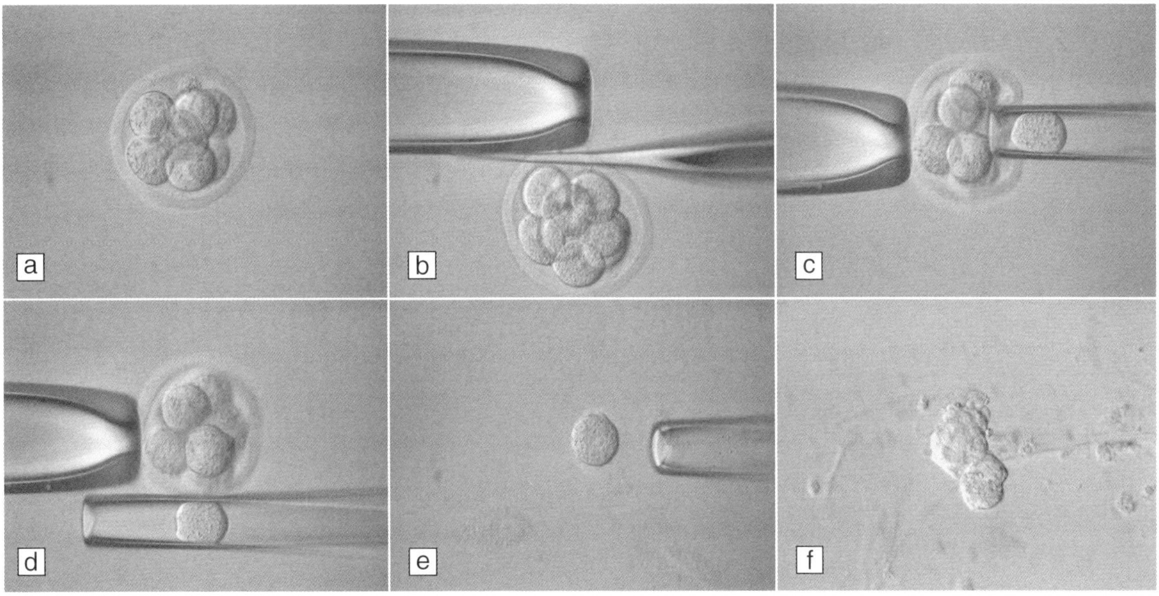

Figure 12.1 Blastomere biopsy procedure. An intact 8-cell-stage mouse embryo (a). Partial zona pellucida dissection by a glass microneedle (b). Single blastomere extraction (c). Isolated blastomere (d), plated on a feeder layer (e). Epiblast-like plaque aggregate on day 5 after plating (f). Original magnifications are 400× (a–e) and 200× (f)

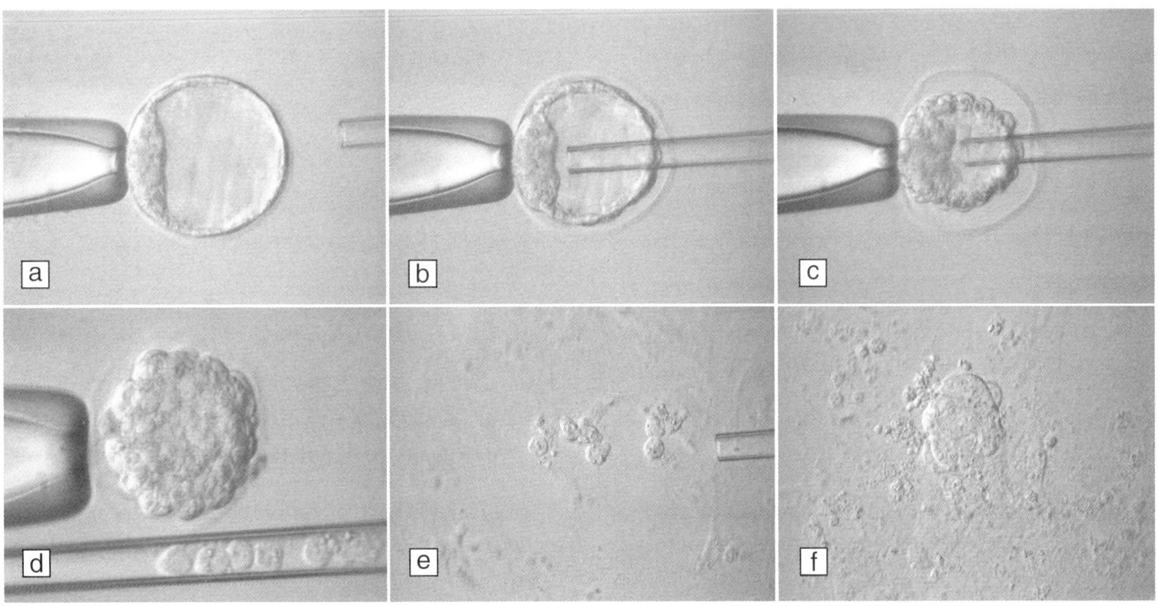

Figure 12.2 Inner cell mass (ICM) cells biopsy procedure. Intact blastocyst (a). A blunt microbiopsy pipette inserted by a piezo device (b). Individual ICM cells are aspirated into the pipette following a brief chemical digestion (c). Five ICM cells in the biopsy needle (d) and on MEF (e). Epiblast-like aggregate on day 3 after plating (f). Original magnifications are 600× (d), 400× (a–c, e) and 200× (f)

The biopsied 8-cell-stage embryos were further cultured to assess their ability to undergo full preimplantation development; on the other hand, the biopsied blastocysts were briefly incubated to assess their ability to restore their blastocoele. To assess in-vivo development, biopsied embryos were transferred to the uteri of pseudo-pregnant CD-1 females. Once live offspring were delivered, their growth, morphological development and behavior were evaluated and compared to those with controls.

Embryonic stem cell generation

Feeder layers of γ-irradiated MEFs were prepared on either 0.1% gelatin treated 4-well culture dishes (Nalge Nunc International, Rochester, NY, USA) or in 30 μl microdrops under oil in tissue culture dishes.[31] Immediately after their isolation, intact blastocysts and biopsied cells were seeded onto a layer of MEF, and cultured in ESC medium in 6% CO_2 at 37°C. The ESC medium consisted of Ko-M with 15% Ko-S containing LIF (2000 IU/ml; Chemicon International, Temecula, CA, USA), 0.1 mmol/l non-essential amino acids (NEAA; Specialty Media), 0.1 mmol/L β-mercaptoethanol (β-ME; Sigma), and 50 U/ml penicillin/50 μg/ml streptomycin (Sigma) and 4 mmol/l L-glutamine (Sigma). Blastomeres, ICM cells and blastocysts were observed every 24 hours for cleavage and attachment on a single MEF layer. On day 4 or 5 after plating, epiblast-like aggregated plaques of at least 50 μm were dissociated using a hand-pulled pipette, followed by trypsinization to promote cell dispersion. After replating in fresh wells, ESC colonies developed in 2 or 3 days, after which they were trypsinized and propagated by passaging them every 2–3 days thereafter.[31]

The established cell lines were tested for the presence of mycoplasma using MycoAlert Mycoplasma Detection Kit (Cambrex, Rockland, ME, USA).

Embryonic stem cell characterization

Morphological characteristics evaluated were cell size, nucleus/cytoplasm ratio and nucleolar patterns. Typically, ESCs were large and had a high nucleus/cytoplasm ratio, with one or more distinct nucleoli. To assess the ploidy of cell lines, DAPI banding was performed on metaphase chromosomes. Pluripotency of derived ESCs was assessed with molecular markers,[31] including alkaline phosphatase (AP) activity and Oct-4. TROMA-1 monoclonal antibody was used as a negative marker. Specimens were fixed, permeabilized and processed for fluorescent marker detection assay as previously described,[31] and were then examined under phase-contrast, fluorescent or, occasionally, laser confocal microscopy.

The pluripotent status of putative ESCs was confirmed by expression of typical marker genes including *Nanog* and *Ttr* (transthyretin – an indicator of early endodermal differentiation). Total RNA was isolated from ESCs, with MEFs serving as a negative control. Primers were custom-designed for the target sequences of *Nanog* and *Ttr* genes, while *Act*-β and *Gapdh* were used as normalizers.[31] Quantitative real-time polymerase chain reaction (qRT-PCR) was performed using SuperScript III Platinum Two-Step qRT-PCR Kit with SYBR Green (Invitrogen). Analysis was carried out using an ABI PRISM 7900HT (Applied Biosystems, Foster City, CA, USA).

In-vitro differentiation

Following trypsinization, cell aggregates of approximately 50–60 ESCs were placed in 20 μl hanging droplets, and cultured for 2 days to allow their aggregation into spheroid embryoid bodies (EBs). On the 3rd day, EBs were transferred to a 60 mm bacteriological Petri dish in 5 ml of DMEM + 20% fetal calf serum (FCS), then after 2 days to gelatin-coated dishes for 5 days.[31,32] Differentiation into cardiomyocytes was monitored according to the appearance of contractility at days 8–9 of culture, at which point the EBs were processed for histological sectioning and transmission electron microscopy (TEM).

In-vivo differentiation and germline transmission

The established cell lines were assessed for their differentiation capability also by inducing testicular teratoma formation. Approximately $1–4 \times 10^6$ undifferentiated cells were injected into the testes of 6- to 8-week-old severe combined immunodeficiency (SCID) mice.[31] At 3–5 weeks later, the resultant tumors were fixed, embedded in paraffin and examined histologically after hematoxylin and eosin staining.

The pluripotency of the mouse ESC lines was assessed by generating chimeric offspring. Host embryos were recovered from stimulated CD-1 females at either the morula stage from the oviducts and cultured overnight, or the blastocyst stage by flushing uterine horns. By micromanipulation, approximately

10 donor ESCs were injected into each blastocyst.[33] Blastocysts were allowed to re-expand in culture before their transfer into the uterine horns of pseudo-pregnant CD-1 foster mothers. Chimeric offspring were identified by eye and coat pigmentation. Chimeric males were test-bred to albino CD-1 females. Germline transmission of the ESC genotype was revealed by the production of heterozygous progeny.

Data analysis

A χ^2 test was utilized for the different comparisons involving blastocyst culture, attachment, ESC derivation and gene expression analysis. A χ^2 two-tailed test was used to assess significance, considered at 5% probability. The qPCR results were plotted by the Sequence Detection System Analysis Software (Version 2.0; Applied Biosystems). Gene expression was reported as a proportion, calculated from the cycle threshold against *Act*-β considered at 100% expression.[34]

Statistical comparisons were reported in text and tables only when significance was reached. In tables, numbers within rows with similar symbols are significantly different. All statistical computations were conducted using StatView 512+ software (BrainPower Inc., Calabasas, CA, USA).

RESULTS

Embryonic stem cell harvest from isolated blastomeres of 8-cell-stage embryos

Single blastomere extraction was successful in all the 8-cell embryos (Figure 12.3). A total of 46 blastomeres isolated from 8-cell embryos ($n = 46$) were plated individually. Of these, 43 (93.5%) underwent at least one division, and after 2 days a total of 22 (47.8%) had attached to the feeder layer. The large majority of each blastomere formed a trophoblastic vesicle of approximately 30–50 μm diameter but then lysed. However, 4 aggregated plaques (8.7%) did develop and after mechanical and enzymatic dissociation the resulting cells were propagated. Finally, 1 ESC line (2.2% per blastomere) was obtained by this method (Figure 12.4). In contrast, when a total of 392 single blastomeres were isolated from 49 embryos and plated in clusters ($n = 49$), 8 ESC lines (16.3% per embryo) resulted (Table 12.1).

Viability of the biopsied 8-cell-stage embryos

The large majority (93.5%) of the biopsied 8-cell embryos developed to blastocysts. After transfer of the biopsied cleaving embryos, 51.2% were delivered

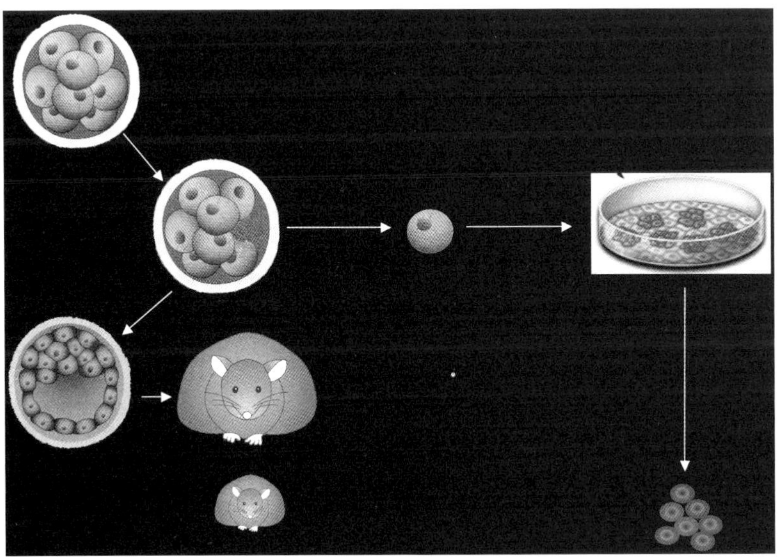

Figure 12.3 Embryo conservation assessment plan by the isolation of a single 8-cell blastomere

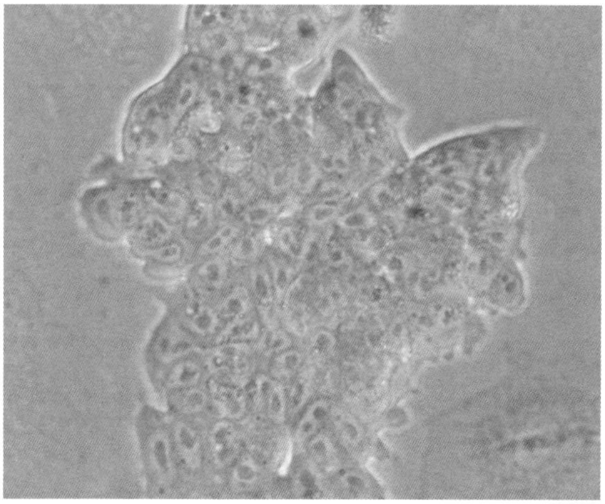

Figure 12.4 Embryonic stem cell colony derived from a single blastomere. Cobblestone cytometric characteristics with large nuclei, nucleoli and high nuclear/cytoplasmic ratio

Table 12.1 Genesis of embryonic stem cells (ESCs) from isolated 8-cell blastomeres

	No. (%)	
Source	*In clusters*	*Individual*
Embryos	49	46
Isolated/plated blastomeres	392	46
Proliferated	49/392[a]	43 (93.5)
Initial aggregates/ embryo	34 (69.4)[b]	4 (8.7)[b]
ESC lines	8 (16.3)[c]	1 (2.2)[c]

[a]Presumed proliferation because of cell clustering
[b,c]χ^2, 2×2, 1 df, effect of single-cell culture on aggregate plaque formation, $p < 0.001$ and ESC colony formation, $p < 0.05$, respectively

alive – comparable to the 56.0% seen in the control group (Table 12.2).

Embryonic stem cell harvest from biopsied inner cell mass cells

In a preliminary experiment, we investigated the feasibility of harvesting ESCs by microsurgically isolating ICM cells from blastocysts (Figure 12.5), and this was performed successfully in 6 out of

Table 12.2 Development of 8-cell-stage embryos following blastomere biopsy

	No. (%)	
Source	*Intact*	*Biopsied*
Embryos	26	46
Successful biopsy		46
Blastocyst development	25 (96.2)	43 (93.5)
Conceptuses transferred	25	43
Foster mother	2	3
Offspring (per transferred embryo)	14 (56.0)	22 (51.2)

10 blastocysts. The 6 groups of sibling ICM-derived cells were plated, and 2 ESC lines were obtained (20% per blastocyst).

Where the intention was to preserve viability of the biopsied blastocysts, the ICM cell biopsy was successful in 13 out of 14 attempts (92.8%). When the respective 13 biopsies (each comprising 5 individual ICM cells) were each plated, they all adhered to the fibroblasts, formed epiblast-like cell aggregates and gave rise to 4 ESC lines (28.6%), compared with 11 ESC lines established from 63 control blastocysts (17.5%) (Table 12.3).

Viability of the biopsied embryos

All the biopsied blastocysts restored their blastocoele cavity during a subsequent 3-hour culture period (Figure 12.6) and, once transferred, 4 offspring (30.8%) were born (Table 12.4). These 4 neonates all developed to adulthood with proven fertility. Their growth pattern, morphological characteristics and behavioral response were all comparable to the controls.

Embryonic stem cell characterization

All the putative ESC lines maintained the morphological features and proliferative ability characteristic of stem cells, they passed bacteriological testing and had a normal karyotype. Furthermore, colony pluripotency was confirmed by molecular markers AP, Oct-4 and TROMA-1 as a negative control for

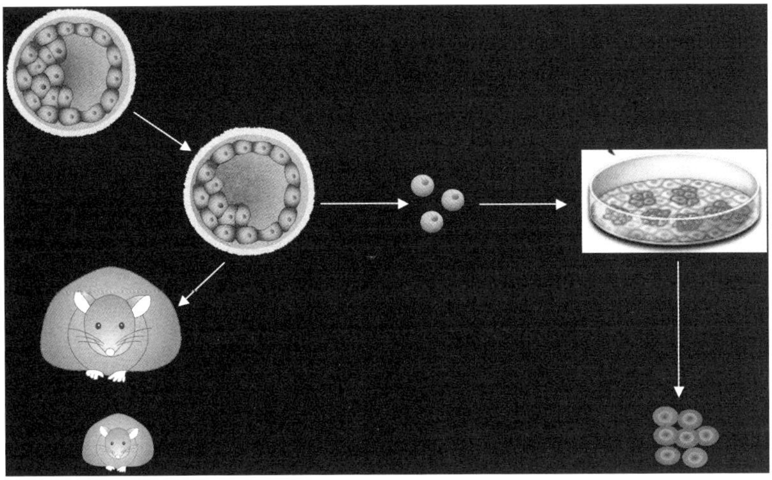

Figure 12.5 Embryo conservation assessment plan by the isolation of individual inner cell mast cells from blastocysts

Table 12.3 Genesis of embryonic stem cells (ESCs) from isolated inner cell mass (ICM) cells

	No. (%)	
Source	*Intact*	*Biopsied*
Blastocysts	63	14
Cell clusters		13 (5 cells)
Plated	63	13[a] (5 cells)
Aggregates	14 (22.2)[b]	8 (57.1)[b]
ESC lines	11 (17.5)	4 (28.6)

[a]Presumed proliferation because of cell clustering
[b]χ^2, 2×2, 1 df, ability of single ICM cells to form epiblast-like aggregates, $p < 0.05$

endodermal and trophoblastic cell contamination. Pluripotency marker assessment was concordant in all ESC colonies. Reverse transcription and qRT-PCR were successful in all cases. As expected, there was a high expression of *Nanog* in ESCs, but not in MEFs, which, however, manifested a higher expression of *Ttr* than the ESC colonies.

Differentiation capability of embryonic stem cells

Culture in the absence of feeder cells and LIF allowed the formation of tight, round aggregates (EBs). About 20% of EBs displayed beating foci typical of cardiomyocyte differentiation by day 9 of culture. Histology and TEM confirmed the presence of cell components related to the embryonic germ layers.

All the testes injected with ESCs developed tumors containing derivatives of all three embryonic germ layers, including mucus-producing columnar epithelium, ciliated columnar epithelium, glandular epithelium arranged in acini, endothelium-lined vessels with intraluminal neutrophils, striated muscle, bone, cartilage, abundant neural tissue often forming rosettes, as shown in Figure 12.7. The chimeric embryos created by injection of ESCs, for all the cell lines including the one from a single 8-cell-stage blastomere and 4 from ICM cells, proved to be capable of producing chimeric offspring at an average rate of 37.5%. Germline transmission in a subsequent generation was proven for at least one cell line in each group.

DISCUSSION

In this study, the efficiency of harvesting ESCs from single 8-cell blastomeres, although slim at about 2%, was similar (3.2%) to that in previous reports where single blastomeres were cultured in clusters[27] or in conjunction with green fluorescent protein (GFP)-labeled ESCs.[28] This limited efficiency can be identified in a prepatterning of the embryo early on in its development, suggesting that already at the 4-cell stage as much as 25–50% of the conceptus, the abembryonic portion, is committed to the production

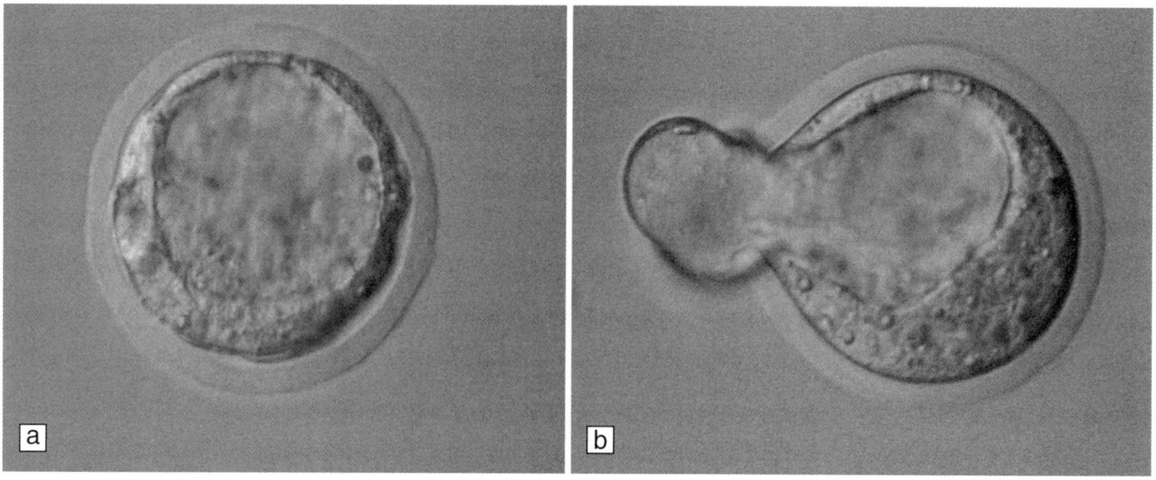

Figure 12.6 Blastocoele re-expansion after 1 hour incubation (a) and 2 hours with herniation through the original zona pellucida gap (b). Original magnifications are 400× (a, b)

Table 12.4 Development of blastocysts following inner cell mass biopsy

	No. (%)	
Source	*Intact*	*Biopsied*
Embryos	13	14
Successful biopsy		13 (92.8)
Restored blastocoele		13
Conceptuses transferred	13	13
Foster mother	1	1
Offspring (per transferred embryo)	8 (61.5)	4 (30.8)

of the germ and trophoblastic cell lineage.[35–38] This view, however, has been challenged by others who question the existence in vertebrates and particularly in mammals of this sort of polarization[39–41] and explain the poor performance of isolated cells as there being an embryonic mass insufficient to sustain development unless supported by other cells.[28,39,42] For the biopsied 8-cell embryo on the other hand, the removal of a blastomere does not interfere to any degree with its survival, as shown by the live birth rate of 51%, a result consistent with the experience coming from preimplantation genetic diagnosis.[43–45]

The removal of 5 ICM cells yielded a harvest rate of about 28%, which is deemed satisfactory in comparison to the individual 8-cell blastomere (Table 12.5). This better performance is possibly related to the fact that ICM cells in a blastocyst are committed to form the embryo proper and not trophoblastic components, in contrast to earlier-stage blastomeres.[39]

Following ICM biopsy, several embryos developed to become healthy offspring. The live birth rate after biopsies both at the cleaving and blastocyst stages was not statistically different from that of the intact control, at least in our experience. However, the implantation potential of the biopsied blastocysts seemed impaired and this may be empirically explained by the fact that in a day 4 blastocyst about 20 cells constitute the ICM,[46] whereas a biopsy on day 3 may involve an embryo with only about 10 ICM cells.[47] Therefore, the removal of 5 cells represents about 50% of the embryo proper vs a 12.5% proportion when the removal is performed on an 8-cell blastomere. Human blastocysts have been biopsied for preimplantation genetic diagnosis (PGD) and have resulted in successful deliveries[48,49] devoid of neonatal malformations. However, these techniques targeted only trophectoderm cells, leaving the animal pole untouched.

Irrespective of the methods of harvesting, all the cell lines obtained here had a typical ESC morphology in the light microscope; they stained strongly for AP activity, and expressed Oct-4[50–52] and *Nanog*,[53,54] all considered stemness markers for their role in

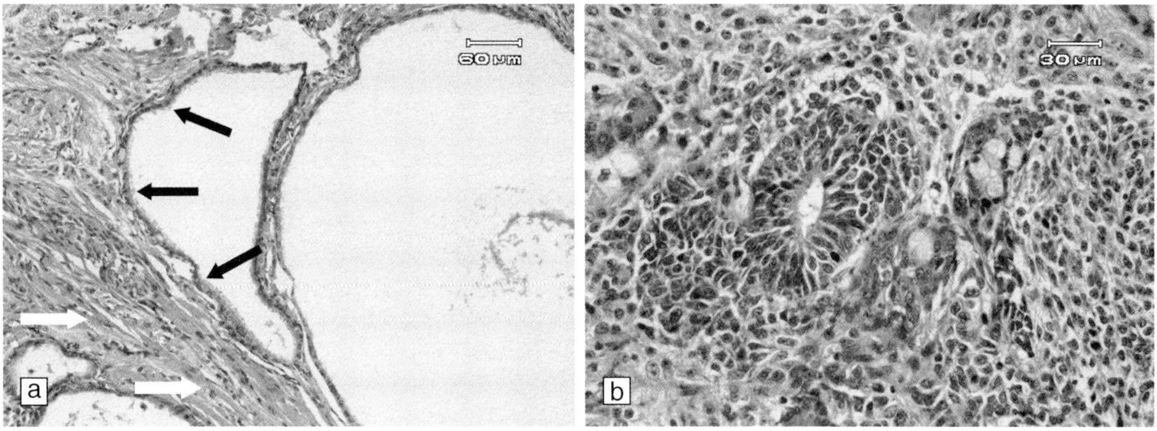

Figure 12.7 In-vivo differentiation assessment. Histological section of a teratoma tumor with representation of the endodermal (ciliated columnar epithelium; black arrows) and mesodermal (striated muscle; white arrows) differentiation (a), and ectodermal (neural rosette) differentiation (b). (See also color plate)

Table 12.5 Embryonic stem cell (ESC) harvest from biopsied cells

	No. (%)	
Source of cells	*8-cell blastomeres*	*ICM cells* 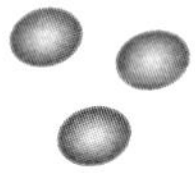
Embryos	46	14
Biopsied/ plated cells	46	13 (5 cells)
Proliferated	43 (93.5)	13[a] (5 cells)
Initial aggregates	4 (8.7)[b]	8 (57.1)[b]
ESC lines	1 (2.2)[c]	4 (28.6)[c]

[a]Presumed proliferation because of cell clustering
[b,c]χ^2, 2×2, 1 df, effect of cell isolation from different embryonic stages on aggregate formation, $p < 0.001$, and ESC colony formation, $p < 0.05$, respectively

regulating pluripotency and self-renewal. Furthermore, testing for trophoblastic markers such as TROMA-1[55,56] and *Ttr*[57,58] served to support the cytometric grading scoring[31] in the derived ESC lines. The development of EBs was an additional sign that the cells harvested and maintained retained the ability to differentiate into the three embryonic disk components. Not least, the fact that all established cell lines gave rise to teratomas in vivo served to demonstrate their true differentiation potential.

The ethical controversy surrounding ESC research has arisen from the apparent necessity to destroy the human blastocyst in order to obtain pluripotent cells that hold the potential utilization for biomedical research and therapy.[18,59] The procedure of embryo biopsy in general and the ICM cell variant in particular may be acceptable to pro-life supporters because the isolated cells from the animal pole of the blastocyst cannot form fetal adnexa (placenta, cord and membranes). This perspective can be compared to the proposal by Hurlbut,[23] and then tested by Meissner and Jaenisch,[24] where they produced an embryo with compromised placentation by a knockdown gene, that needs to be reinstalled to produce true pluripotent stem cells. However, although *Cdx2* is expressed in the trophectoderm of human blastocysts[60] and in derivatives of hESCs,[61] its role in the human placenta has not been determined. Moreover, the approach requires additional manipulation of the donor cells that may complicate the logistics of production and safety assessment of patient-specific ESC lines for therapy.

The embryo biopsy approach differs in that the embryo's dignity is maintained.[18] In fact, the embryo is not used as a mere means: the embryo conservation procedure aims at retrieving ESC precursors from the ICM, still granting embryonic health on one hand and on the other hand providing a sort of insurance policy to support the health of the embryo or the individual through its development/life, enacting a situation similar to the storage of cord blood at child birth. This would all together establish the premises for ESC banking and limit the need for nuclear transplantation procedures (therapeutic cloning), being in fact these genotyped ESC.

CONCLUSIONS

The isolation of individual cells from cleaving embryos or from blastocysts allows the establishment of ESC lines of comparable quality to those derived from intact blastocysts or from whole ICMs. Although postimplantation development of the biopsied blastocysts sometimes seemed impaired, this approach has proved crucial in pursuing embryo conservation and provides a foundation for systematic banking of genotyped ESCs.

Because the present ways of obtaining hESCs involve destroying the embryo, hESC research is under attack and, in some countries (including the USA) it runs the risk of being banned. Compromise solutions such as parthenogenesis, the use of defective embryos, genetic manipulation to create a pseudo-embryo that cannot form a placenta and determining its developmental arrest have been proposed. Although these procedures, and indeed the embryo biopsy method discussed here, could meet current ethical objections, at the same time they may give rise to the fear in the pro-choice community that they will act to delay the advent of the therapeutic benefits that this research promises. However, because of its ethical acceptability, not least for investors, the pursuit of the biopsy approach in the cleaving embryo or blastocyst may hasten the therapeutic benefits of hESCs.

Acknowledgments

We wish to thank Dr Matthew Lios and Professor Alan Trounson for contributing to the study design. We are grateful to Professor J Michael Bedford for his critical reading of the manuscript. The TROMA-1 antibody developed by Brulet et al[55] was obtained from the Developmental Studies Hybridoma Bank under the auspices of the NICHD and maintained by the University of Iowa, Department of Biological Sciences, Iowa City, IA, USA.

REFERENCES

1. Reubinoff BE, Itsykson P, Turetsky T et al. Neural progenitors from human embryonic stem cells. Nat Biotechnol 2001; 19: 1134–40.
2. Zhang SC, Werning M, Duncan ID et al. In vitro differentiation of transplantable neural precursors from human embryonic stem cells. Nat Biotechnol 2001; 19: 1129–33.
3. Kehat I, Kenyagin-Karsenti D, Snir M et al. Human embryonic stem cells can differentiate into myocytes with structural and functional properties of cardiomyocytes. J Clin Invest 2001; 108: 407–14.
4. Kim JH, Auerbach JM, Rodriguez-Gomez JA et al. Dopamine neurons derived from embryonic stem cells function in an animal model of Parkinson's disease. Nature 2002; 418: 50–6.
5. Lumelsky N, Blondel O, Laeng P et al. Differentiation of embryonic stem cells to insulin-secreting structures similar to pancreatic islets. Science 2001; 292: 1389–94.
6. Kaufman DS, Hanson ET, Lewis RL et al. Hematopoietic colony-forming cells derived from human embryonic stem cells. Proc Natl Acad Sci USA 2001; 98: 10716–21.
7. Evans MJ, Kaufman MH. Establishment in culture of pluripotential cells from mouse embryos. Nature 1981; 292: 154–6.
8. Williams RL, Hilton DJ, Pease S et al. Myeloid leukaemia inhibitory factor maintains the developmental potential of embryonic stem cells. Nature 1988; 336: 684–7.
9. Smith AG, Heath JK, Donaldson DD et al. Inhibition of pluripotential embryonic stem cell differentiation by purified polypeptides. Nature 1988; 336: 688–90.
10. Robertson EJ. Embryo-derived stem cell lines. In: Robertson EJ, ed. Teratocarcinomas and Embryonic Stem Cells: a Practical Approach. Oxford, UK: IRL Press, 1987: 71–112.
11. Solter D, Knowles BB. Immunosurgery of mouse blastocyst. Proc Natl Acad Sci USA 1975; 72: 5099–102.
12. Martin GR. Isolation of a pluripotent cell line from early mouse embryos cultured in medium conditioned by teratocarcinoma stem cells. Proc Natl Acad Sci USA 1981; 78: 7634–8.
13. Thomson JA, Itskovitz-Eldor J, Shapiro SS et al. Embryonic stem cell lines derived from human blastocysts. Science 1998; 282: 1145–7.
14. Reubinoff BE, Pera MF, Fong CY et al. Embryonic stem cell lines from human blastocysts: somatic differentiation in vitro. Nat Biotechnol 2000; 18: 399–404.

15. Lanzendorf SE, Boyd CA, Wright DL et al. Use of human gametes obtained from anonymous donors for the production of human embryonic stem cell lines. Fertil Steril 2001; 76: 132–7.

16. Sjogren A, Hardarson T, Andersson K et al. Human blastocysts for the development of embryonic stem cells. Reprod Biomed Online 2004; 9: 326–9.

17. Kim SJ, Lee JE, Park JH et al. Efficient derivation of new human embryonic stem cell lines. Mol Cells 2005; 19: 46–53.

18. Liao SM. Rescuing human embryonic stem cell research: the Blastocyst Transfer Method. Am J Bioeth 2005; 5: 8–16.

19. Lin H, Lei J, Wininger D et al. Multilineage potential of homozygous stem cells derived from metaphase II oocytes. Stem Cells 2003; 21: 152–61.

20. Landry D, Zucker H. Embryonic death and the creation of human embryonic stem cells. J Clin Invest 2004; 114: 1184–6.

21. Alikani M, Willadsen SM. Human blastocysts from aggregated mononucleated cells of two or more non-viable zygote-derived embryos. Reprod Biomed Online 2002; 5: 56–8.

22. Byrne A, Smonsson S, Gurdon J. From intestine to muscle: nuclear reprogramming through defective cloned embryos. Proc Natl Acad Sci USA 2003; 99: 6059–63.

23. Hurlbut WB. Altered nuclear transfer as a morally acceptable means for the procurement of human embryonic stem cells. Perspect Biol Med 2005; 48: 211–28.

24. Meissner A, Jaenisch R. Generation of nuclear transfer-derived pluripotent ES cells from cloned Cdx2-deficient blastocysts. Nature 2006; 439: 212–15.

25. Sills ES, Takeuchi T, Tanaka N et al. Identification and isolation of embryonic stem cells in reproductive endocrinology: theoretical protocols for conservation of human embryos derived from in vitro fertilization. Theor Biol Med Model 2005; 2: 25–32.

26. Amit M, Carpenter MK, Inokuma MS et al. Clonally derived human embryonic stem cell lines maintain pluripotency and proliferative potential for prolonged periods of culture. Dev Biol 2000; 227: 271–8.

27. Delhaise F, Bralion V, Schuurbiers N et al. Establishment of an embryonic stem cell line from 8-cell stage mouse embryos. Eur J Morphol 1996; 34: 237–43.

28. Chung Y, Klimanskaya I, Becker S et al. Embryonic and extraembryonic stem cell lines derived from single mouse blastomeres. Nature 2006; 439: 216–19.

29. Wang A, Takeuchi T, Tanaka N et al. Disaggregation of the inner cell mass enhances the harvesting of pluripotent cells. Hum Reprod 2005; 20 (Suppl 1): i162.

30. Takeuchi T, Rosenwaks Z, Palermo GD. A successful model to assess embryo development after transplantation of prophase nuclei. Hum Reprod 2004; 19: 975–81.

31. Tanaka N, Takeuchi T, Neri QV, Sills ES, Palermo GD. Laser-assisted blastocyst dissection and subsequent cultivation of embryonic stem cells in a serum/cell free culture system: applications and preliminary results in a murine model. J Transl Med 2006; 4: 20.

32. Wobus AM, Wallukat G, Hescheler J. Pluripotent mouse embryonic stem cells are able to differentiate into cardiomyocytes expressing chronotropic responses to adrenergic and cholinergic agents and Ca^{2+} channel blockers. Differentiation 1991; 48: 173–82.

33. Bradley A. Production and analysis of chimeric mice. In: Robertson EJ, ed. Teratocarcinomas and Embryonic Stem Cells: a Practical Approach. Oxford, UK: IRL Press, 1987: 113–52.

34. Takeuchi T, Neri QV, Katagiri Y et al. Effect of treating induced mitochondrial damage on embryonic development and epigenesis. Biol Reprod 2005; 72: 584–92.

35. Gardner RL. The early blastocyst is bilaterally symmetrical and its axis of symmetry is aligned with the animal-vegetal axis of the zygote in the mouse. Development 1997; 124: 289–301.

36. Gardner RL. Specification of embryonic axes begins before cleavage in normal mouse development. Development 2001; 128: 839–47.

37. Edwards RG, Beard HK. Oocyte polarity and cell determination in early mammalian embryos. Mol Hum Reprod 1997; 3: 863–905.

38. Edwards RG, Hansis C. Initial differentiation of blastomeres in 4-cell human embryos and its significance for early embryogenesis and implantation. Reprod Biomed Online 2005; 11: 206–18.

39. Kelly SJ. Studies of the developmental potential of 4- and 8-cell stage mouse blastomeres. J Exp Zool 1977; 200: 365–76.

40. Fujimori T, Kurotaki Y, Miyazaki J-I et al. Analysis of cell lineage in two- and four-cell mouse embryos. Development 2003; 130: 5113–22.

41. Hiiragi T, Solter D. First cleavage plane of the mouse egg is not predetermined but defined by the topology of the two apposing pronuclei. Nature 2004; 430: 360–4.

42. Tarkowski AK, Ozdzenski W, Czolowska R. Identical triplets and twins developed from isolated blastomeres of 8- and 16-cell mouse embryos supported with tetraploid blastomeres. Int J Dev Biol 2005; 49: 825–32.

43. Handyside AH, Kontogianni EH, Hardy K et al. Pregnancies from biopsied human preimplantation embryos sexed by Y-specific DNA amplification. Nature 1990; 344: 768–70.

44. Verlinsky Y, Tur-Kaspa J, Cieslak J et al. Preimplantation testing for chromosomal disorders improves reproductive outcome of poor prognosis patients. Reprod Biomed Online 2005; 11: 219–25.

45. Munne S, Fischer J, Warner A et al. Preimplantation genetic diagnosis significantly reduces pregnancy loss in infertile couples: a multicenter study. Fertil Steril 2006; 85: 326–32.

46. Thouas GA, Korfiatis NA, French AJ et al. Simplified technique for differential staining of inner cell mass and trophectoderm cells of mouse and bovine blastocysts. Reprod Biomed Online 2001; 3: 25–9.

47. Saburi S, Azuma S, Sato E et al. Developmental fate of single embryonic stem cells microinjected into 8-cell stage mouse embryos. Differentiation 1997; 62: 1–11.

48. Veiga A, Sandalinas M, Benkhalifa M et al. Laser blastocyst biopsy for preimplantation diagnosis in the human. Zygote 1997; 5: 351–4.

49. de Boer KA, Catt JW, Jansen RPS, Leigh D, McArthur S. Moving to blastocyst biopsy for preimplantation genetic diagnosis and single embryo transfer at Sydney IVF. Fertil Steril 2004; 82: 295–8.

50. Nichols J, Zevnik B, Anastassiadis K et al. Formation of pluripotent stem cells in the mammalian embryo depends on the POU transcription factor Oct 4. Cell 1998; 95: 379–91.

51. Okamoto K, Okazawa H, Okuda A et al. A novel octamer binding transcription factor is differentially expressed in mouse embryonic cells. Cell 1990; 60: 461–72.

52. Rosner MH, Vigano MA, Ozato K et al. A POU-domain transcription factor in early stem cells and germ cells of the mammalian embryo. Nature 1990; 345: 686–92.

53. Chambers I, Colby D, Robertson M et al. Functional expression cloning of Nanog, a pluripotency sustaining factor in embryonic stem cells. Cell 2003; 113: 643–55.

54. Mitsui K, Tokuzawa Y, Itoh H et al. The homeoprotein Nanog is required for maintenance of pluripotency in mouse epiblast and ES cells. Cell 2003; 113: 631–42.

55. Brulet P, Babinet C, Kemler R et al. Monoclonal antibodies against trophectoderm-specific markers during mouse blastocyst formation. Proc Natl Acad Sci USA 1980; 77: 4113–7.

56. Kemler R, Brulet P, Schnebelen MT, Gaillard J, Jacob F. Reactivity of monoclonal antibodies against intermediate filament proteins during embryonic development. J Embryol Exp Morphol 1981; 64: 45–60.

57. Soprano DR, Soprano KJ, Goodman DS. Retinol-binding protein and transthyretin mRNA levels in visceral yolk sac and liver during fetal development in the rat. Proc Natl Acad Sci USA 1986; 83: 7330–4.

58. Makover A, Soprano DR, Wyatt ML, Goodman DS. An in situ-hybridization study of the localization of retinol-binding protein and transthyretin messenger RNAs during fetal development in the rat. Differentiation 1989; 40: 17–25.

59. Melton DA, Daley GQ, Jennings CG. Altered nuclear transfer in stem-cell research – a flawed proposal. N Engl J Med 2004; 351: 2791–2.

60. Adjaye J, Huntriss J, Herwig R et al. Primary differentiation in the human blastocyst: comparative molecular portraits of inner cell mass and trophectoderm cells. Stem Cells 2005; 23: 1514–25.

61. Hyslop L, Stojkovic M, Armstrong L et al. Downregulation of NANOG induces differentiation of human embryonic stem cells to extraembryonic lineages. Stem Cells 2005; 23: 1035–43.

CHAPTER 13

Embryo-friendly approaches to human embryonic cell derivation

Irina Klimanskaya

INTRODUCTION

The topic of this chapter has obviously been inspired by heated debates in society about the ethics of using leftover in-vitro fertilization (IVF) embryos for derivation of embryonic stem (ES) cell lines. ES cells, first derived in 1981 by Evans and Kaufman,[1] have been studied extensively as a model of development and differentiation. Isolation of human ES (hES) cells from leftover IVF embryos in 1998[2] boosted the research in this field, leading to great hopes for approaching the era of cell therapies. ES cells, the progeny of the inner cell mass (ICM) of a blastocyst, remain pluripotent, maintain normal karyotype through multiple passages in culture and can differentiate into derivatives of all three germ layers in vitro and in vivo, making teratomas in laboratory animals.[3–5] Among their differentiation derivatives that can be produced in vitro are such sought-after cells as cardiomyocytes, neurons, oligodendrocytes, retinal pigment epithelium, and insulin-producing cells.[4,6–11] Such cells and tissues, if robustly produced from ES cells, would satisfy an unmet medical need for tissue and organ repair and could be generated to decrease the risk of immune rejection either through banking a variety of genetically diverse cell lines or via patient-specific nuclear transfer technology.

However, ES cell research has been somewhat impeded by the controversy surrounding the use of leftover IVF embryos for generation of ES cells and donation of oocytes, which are intended not for fertilization and pregnancy but for alternative approaches to produce patient immune-compatible cells for regenerative medicine applications.[12–14] These debates have resulted in several bills being passed by the legislators of different countries that put a number of restrictions on embryonic stem cell research, including limitations on the available state funds, along with strict guidelines on oocyte and leftover embryo use, which don't add momentum to advancements in this field.[15]

Finding an alternative to using embryos for sourcing cells and tissues for regenerative medicine applications would add vigor to embryonic stem cell research and satisfy its most zealous opponents. While currently all published human ES cell lines were derived from IVF embryos, several approaches are being developed which could potentially allow the creation of ES cells without embryo destruction. Athough several such techniques have so far been mere proof of principle (and others haven't even reached that stage), there is a lot of potential that currently depends on the reproducibility and reliability of such technologies. At present, there are following possibilities of generating ES cells without embryo destruction: transdifferentiation or reprogramming[16–18] of somatic cells into another somatic cell type, fusion,[19,20] deriving ES cells from activated oocytes, or parthenotes which have no potential to develop into whole organisms,[21,22] or making ES cells from one or two biopsied blastomeres (the same technique that is widely used for preimplantation diagnostics of genetic diseases), which leaves the embryo alive.[23] Although no naturally fertilized embryos are used for somatic cell nuclear transfer (SCNT), this procedure remains controversial, as an artificially created embryo can possibly develop to term, at least, in animal experiments.[24] Still, an approach called 'altered nuclear transfer' has been proposed to create genetically modified non-viable embryos for generation of ES cells.[25] In addition to making new ES cell lines, another embryo-friendly way of deriving a variety of somatic cells would be to use existing ES cell lines for research or even therapy (if their safety can be ascertained) or adult stem or germ cells which can differentiate into a broad range of cell types.

TRANSDIFFERENTIATION USING CELL LYSATES

The old dogma stating that after a cell undergoes terminal differentiation it is committed to this fate, or, in other words, that terminal differentiation is terminal, is now being reassessed as more and more studies appear that show the possibility of reprogramming (aside from SCNT) the genome of an adult somatic – or 'terminally' differentiated – cell. The prospect of turning one differentiated cell into another is very attractive, as this would allow one to create patient-specific cell types on demand without using embryos to create ES cells and developing technologies to differentiate them. The possible variations of this technology would be either direct transdifferentiation of a somatic cell to another somatic cell or to a progenitor or an ES cell that could then be differentiated into the desired cell type. The pioneering works of a Norwegian group led by Philipp Collas[16–18] used the bacterial toxin streptolysin-O to permeabilize the cellular membrane in the absence of calcium so that these permeabilized cells could be loaded with cellular extracts of another cell type (Figure 13.1).

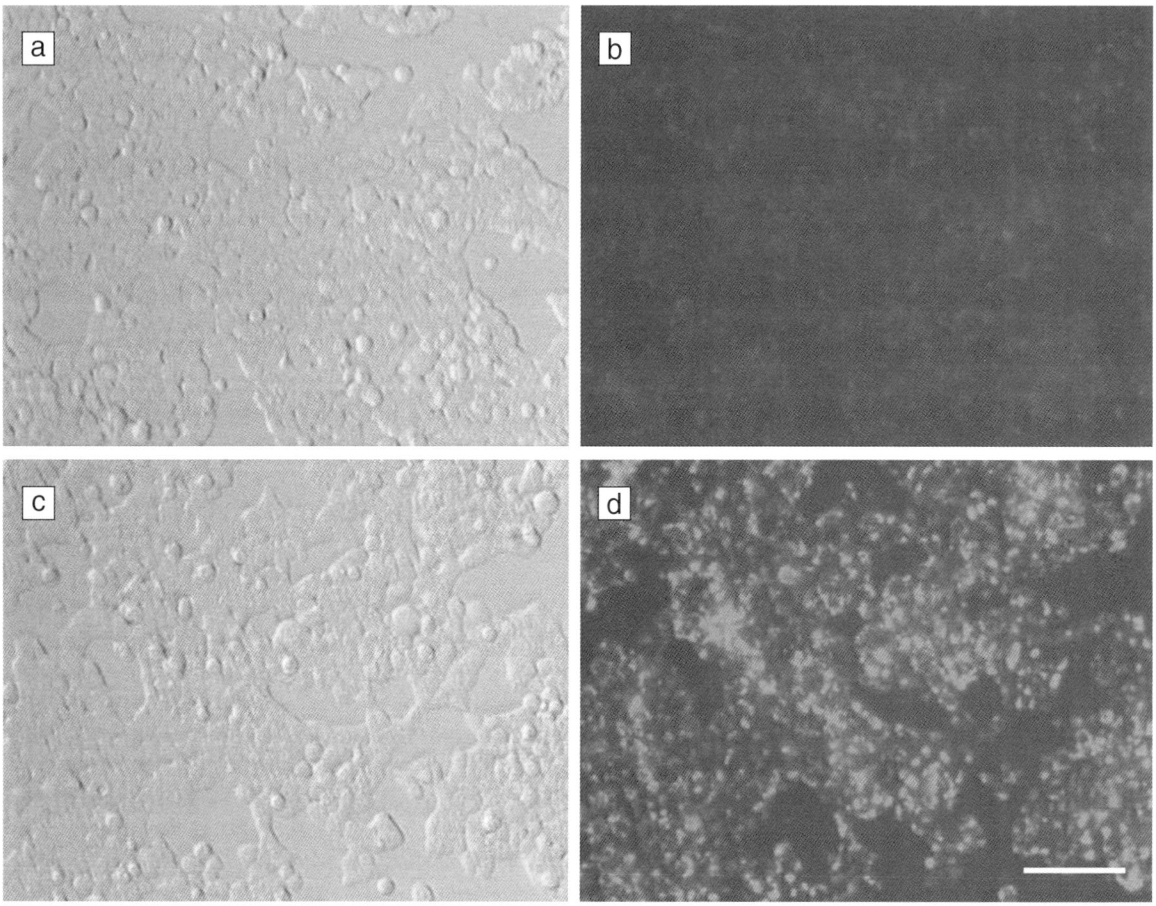

Figure 13.1 Uptake of rhodamine-albumin by unpermeabilized (a,b) and permeabilized (c,d) 293T cells in the presence of cell extracts: (a,c) phase contrast; (b,d) fluorescence. Scale bar, 100 μm. (Images courtesy of Dr Sadhana Agarwal, Advanced Cell Technology, Inc.) (See also color plate)

After the procedure, the cellular membrane can be resealed in the presence of calcium, and the reprogramming of the recipient cell is achieved by the cytoplasmic 'cocktail' of the donor cells. Such experiments were originally performed using 293T and skin fibroblasts that were loaded with extracts of human T cells and were shown to upregulate T-cell-specific receptors and assemble the interleukin-2 receptor in response to activation of the T-cell receptor CD3 complex.[17] Recently, the same group[16] reported reprogramming of 293T cells by extracts of the human embryonic carcinoma cell line NCCIT to acquire characteristics of pluripotency which could be retained through multiple passages in culture. Such state of pluripotency was characterized by changes in morphology, induction of pluripotency-associated genes such as *Oct-4*, *Sox2*, *Nanog* or *Rex1*, down-regulation of *293T* gene expression over time, as well as acquisition of the ability to differentiate in an embryonic carcinoma-like manner. Such reprogrammed cells were induced to differentiate along the neural lineage and into adipocytes, osteoblasts and endothelial cells. It still needs to be determined how stable such transdifferentiated cell lines are over time, whether they maintain normal karyotype and how safe they are, considering that an embryonic carcinoma cell line was used for reprogramming, and more studies of their differentiation derivatives beyond initial analysis of a few markers would be needed to evaluate them in comparison to their ES-derived and in-vivo counterparts. It is also important that such reprogramming technology could be applied to other somatic cell types that can be easily obtained from a patient, such as skin fibroblasts or lymphocytes, so that desired patient-specific cell types could be produced on demand.

REPROGRAMMING VIA FUSION OF EMBRYONIC STEM CELLS WITH SOMATIC CELLS

The work done in the USA at Harvard University[20] showed that if hES cells and adult fibroblasts are fused, the resulting hybrid cells acquire the phenotype of ES cells. The authors fused GFP (green fluorescent protein)-positive, hygromycin-resistant hES cells with puromycin-resistant fibroblasts, and the resulting hygromycin/puromycin-resistant and GFP-positive hybrids exhibited the properties of ES cells rather than those of fibroblasts, expressing ES cell-specific markers. The authors also showed by introducing into the genome of fibroblasts a reporter construct, GFP under the control of a mouse Rex-1 gene, and fusing them with GFP-negative ES cells, that the ES-specific genes of fibroblasts were activated, as judged by GFP expression of the hybrid cells. The main conclusion made by the authors was that ES cells have the capacity to reprogram the genome of an adult somatic cell, which is in agreement with the earlier studies showing that ES and embryonic germ (EG) cells have the potential to reprogram the nuclei of somatic cells.[19,26,27] Tada and co-authors[26] showed that mouse thymocytes fused with ES cells begin to express Oct-4 and such hybrids can contribute to all three germ layers in an embryo. Do and Scholer[27] addressed the question whether the reprogramming signals are located in the cytoplasm or nuclei of ES cells. They separated cytoplasts and karyoplasts of ES cells through centrifugation on a Ficoll gradient and also used mitotically arrested with mitomycin C ES cells, then used each type for fusion with neurosphere cells. In their experiments only karyoplasts and mitomycin C-inactivated ES cells showed the reprogramming ability and induced Oct-4 expression in cells of neurospheres, so the authors concluded that such Oct-4 reprogramming cues reside in the ES cell karyoplast. However, all these studies, although of academic interest, are still far from therapeutic applications, or, at least, will depend on the development of techniques that allow separation of chromosomes of ES cells and somatic cells, either before or after the fusion.

Contrary to the results of the latter work, the group at the Reproductive Genetics Institute in Chicago[28] has published a report on successful reprogramming of human somatic cells with cytoplasts. They enucleated human ES cells by upside-down centrifugation of cells on cover slips at 25 000 *g* for 50 minutes and fused them using polyethylene glycol (PEG) with lymphocytes or fibroblasts. They claim to have achieved reprogramming of the adult somatic cells, which acquired ES colony morphology, expressed Oct-4 and could be passaged. They didn't, however, provide better characterization of the 'cybrids', such as evidence of other markers of pluripotency, retention of such markers over passaging, differentiation, at least, in vitro, into derivatives of three germ layers or statistics on the efficacy of this method. Yet the major hindrance to this approach is the presence of all participants of the procedure in the mixed resulting cultures – ES cells, 'cybrids' and tetraploid cells – coming from fusion with remaining non-enucleated ES cells, so development of a technique for isolation of reprogrammed cells is still in order.

With only a few reports on the accomplished reprogramming of somatic cells and very limited data, these experiments are still at the phase of academic research rather than technology development and will require more experimentation and proof of reproducibility by other laboratories. Such techniques largely depend on fine-tuning conditions of the system and the experimentator's skills set, so making this approach robust would require more studies in order to find key factors and conditions contributing to success.

DERIVATION OF EMBRYONIC STEM CELLS FROM GENETICALLY MODIFIED EMBRYOS

SCNT is regarded as a powerful technology for creating patient-specific ES cells and, subsequently, somatic cells. Aside from bogus SCNT patient-specific ES cell lines[29–32] no such lines have been established to date. This approach is not free from controversy: no genetically different human being is created, so some see it as sidestepping the ethical issues;[14] on the other hand, because cloned animals can be healthy and normal,[24] opponents of cloning regard it as a new life being created and destroyed. A high-tech approach developed in the laboratory of Dr Rudolf Jaenisch at Massachusetts Institute of Technology[25] tried to address this controversy. The researchers used a combination of SCNT and gene-targeting techniques, which they called altered nuclear transfer, or ANT, to create embryos to generate mouse blastocysts with a knocked-out *cdx2* gene that resulted in abnormal trophoblasts, so such embryos were unable to implant and, therefore, develop. The defective blastocysts, however, generated pluripotent ES cells, so the authors proposed this technique as a way of generating ES cells without embryo destruction. This approach may need more investigation of human-specific trophoblast genes before this technology is transferred to human embryos. The other concern the authors raise is the use of retroviral vectors which would bring up safety issues, if applied to human embryos. Another less-scientific but rather ethical issue is that in order to avoid destroying human embryos for ES cell generation, defective human embryos are being created and destroyed, and this could raise concerns among those who see preimplantation embryos as human beings, because the boundary between the destruction of non-viable embryos and refusal to support life may be too thin. Therefore, such technologies need to be approached with caution because they may result in creating even more controversy at the least.

SINGLE-BLASTOMERE-DERIVED EMBRYONIC STEM CELLS

In our laboratory we developed an approach to derive ES cells without embryo destruction using the single-blastomere biopsy procedure[23] similar to what is routinely used for preimplantation genetic diagnosis (PGD). In IVF clinics such procedures have become routine, and one or two blastomeres are removed and analyzed without depriving the embryo of its developmental potential. Such biopsied embryos remain fully viable and have produced many babies.[33] Multiple studies exploring the developmental potential of a single blastomere showed that it can contribute to all tissues and organs if aggregated with other blastomeres in a mouse embryo.[34,35] However, the recent data have shown that there is possible predisposition of blastomeres to trophoblast or ICM fate even at the 2-cell stage[36–38] that depends on the spatial arrangement and order of their second cleavage divisions; therefore, the potential of blastomeres to form all tissues may depend on them being in the proper environment, i.e. surrounded by other blastomeres. In our experiments single blastomeres from 129/Sv-*ROSA26:LacZ* were aggregated in microdepressions (similar to what is used for making aggregation chimeras) with GFP-labeled ES cells which seemed to support their division. In a day or two GFP-negative 'buds' were observed on the sides of GFP-positive cell clumps, which were separated from GFP-positive cells under a fluorescent microscope[23] either at this stage or later after such mixed clumps were plated on mitomycin C-inactivated mouse embryonic fibroblasts (MEFs) and produced a mixed outgrowth (Figure 13.2). Using mechanical passaging controlled under the fluorescent microscope, GFP-negative cells were selected and mechanically passaged until a pure population of GFP-negative ES cells was obtained. Several ES cell lines were generated that showed normal karyotype, expressed Oct-4, nanog, SSEA-1, stained positive for alkaline

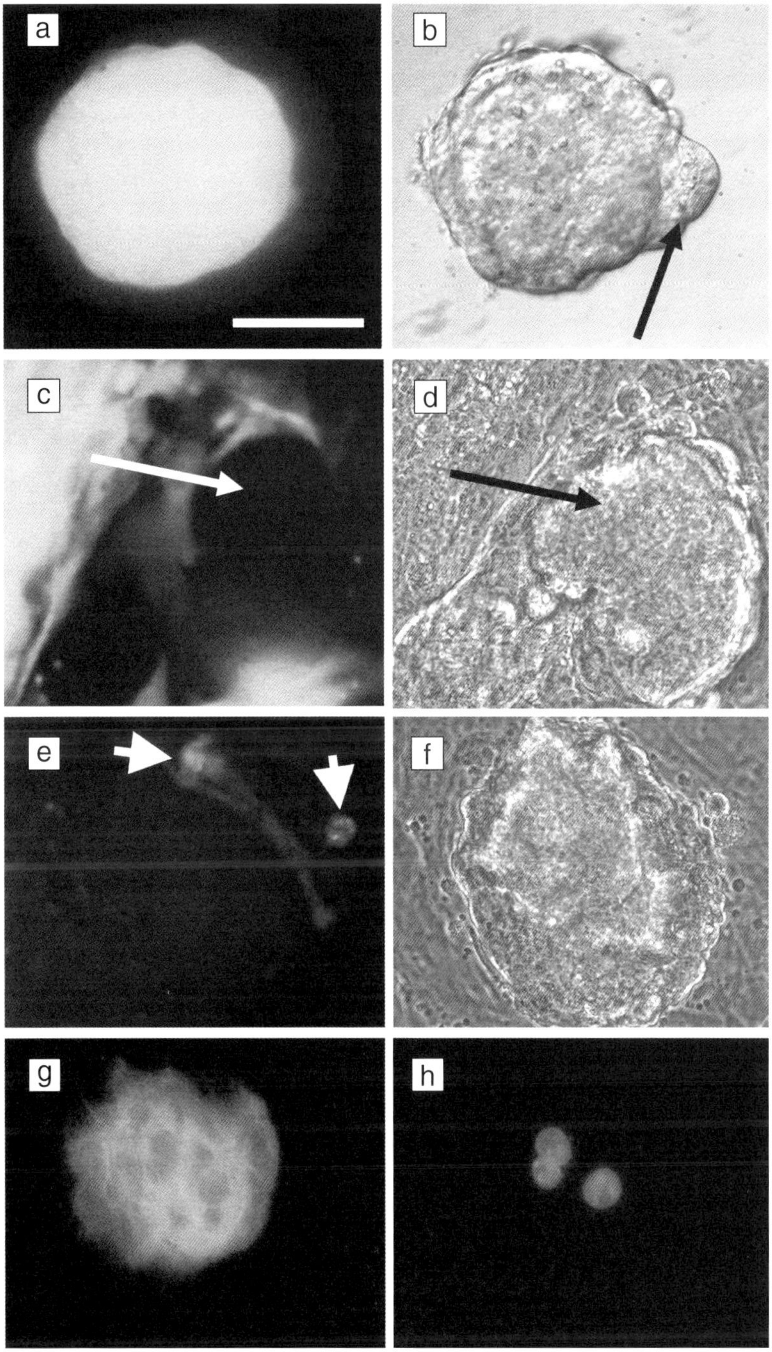

Figure 13.2 Stages of single blastomere growth in the presence (a–f) or absence (g,h) of mouse embryonic stem (mES) cells: (a,c,e) green fluorescence; (b) Hoffman modulation optics; (d,f) phase contrast. (a,b) Clump of GFP-positive mES cells 48 hours after aggregation with single blastomeres; arrow shows a protruding cluster of GFP-negative cells. (c,d) Outgrowth of GFP-negative cells aggregated with GFP^+ mES cells, after being plated on MEF; arrows point to GFP-negative cells. (e,f) Passage 1 of the outgrowth; arrows show remaining GFP^+ mES cells. (g,h) Single blastomere outgrowth on MEF for 4 days without ES cells, stained with Troma-1 and DAPI. Scale bar, 100 μm. (Reproduced from Chung et al,[23] with permission) (See also color plate)

phosphatase activity, and contributed to germline transmission, generating normal mouse pups in the second generation. The origin of these ES cells was confirmed by positive Lac-Z labeling and negative DNA polymerase chain reaction (PCR) for GFP.

The efficiency of the single blastomere approach for deriving mouse ES cells was lower (<10%) than in conventional approaches that use whole blastocysts. This efficiency can possible be increased by optimization of culture conditions and blastomere biopsy procedure. However, considering the data on early commitment of blastomeres to ICM or trophoblast fate,[36–38] such specification may be a limiting factor for the efficiency when 8-cell embryos are used. In our experiments, trophoblast stem cell lines were also produced from blastomeres coming from the same batches of dissociated embryos.[23]

Recently our group accomplished derivation of two human ES cell lines from single blastomeres using a slight modification of the approach described above.[24a] Developing single human blastomeres were placed into microdrops which were merged with other microdrops containing colonies of GFP-labeled hES cells. The blastomeres formed ES-cell-like outgrowths which were later passed mechanically, ensuring that no GFP-positive cells were selected. Two lines of hES cells derived using this technique from single blastomeres contained no presence of GFP-labeled ES cells as was shown by genomic DNA PCR and microsatellite analysis. The hES cells maintained normal karyotype, expressed hES markers Oct-4, nanog, SSEA-3, SSEA-4, TRA-1-60, TRA-1-61, stained for alkaline phosphatase and differentiated into the derivatives of all three germ layers in teratomas and *in vitro*. Because of the relatively low success rate this technique needs further development to progress from proof of principle to a clinical approach. 16 embryos or total of 91 blastomeres were used, but only six of them were grade I/II, and only 53 blastomeres divided. Nineteen ES-like outgrowths were produced initially and later lost to differentiation, so optimization of the culture conditions at the crucial early stages of blastomere outgrowth could further increase the success rate as well as selection of higher quality embryos. Possible blastomere commitment to ICM or trophoblast may be another explanation of the low success rate,[36–38] but at this time there is not enough known about early commitment of human blastomeres to be able to identify and select desirable blastomeres. If single-blastomere hES cell derivation technique gets further developed, so that hES cells can be produced more efficiently, it would allow to create hES cell lines without embryo destruction, which would probably qualify them for government funding worldwide and enable the production of syngeneic hES lines for the babies born through the IVF.

ES cells via parthenogenesis

One attractive possibility to overcome the problem of immune compatibility is the generation of ES cells and their derivatives from activated non-fertilized oocytes, or parthenotes that would only carry maternal *HLA* genes and thus allow reduction of the variability and number of lines required for immune matching the patients. Owing to genetic imprinting and deficiencies of maternal and paternal haploid gene sets, their combined action is required for normal development of an embryo, so parthenote mammalian embryos are unable to develop to birth. However, primate pluripotent cells were produced from such parthenote embryos[21] and seem to have the same phenotype, behavior and differentiation potential as 'normal' ES cells.[21,39] No such lines have yet been established from human oocytes, although there were attempts that produced proliferating cells that survived two passages.[22] It is unclear if such human lines will be eventually produced with further optimization of the technology and more oocytes available for research, which are generally in limited supply, or maternal imprinting may be involved, so modification of oocytes may be required in order to compensate for maternally silenced genes. From the ethical viewpoint, parthenote ES cells may be less controversial because no life is destroyed, and such embryos or ES cells can be seen as advanced derivatives of an ovarian teratoma which is an in vivo analog of a parthenote.

GERM CELLS

Embryonic germ cells derived from the primordial germ ridge could be an alternative to ES cells,[40,41] owing to their ability to retain pluripotency in culture and differentiate into derivatives of three germ layers, but, by the same token – their embryonic origin – their use for research or therapy is controversial. However, a group in Germany[42] has isolated multipotent adult germline cells (maGSCs) from mouse testes which meet all the criteria for ES cells, including germline transmission. If such cells were established from human testicular biopsies, they could become an excellent source of patient-specific cells for therapy without all the ethical problems surrounding ES cells. Another interesting approach was developed by Primegen, Biotech LLC, a Californian cell therapy company (press-release on www.primegenbiotech.com), who claim to have developed a technique to reprogram adult male germ cells into a pluripotent state. Another Californian company, Moraga, Moraga Biotechnology Corporation http://www.moragabiotech.com has announced that they isolated blastomere-like totipotent stem cells from somatic tissues which could differentiate into all tissues of the body. Although there is no publication of these findings, if these techniques hold true and could be reproducibly applied to isolation of pluripotent human cells, this could be a solution to the ES cell controversy.

In conclusion, there is currently no efficient and controversy-free technology to produce embryonic stem cells – or their differentiation derivatives – without embryo destruction (with a possible exception of single blastomere approach which still needs to be fine tuned to improve efficiency). The few approaches described above are still in infancy, and more research and optimization of these techniques is needed before any of them can move into application stage.

Acknowledgments

I would like to thank Dr Sadhana Agarwal for providing the photographs (Figure 13.1) to illustrate cell permeabilization with streptolysin-O and for a critical review of the manuscript and Drs Matvey Lukashev and Maria Mileikovskaya for their helpful comments.

REFERENCES

1. Evans MJ, Kaufman MH. Establishment in culture of pluripotential cells from mouse embryos. Nature 1981; 292: 154–6.
2. Thomson JA, Itskovitz-Eldor J, Shapiro SS, et al. Embryonic stem cell lines derived from human blastocysts. Science 1998; 282: 1145–7.
3. Carpenter MK, Rosler E, Rao MS. Characterization and differentiation of human embryonic stem cells. Cloning Stem Cells 2003; 5(1): 79–88.
4. Lanza R, Gearhant J, Hogan B et al. Handbook of Stem Cells, Vol 1: Embryonic Stem Cells. Amsterdam: Elsevier 2004.
5. Hoffman LM, Carpenter MK. Characterization and culture of human embryonic stem cells. Nat Biotechnol 2005; 23(6): 699–708.
6. Smith AG. Embryo-derived stem cells: of mice and men. Annu Rev Cell Dev Biol 2001; 17: 435–62.
7. Passier R, Denning C, Mummery C. Cardiomyocytes from human embryonic stem cells. Handb Exp Pharmacol 2006; 174: 101–22.
8. Ben-Hur T. Human embryonic stem cells for neuronal repair. Isr Med Assoc J 2006; 8(2): 122–6.
9. Klimanskaya I, Hipp J, Rezai KA et al. Derivation and comparative assessment of retinal pigment epithelium from human embryonic stem cells using transcriptomics. Cloning Stem Cells 2004; 6(3): 217–45.
10. Olivier EN, Rybicki AC, Bouhassira EE. Differentiation of human embryonic stem cells into bipotent mesenchymal stem cells. Stem Cells 2006; 24(8): 1914–22.
11. Kania G, Blyszczuk P, Wobus AM. The generation of insulin-producing cells from embryonic stem cells – a discussion of controversial findings. Int J Dev Biol 2004; 48(10): 1061–4.
12. Hug K. Sources of human embryos for stem cell research: ethical problems and their possible solutions. Medicina (Kaunas) 2005; 41(12): 1002–10.
13. Hug K. Therapeutic perspectives of human embryonic stem cell research versus the moral status of a human embryo – does one have to be compromised for the other? Medicina (Kaunas) 2006; 42(2): 107–14.
14. Evans M. Ethical sourcing of human embryonic stem cells – rational solutions? Nat Rev Mol Cell Biol 2005; 6(8): 663–7.
15. Lanza RP, Cibelli JB, West MD et al. The ethical reasons for stem cell research. Science 2001; 292(5520): 1299.
16. Taranger CK, Noer A, Sorensen AL et al. Induction of dedifferentiation, genomewide transcriptional programming, and epigenetic reprogramming by extracts of carcinoma and embryonic stem cells. Mol Biol Cell 2005; 16(12): 5719–35.
17. Hakelien AM, Gaustad KG, Taranger CK et al. Long-term in vitro, cell-type-specific genome-wide reprogramming of gene expression. Exp Cell Res 2005; 309(1): 32–47.
18. Hakelien AM, Landsverk HB, Robl JM, Skalhegg BS, Collas P. Reprogramming fibroblasts to express T-cell functions using cell extracts. Nat Biotechnol 2002; 20(5): 460–6.
19. Tada M, Tada T, Lefebvre L, Barton SC, Surani MA. Embryonic germ cells induce epigenetic reprogramming of somatic nucleus in hybrid cells. EMBO J 1997; 16(21): 6510–20.

20. Cowan CA, Atienza J, Melton DA et al. Nuclear reprogramming of somatic cells after fusion with human embryonic stem cells. Science 2005; 309(5739): 1369–73.

21. Cibelli JB, Grant KA, Chapman KB et al. Parthenogenetic stem cells in nonhuman primates. Science 2002; 295(5556): 819.

22. Lin H, Lei J, Wininger D et al. Multilineage potential of homozygous stem cells derived from metaphase II oocytes. Stem Cells 2003; 21(2): 152–61.

23. Chung Y, Klimanskaya I, Becker S et al. Embryonic and extraembryonic stem cell lines derived from single mouse blastomeres. Nature 2006; 439(7073): 216–19.

24. Lanza RP, Cibelli JB, Faber D et al. Cloned cattle can be healthy and normal. Science 2001; 294(5548): 1893–4.

24a. Klimanskaya I, Chung Y, Becker S, Lu S-J, Lanza R. Human embryonic stem cell lines derived from single blastomeres. Nature: advance online publication; 23 August 2006.

25. Meissner A, Jaenisch R. Generation of nuclear transfer-derived pluripotent ES cells from cloned Cdx2-deficient blastocysts. Nature 2006; 439(7073): 212–15.

26. Tada M, Takahama Y, Abe K et al. Nuclear reprogramming of somatic cells by in vitro hybridization with ES cells. Curr Biol 2001; 11(19): 1553–8.

27. Do JT, Scholer HR. Nuclei of embryonic stem cells reprogram somatic cells. Stem Cells 2004; 22(6): 941–9.

28. Strelchenko N, Kukharenko V, Shkumatov A et al. Reprogramming of human somatic cells by embryonic stem cell cytoplast. Reprod Biomed Online 2006; 12(1): 107–11.

29. Hwang WS, Ryu YJ, Park JH et al. Evidence of a pluripotent human embryonic stem cell line derived from a cloned blastocyst. Science 2004; 303(5664): 1669–74. Retraction in: Kennedy D. Science 2006; 311(5759): 335. Erratum in: Science 2005; 310(5755): 1769.

30. Hwang WS, Roh SI, Lee BC et al. Patient-specific embryonic stem cells derived from human SCNT blastocysts. Science 2005; 308(5729): 1777–83. Retraction in: Kennedy D. Science 2006; 311(5759): 335. Erratum in: Science 2005; 310(5755): 1769.

31. Civin CI. Cloned photomicrographs, not cloned cells. Stem Cells 2005 Dec 28; [Epub ahead of print].

32. Martin TJ. Reactions to the Hwang scandal. Science 2006; 311(5761): 606–7.

33. Handyside AH, Kontogianni EH, Hardy K, Winston RM. Pregnancies from biopsied human preimplantation embryos sexed by Y-specific DNA amplification. Nature 1990; 344: 768–70.

34. Kelly SJ. Studies of the developmental potential of 4- and 8-cell stage mouse blastomeres. J Exp Zool 1977; 200(3): 365–76.

35. Pedersen RA. Potency, lineage and allocation in preimplantation mouse embryos. In: Rossant J, Pedersen RA, eds. Experimental Approaches to Mammalian Embryonic Development. New York: Cambridge University Press, 1988: 3–33.

36. Piotrowska K, Wianny F, Pedersen RA et al. Blastomeres arising from the first cleavage division have distinguishable fates in normal mouse development. Development 2001; 128(19): 3739–48.

37. Piotrowska-Nitsche K, Zernicka-Goetz M. Spatial arrangement of individual 4-cell stage blastomeres and the order in which they are generated correlate with blastocyst pattern in the mouse embryo. Mech Dev 2005; 122(4): 487–500.

38. Piotrowska-Nitsche K, Perea-Gomez A, Haraguchi S et al. Four-cell stage mouse blastomeres have different developmental properties. Development 2005; 132(3): 479–90.

39. Vrana KE, Hipp JD, Goss AM et al. Nonhuman primate parthenogenetic stem cells. Proc Natl Acad Sci USA 2003; 100 (Suppl 1): 11911–16. Erratum in: Proc Natl Acad Sci USA 2004; 101(2): 693.

40. Shamblott MJ, Axelman J, Wang S et al. Derivation of pluripotent stem cells from cultured human primordial germ cells. Proc Natl Acad Sci USA 1998; 95(23): 13726–31. Erratum in: Proc Natl Acad Sci USA 1999; 96(3): 1162.

41. Shamblott MJ, Axelman J, Littlefield JW et al. Human embryonic germ cell derivatives express a broad range of developmentally distinct markers and proliferate extensively in vitro. Proc Natl Acad Sci USA 2001; 98(1): 113–18.

42. Guan K, Nayernia K, Maier LS et al. Pluripotency of spermatogonial stem cells from adult mouse testis. Nature 2006; 440(7088): 1199–203.

CHAPTER 14

Human embryonic stem cell culture in feeder-free, xeno-free conditions

Amparo Galán, Antonio Pellicer and Carlos Simon

INTRODUCTION

The report of the derivation of the first human embryonic stem cell (hESC) lines[1] represented a revolutionary discovery, since its biological characteristics were both enormously promising therapeutically and heralded important regulatory challenges. hESCs are derived from the inner cell mass (ICM) of embryos cultured to the morula or blastocyst stage. Their most significant properties are their robust proliferative capacity for self-renewal and their pluripotency, by which they are capable of differentiating into virtually any cell type under the right conditions. These unique characteristics of hESCs make them suitable for future application in humans, as their lines may constitute an unlimited source of all cell types to be used in cell-based regenerative medicine therapies, and also in human developmental studies, tissue engineering, in-vitro gene therapy models[2] and as a screening tool for the pharmaceutical industry.

These undifferentiated cells display typical surface markers of SSEA-3, SSEA-4, TRA-1-60 and TRA-1-81 antibodies, and alkaline phosphatase enzymatic activity. In addition, molecular gene expression analysis have detected positive amplification for the undifferentiation markers Oct-3/4,[3] Sox2, Rex-1[4] Foxd3,[5] Fgf4, Cripto, Thy-1, LeftyA[6] and Nanog[7] and negative amplication for differentiation markers from the ectoderm (Dbh), mesoderm (Matn1) and endoderm (Amy).[3] hESCs also display normal karyotypes all along passages, and telomerase activity characteristic of immortal cells. Their pluripotency has been demonstrated by spontaneous differentiation both in vitro by embryoid bodies formation, and in vivo by teratoma formation when injected into severe combined immunodeficiency (SCID) mice.[1,8]

Initial derivations of hESCs were performed in Thomson's laboratory using the ICMs of human blastocysts placed on inactivated murine feeder cells (mouse embryonic fibroblasts [MEF]).[1] More than 78 hESC lines are available on the National Institutes of Health (NIH) registry, but all have been derived and propagated on MEF (xenosupports) in the presence of animal-based proteins (xenoproteins). The use of feeders from mice and products from animal sources raises the possibility of zoonosis. To avoid the presence of animal cells in the culture process, feeder-free conditions were developed based on the use of extracellular matrix (ECM) from mice and conditioned medium either from animal or human fibroblasts. Nevertheless, these approaches did not rule out the risk of animal contamination. Contamination by animal products represented less of a theoretical concern when it was found that hESCs cultured with animal cells or serum products could take up Neu5Gc, a non-human sialic acid that is immunogenic in cells used for human transplantation.[9]

In order to overcome this problem, many laboratories have developed xeno-free systems to derive and propagate hESCs, thereby minimizing contact with animal cells/products/proteins.[10] These systems employ human feeder cells, and even autogeneic feeders from hESC lines,[11–14] whereas acid Tyrode's solution rather than pronase or immunosurgery is employed for the removal of the zona pellucida of the embryo,[13,15] and culture media are composed of serum replacement (SR) rather than products of an animal origin.[10] However, experience with organ and tissue allotransplantation has shown that diseases and infectious agents can be transmitted from human donor cells to the recipient, thus making necessary an extensive and time-consuming microbiological analysis of human feeder cell lines prior to their use, and in addition, the media used currently for culture conditions are poorly defined, with some animal origin proteins. Attempts to improve derivation and propagation conditions have led to the derivation of the first hESC line in feeder-free conditions, in the presence of ECM from mice and SR instead of conditioned medium.[16] The latest breakthrough has been achieved by Ludwig and colleagues, who have derived two hESC lines in feeder-free conditions, using a human matrix, and with a complete defined medium containing recombinant proteins and molecules.[17]

Until now, the specific factors that promote initial hESC self-renewal and maintenance have represented the greatest enigma in this process. Moreover, we do not know whether these factors are soluble or whether they act through direct ECM ligand–receptor binding or through a cooperative action. The molecular signaling pathways involved in stemness are still unknown, and research will strive to move forward progressively through a trial-and-error strategy until these basic questions are answered.

The expectations raised by these breakthroughs with regard to future clinical applications in humans are impulsing the need for further tuning. Regulations in many countries (e.g. US Food and Drug Adminstration [FDA] regulations) are based on the possible contamination of hESCs with mouse cells or by-products/contaminants, which rules out the use of these lines in regenerative medicine. As previously mentioned, zoonosis, the transmission of pathogens from animals to humans, is a serious concern within the medical field. In fact, the term 'research grade versus clinical grade' has been coined to distinguish between hESC lines derived in the presence or absence of animal 'cells/products/contaminants'.

According to new EU directives (2003/94/EC and 2004/24/EC), hESCs for transplantation must be cultured under conditions of good manufacturing practice (GMP) so as to guarantee the safety and quality of the cells.[18,19] Incorporating GMP conditions implies impeccable record keeping, qualified personnel, high sanitary standards, equipment verification, validation of processes and complaint management. In addition, conditions must be closely controlled and xeno-free, in order to avoid the risk of zoonosis, and feeder-free systems must allow for large-scale production.[20] The aforementioned European directive refers to cellular stem-cell-derived materials that are intended for human application, but not to the preceding in-vitro research. The directive was agreed in March 2004 and member states have been obliged to implement it by April 2006. The standards for processing, preservation, storage and distribution to be met will, in broad terms, be the same as those for donated and processed cells and tissues, which must be thoroughly tested and characterized.

The extreme flexibility and growth capacity of hESCs make them ideal for producing large quantities of differentiated cells for therapeutic applications. However, there is an urgent need for a reliable process through which further hESC lines of therapeutic grade may be derived and propagated. This chapter offers an historical overview of the different strategies that have been undertaken in this field, ranging from the hESC lines that were grown in the presence of human feeders to the evolution from animal serum to serum replacement, and from feeder to feeder-free conditions to completely animal-free, feeder-free and culture-defined conditions and the derivation and propagation of hESC lines for clinical applications.

HUMAN FEEDERS

The first attempts to use human feeders in order to avoid zoonosis involved fetal tissues, fetal muscle (FM) and fetal skin (FS) cells. Cultures of FM and FS cells were established as feeders and were supported by human serum (screened for human immunodeficiency virus [HIV]-1 and HIV-2, and hepatitis B). These cell types were reported to maintain existing HES-3 and HES-4 (ES Cell International, Singapore) lines for more than 20 passages, in the presence of human serum.[11] However, the use of fetal fibroblasts is problematic in terms of the restricted availability of tissues, ethical concerns surrounding the use of cells from human aborted fetuses and the need to screen cell sources for potential pathogens.

In a later study, the same group evaluated a panel of 11 different human adult, fetal and neonatal feeders with respect to their capacity to maintain hESCs, in an attempt to develop feeder layers composed of fibroblasts from adult biopsies.[19] HES-3 and HES-4 were able to grow in an undifferentiated stage for a long period in the presence of SR in adult skin fibroblasts, which were consequently presented as the first adult tissue that could be used as a feeder layer. Nevertheless, fetal fibroblasts were clearly superior to the other fibroblast feeders,[19] confirming the general view that fetal or embryonic tissues are more supportive than adult tissues in vitro, and more importantly highlighting the differences in feeding conditions between human cell types and sources.

The human endometrial epithelium (hUEC) directly interacts with human embryos through several systems and aids embryonic development in vitro, thus constituting the basis of the clinical program of endometrial co-culture for the development of human blastocysts in in-vitro fertilization (IVF).[21,22] As previously demonstrated, the molecular crosstalk between the human embryo and the endometrium is essential,[23] thus making it an ideal supporter of hESC lines. In this context, Richards and colleagues[19] attempted to develop various hUEC lines, initially without success. However, in later attempts, both hUECs and parenchymal cells were shown to support the hESC line Miz-hES1[24] and the hUECs' capacity as suitable feeder layers were demonstrated with the derivation of three new lines (Table 14.1).[25] The variability in the supporting capacity of hUECs seems to be because the endometrial cells were obtained at different phases of the menstrual cycle.

An interesting approach to manage new feeders involves the use of postnatal human skin fibroblasts to generate a proper cell layer. In 2003, a report described the first production of fibroblast cell lines using foreskin to support I-6, I-3[26] and H-9[1] by employing either fetal borine serum (FBS) SR or human serum (HS).[27] A significant step forward was achieved by Hovatta et al, when they derived their first hESC lines (HS181 and HS207) using postnatal, commercially available foreskin fibroblasts with fetal calf serum (FCS) as the growing medium.[28]

In a more recent study, Choo et al[29] tested three commercially available human foreskin feeders in an attempt to eliminate animal components in the culture conditions. HES-3 and HES-4, grown in the presence of serum or serum replacement (KO-serum, SR), expanded undifferentiated for more than 30 passages and showed pluripotency markers and normal

Table 14.1 Human feeders used for human embryonic stem cell (hESC) derivation

Feeder type[a]	*Inactivation*	*hESC line derived*	*Culture composition*[b]	*Reference*
Miz-Endo-1 (hUEC)	Mitomycin-C	Miz-hES-9 Miz-hES-14 Miz-hES-15	SR	25
CRL-2429 (FSK)	Irradiation	HS181 HS207	FCS	28
CRL-2429 (FSK)	Irradiation	HS293	SR	30
CRL-2429 (FSK)	Irradiation	HS306	SR	30
8B (Placenta)	Irradiation	UCSF1 UCSF2	SR	12
8B (Placenta)	Irradiation	VAL-1 VAL-2	SR	13
EDF-H1 EDF-SH1 EDF-SH2	Irradiation	SH7	SR	32

[a]hUEC, uterine endometrium; FSK, foreskin; EDF, hESC derived fibroblast feeder
[b]SR, serum replacement; FCS, fetal calf serum
Data from Galán et al[10]

morphology in the presence of SR. An improvement to the derivation process consisted of the establishment of two hESC lines, HS293 and HS306, using commercially available human foreskin fibroblasts (CRL-2429, ATCC) as feeders and SR medium instead of conventional FCS.[30] Both lines have surpassed passage 56 and 41, respectively. The lines express typical markers of pluripotency and are able to form embryoid bodies in vitro and teratomas in SCID mice in vivo. SR is an important step forward, allowing the use of human feeders in xeno-free conditions.

Since in-vivo undifferentiated hESCs are surrounded by the trophoectoderm during development, the use of human placental fibroblast lines as a feeder layer in the hESC derivation process is an approximation to the in-vivo stem cell environment.[12,13] In this context, two recent reports have shown that early-gestation placental fibroblasts can be used as feeders to propagate established hESC lines and derive new ones such as UCSF1 and UCSF2,[12] and VAL-1 and VAL-2 (Figure 14.1).[13] In these reports, the derivation process was designed to minimize contact with animal cells/products/proteins.[13] The zona pellucida was removed using acid Tyrode's solution rather than pronase, and without performing immunosurgery, thereby eliminating exposure to animal antibodies and complement factors. The derivation and culturing processes took place in SR rather than FCS. As the placental fibroblasts were screened for animal and human pathogens, and no serum was used during the derivation process, the risk of zoonosis was greatly reduced, and thus a therapeutic grade line was approached. However, it is important to note that animal components were used in the establishment

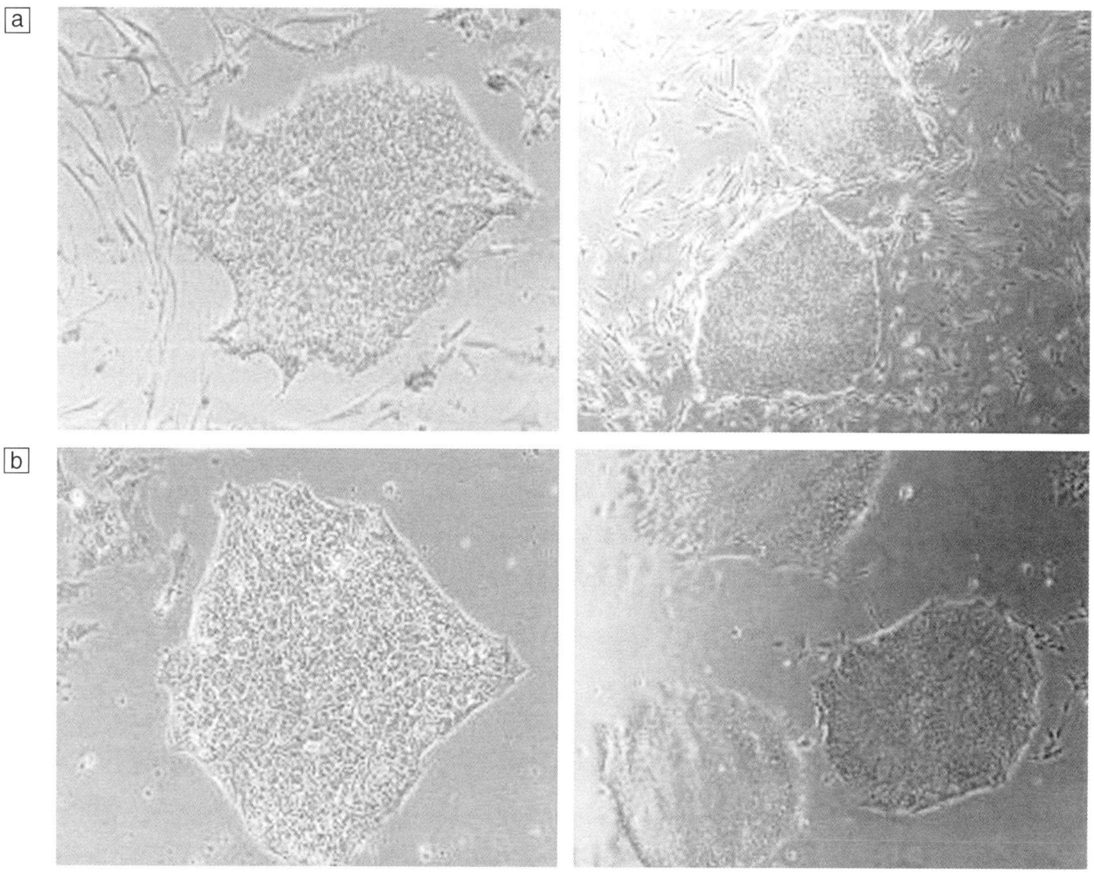

Figure 14.1 Morphological features of VAL-1 and VAL-2 colonies in the presence of feeders (a) and in feeder-free conditions (b). Colonies are typically flattened with defined borders all throughout passages

and propagation of the human placental fibroblast feeders, making necessary further experiments to derive both feeders and hESCs in the absence of serum and animal proteins.[13,15]

It should be taken into account that the use of feeder cells for the derivation and culture of hESCs limit their medical application, as allogeneic feeders carry the risk of interspecies virus transfer.[11,14,28,31] For this reason, the recent approach of using fibroblast-like cells differentiated from hESC as feeder cells has brought us closer to the therapeutic application of hESCs.[14,32] The idea behind this new human feeder source is that fibroblast-like cells differentiated from hESCs may also support the stemness of the same or different hESC lines. Two recent studies have explored the possibility of creating an autogeneic fibroblast feeder,[14,32] and have successfully concluded that this system could facilitate large-scale production of hESC lines with a genotypically homogeneous system in a standardized, animal pathogen-free environment. In the first study, fibroblasts were obtained from spontaneous differentiation of hESC lines H1[1] and hES-NCL1[14] after being grown in feeder-free conditions for 1 week. Cells from hES-NCL1 with a fibroblast-like morphology were successfully used in the autogeneic propagation of hES-NCL1 and the allogeneic support of H1 cells.[14] In the second study, three hESC lines – H1, SH1 and SH2[32] – were used to derive fibroblast feeders (EDFs). Eleven EDF subcultures were established from these lines, and have been shown to support the sustained growth of hESCs. In addition, a new hESC line, SH7, has been derived using EDFs as a support.[32] This feeder cell system, derived from hESCs, successfully prolongs the growth of undifferentiated and cytogenetically stable colonies, and eliminates risk factors and concerns surrounding the use of xenogeneic or unknown allogeneic factors. However, this differentiation into fibroblasts may not be definitive, and some remaining undifferentiated cells may divide again, leading to a mix of colonies of different origins.[10,20]

EXTRACELLULAR MATRICES FOR HUMAN EMBRYONIC STEM CELL DERIVATION AND EXPANSION

The use of feeder layers limits stem cell research designs, since data obtained from experiments might result from a combined response of hESCs plus feeder cells to various stimuli. Besides, a feeder-free culture system would allow simplification of the analysis of the environmental factors that are involved in the undifferentiation, pluripotency and self-renewal of hESCs. This implemented system would also simplify hESC-based in-vitro models for the study of early embryogenesis. Finally, the introduction of feeder-free systems in gene transfer protocols will be necessary for the genetic manipulation of hESCs in gene therapy studies and embryology, since the presence of feeder cells may interfere in all the genetic modifications of hESCs.[2,33] In addition, experience with organ and tissue allotransplantation has shown that HIV-1, HIV-2, Creutzfeldt–Jakob disease, hepatitis B or C viruses and other infectious agents can be transmitted from human donor cells to the recipient.[15]

Culture in feeder-free conditions consists of an in-vitro system where hESCs can be grown in the absence of any other cell type. Because of the special requirements of hESCs, many groups have developed feeder-free systems using different sources. Most of the systems use ECM extracted from murine or human sources supplemented with conditioned medium (medium harvested from a culture of feeder cells, at 24 hours, rich in released growth factors) from feeders and/or additional growth factors.

The ECM provides structural support in a multicellular layer, as well as important regulatory signals governing cell growth, metabolism and differentiation. Throughout these various cell–biological processes, the ECM can act both as a structural scaffolding for cell adhesion and migration and as a trigger for signaling through its receptors.[34] One of the most important properties of the ECM is its functional diversity:[35] some components are designed to be rigid, others elastic, some wet, others sticky. All have modular designs that impart diverse roles, yet allow for highly specialized functions. Most components of the ECM involve structural proteins, adhesive glycoproteins, matricellular proteins and proteoglycans.

Referring to structural proteins, collagen is the most ubiquitous ECM protein and is responsible for its structure and resiliency in tissues. Elastin is a predominant component of the elastic fiber, and fibrillin plays key roles in microfibrillar structures. With regard to adhesive glycoproteins, ECM is mainly composed of fibronectin, vitronectin, laminin and basement membranes. Both fibronectin and vitronectin can be purified by affinity chromatography from human plasma, providing large quantities of an individual adhesive protein useful for cell culture studies. Matricellular proteins include a group of extracellular proteins that function by binding to matrix proteins and to cell surface receptors but do not contribute to the structural integrity of the ECM; these proteins include SPARC (osteonectin), thrombospondin, tenascin and other molecules that function to modulate a wide range of biological responses to the ECM.[36] Finally, proteoglycans are a major class of diverse ECM molecules that are implicated in signal transduction, adhesion and ECM structure. Components of the ECM are not static, but, instead, are in a dynamic balance between synthesis and degradation. The continuous turnover and active remodeling of the ECM in embryonic development depends critically on carefully regulated degradation by proteolytic enzymes, particularly by the matrix metalloproteinases (MMPs).[34] It is not possible to ascertain the functional properties of a complex matrix such as basement membrane without studying its individual components. It is also clear that the functional complexity of the assembled three-dimensional membrane is greater than the sum of the isolated component.

The first steps towards a feeder-free system in hESCs were taken by the group of Xu and collaborators[37] who established the first protocol for feeder-free hESC propagation that is still now the basis for many studies in several groups.[38–42] In the original paper,[37] several ECMs were evaluated to support hESC growth in an undifferentiated stage. Matrigel and laminin were found to give the best conditions for hESC culture and maintenance when supplemented with MEF-conditioned medium.[1,8] Matrigel is an animal basement membrane preparation extracted from Engelbreth–Holm–Swarm mouse sarcoma, a tumor rich in ECM proteins: laminin, collagen IV, heparan sulfate proteoglycans, entactin, and nidogen 1. Unfortunately, Matrigel or MEF-conditioned medium is not a good resource for potential medical application of hESCs, as xenogeneic pathogens may be transmitted.[9,19,43]

In mouse ESC cultures, the feeder layer can be replaced by the addition of the cytokine leukemia inhibitory factor (LIF) to the growth medium, keeping cells pluripotent and undifferentiated.[44,45] Nevertheless, LIF does not have this effect in hESCs and, currently, the most useful molecule preventing hESC differentiation is the human basic fibroblast growth factor (bFGF) added to the conditioned media.[27,46]

Large-scale gene expression profiling of hESCs reveals that components of several signal transduction pathways are transcriptionally enriched in the undifferentiated state, allowing a prioritization of the pathways and possible factors to be studied. Following these premises, it was detected that the main components of the canonical Wnt pathway were present in undifferentiated hESCs.[47] Furthermore, the potential use of the pharmacological component 6-bromoindirubin-3′-oxime (BIO),[48] has been proven to maintain the undifferentiated phenotype in hESCs and sustain the expression of the pluripotent state-specific transcription factors. Furthermore, BIO-mediated Wnt activation is functionally reversible,[43] which could be potentially of great clinical value.

Other researchers have reported different methodologies for the maintenance of hESCs in the absence of a feeder cell layer. These studies have identified a number of polypeptide factors, including transforming growth factor-β (TGF-β), Wnt3a, nodal and other factors that appear to enhance stem cell renewal under different culture conditions.[49,50] However, none of these factors eliminates the use of animal products or supports efficient clonal growth of the cells.

In an attempt to overcome the problem with xenosupports, xenoproteins and conditioned media, Amit and collaborators[51] demonstrated the feasibility of a defined serum- and feeder layer-free culture system based on the use of SR, TGF-β_1, LIF, bFGF and human fibronectin matrix as a substitute for the Matrigel of animal origin. In these conditions, hESCs have been able to grow and remain undifferentiated after prolonged culture. However, this system has not avoided completely the contact between hESC and animal derivatives, just reduced their exposure.

Of the most satisfactory systems for feeder-free propagation developed, those by Wang,[40] Xu,[41] and Xu[42] and collaborators stand out. The first system is based on adding noggin and bFGF to the media,[40] the second involves the combination of several factors with bFGF and the third also utilizes the addition of noggin to the culture medium along with an increase of the dose of bFGF.[42] However, although the culture conditions are improved, these systems still involve the use of Matrigel of animal origin for the expansion of hESC lines.

In an approach to improve xeno-free hESC cultures, Stojkovic and colleagues[52] have developed a system that employs HS as a matrix and conditioned medium from hES-dF for the growth of hESC (see above). Several studies have previously described the use of HS as a supplement to grow hESC. Richards et al[19] reported the possibility of growing hESCs on human fibroblasts in media supplemented with HS for at least 10 passages. However, the use of HS in culture media was not beneficial for prolonged cultures of hESCs, as increased differentiation rates were observed.[19] In this context, the method described by Stojkovic and colleagues really means a breakthrough, as this system successfully works for the attachment and long-term growth of undifferentiated hESCs (Figure 14.2). Therefore, replacement of Matrigel ECM derived from MEF, or MEF-conditioned medium[40,41,42,53] by HS and hES-dF-conditioned medium, provides a safer direction towards completely animal-free conditions and for application, handling and understanding of hESC biology.

In the next decade, the field of hESC research will center its efforts on overcoming obstacles such as the need to develop consistent feeder-free and xeno-free systems that will ensure the clinical grade of newly derived hESC lines. All the above-mentioned methods have been demonstrated to support hESC growth in an undifferentiated stage, but have not been able to derive any new hESC line.

In an important step forward, Klimanskaya et al[16] have been able, for the first time, to derive a new hESC line, ACT-14, under feeder-free conditions. For that purpose, ECM components derived from MEF extracts (Matrigel)[55] and SR instead of conditioned medium were used. Handpicked colonies of hESCs were plated onto ECM-coated plates, and subsequently passaged with either mechanical or enzymatic maintenance techniques. For growth and expansion, usual medium containing SR, LIF and bFGF was used.[16] After more than 20 passages on ECM, ACT-14 retained the markers of pluripotency, a normal female karyotype along the passages and retained their capacity to form differentiated cell types of all three germ layers.[16]

The ECM was obtained from plated and irradiated MEF and SR was used. Preliminary studies indicate that the plates could be dehydrated, treated with paraformaldehyde, heat-pasteurized or gamma-irradiated, besides other conventional treatment and sterilization processes, without substantial changes in hESC performance, and thus, eliminating the infectivity of viral structures and other possible infectious agents. This is the first report that describes a complete derivation and expansion of an hESC line under feeder-free conditions;[16] however, the immunogenicity of the xenocomponents of the extracellular matrix from MEF still remains. This difficulty will be hopefully overcome in the near future.[54]

One of the main problems is that the extrinsic factors necessary for maintaining hESC pluripotency and self-renewal are currently poorly understood, because of complex culture conditions that include both growth of inactivated feeder cells and SR, a cocktail of proteins and soluble factors. The ECM is a three-dimensional molecular complex that varies in composition and diversity, and consists of basic components such as fibronectin, collagens and other glycoproteins, hyaluronic acid, proteoglycans and elastins; it also harbors and presents molecules such as growth factors and hormones,[56,57] although many of these molecules would be inactivated during heat pasteurization or sterilization. Further studies will be needed to determine which of these ECM molecules or their spatial organization are crucial for the maintenance of the undifferentiated hESC phenotype, as well as the identification of the target proteins and components included in the growing media necessary for this process.[16,54]

DERIVATION AND GROWTH OF HUMAN EMBRYONIC STEM CELLS IN DEFINED MEDIUM

Widespread therapeutic application of hESCs requires reliable scaled production of well-characterized cell lines. As an alternative to xenogeneic and allogeneic cultures, SR is now used by most of the groups that culture hESC lines, but these media continue to contain animal proteins rather than solely human proteins, and preferably clonal recombinant proteins. Also, most groups use conditioned media for the propagation of hESCs in feeder-free conditions; these media are composed of proteins and molecules of different origin and heterogeneity, thus highlighting the necessity of defined media for further applications.[10,15,54]

Initial attempts to develop a defined medium led to the identification of a number of polypeptide factors, including TGF, Wnt-3a, nodal and other factors, which, when added to the growing medium, enhanced stem cell renewal under different culture conditions. However, none of these factors permits animal

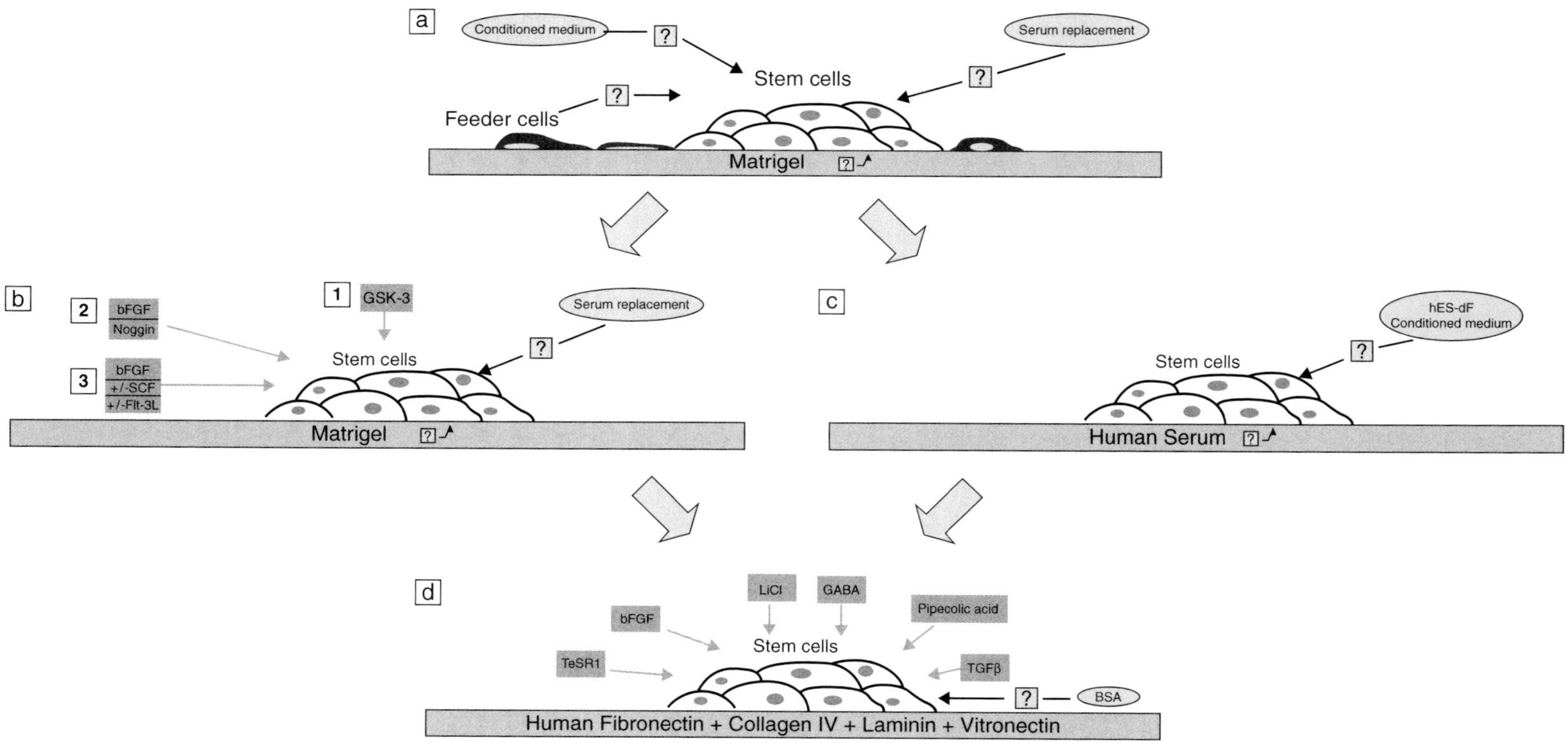

Figure 14.2 Evolution of hESC culture in vitro through defined growing conditions. (a) Foreign, unknown or potentially biohazardous components are introduced by conditioned medium, serum replacement (SR), feeder cells or Matrigel.[1,6,10,37] (b) GSK-3 (**1**),[43] bFGF alone or in the presence of noggin, or other growth components (**2** and **3**) can replace some of the unknown components; yet, SR is still used in most conditions[40–42] and animal origin Matrigel. (c) Using conditioned medium obtained from autogeneic feeders and human serum as matrix.[52] (d) Approaching an ideal defined culture condition. TeSR1-defined medium supplemented by five growth factors, growing on a synthetic matrix. Only the HSA component is not fully defined

products to be completely substituted or supports efficient clonal growth of the cells.[49,50,58]

The main objective at present is to determine the minimal combination of growth factors that maintains the proliferation and pluripotency of undifferentiated hESCs without the need for feeder cells or conditioned medium. In this context, three new types of medium that minimize animal exposure and improve culture definition have evolved. The first was developed by Wang and collaborators[40] and employs a feeder-free system based on Matrigel, nogging and bFGF. They have demonstrated that noggin (an antagonist of bone morphogenetic protein [BMP]) is critical for preventing the differentiation of hESCs in culture, and that a combination of noggin and bFGF maintains the prolonged growth of hESCs in feeder-free conditions without the need for a conditioned medium.[40]

A similar conclusion was achieved by Xu and colleagues,[42] who reported that, when noggin is added to the culture medium, and the dose of bFGF is increased, hESCs can be grown without a feeder cell layer or conditioned medium. In this way, the group used SR-containing medium and Matrigel as the ECM, demonstrating that increased doses of bFGF reduce the differentiation signaling pathway controlled by BMP, and that they are necessary to sustain self-renewal and developmental potential of hESCs.[42]

In the third study, cumulative data collected by Xu and colleagues showed that growth of hESCs was supported by SR non-conditioned medium containing bFGF or bFGF in combination with other growth factors such as SCF, Flt3L, TPO or LIF.[41] In contrast, the addition of all the other factors (alone or in combination) without FGF did not maintain the growth of undifferentiated cells. Another possible source of molecules for undifferentiated hESC propagation could be the hESC growth factors produced during culture. However, it is unlikely that the autocrine and paracrine factors produced by hESCs can adequately support the growth of these cells in long-term culture.[41]

It has been demonstrated that high concentrations of bFGF support hESCs in the absence of fibroblasts and that bFGF supports clonal growth on fibroblasts in the presence of a commercially available serum substitute.[16,17,42,59] However, in all the cited reports, poorly defined SR and matrigel are used, which means that animal components and undefined substances were still present in the culture environment. For further applications it will be necessary to improve all these conditions through accurately defined parameters.

A recent report presented a feeder-independent method that permits hESC culture and novel derivations, including protein components derived solely from recombinant sources from human materials (Table 14.2 and Figure 14.2).[17] For that purpose a defined medium was synthesized and a human matrix combining collagen IV, fibronectin, laminin and vitronectin was developed.[17]

The resulting medium (TeSR1) is composed of the standard base (DMEM/F12) supplemented with human serum albumin (HSA), vitamins, antioxidants, trace minerals, specific lipids and cloned growth factors, all perfectly quantified. Analysis of physicochemical culture conditions suggested that undifferentiated hESC proliferation was optimal at a pH 7.2, an osmolarity of 350 mOsmol and an atmosphere of 10% CO_2 and 5% O_2; these conditions were recreated in the subsequent media. To define the growth factors to be added, an initial test was performed based on receptors expressed by hESC.[58] Five molecules found to have a positive effect on undifferentiated proliferation – bFGF, lithium chloride (LiCl), γ-aminobutyric acid (GABA), pipecolic acid and TGF-β – were eventually included in TeSR1. Removal of any one of the five factors significantly decreased some parameter of culture performance, but only the removal of bFGF had a dramatic effect on both the total number of cells and the percentage of cells expressing ESC markers.[17]

Using TeSR1 medium on the four human matrix components, Thomson's group derived two new hESC lines, WA15 and WA16. Both lines display typical characteristics and, at the time of publication, have been continuously in culture for more than 7 months.[17] Unfortunately, both lines presented chromosomal abnormalities. After 4 months in culture, WA16 was shown to be XXY (Klinefelter's syndrome) and WA15 was karyotypically normal (XY). Klinefelter's syndrome is the most common human chromosomal abnormality, and it is unclear whether it was present in the embryo itself or was acquired during culture. The new hESC line WA15 was initially normal, but converted to trisomy 12 between months 4 and 7 of culture, probably owing to the enzymatic dissociation used to passage the cells. The emergence of abnormal karyotype 12 in hESCs has been described previously,[43] and is usually associated with clonal events.[17]

Table 14.2 Chronology of the derivation and propagation of human embryonic stem cell (hESC) lines. From feeder-free to animal-free and defined medium conditions. Evolution from the first lines propagated in feeder-free conditions up to the ones derived and propagated in feeder-free, animal-free and defined conditions

Matrix	*Culture medium*	*hESC lines propagated*	*hESC lines derived*	*Reference*
Matrigel (A)	MEF CM	H1, H7, H9, H14		37
Human Fibronectin (H)	SR + TGF-β_1 + LIF + bFGF	I-6, I-3, H9		51
Matrigel (A)	+ GSK-3	H1, BGN-1, BGN-2		43
Matrigel (A)	KSR + bFGF	H1, H9		40
Matrigel (A)	+ KSR + bFGF + noggin or bFGF at high concentrations	H1, H9, H14		42
Matrigel (A)	+ KSR + bFGF +/– SCF +/– Flt-3L	H7, H9		41
Human Serum (H)	HES-dF CM	H1, hES-NCL1		52
MEF ECM (A)	SR		ACT-14	16
Human fibronectin + collagen IV + laminin + vitronectin (H)	TeSR1 + bFGF + LiCl + GABA + pipecolic acid + TGF-β	H1, H9	WA15, WA16	17

MEF CM, mouse embryonic fibroblasts conditioned medium; SR, serum replacement; TGF-β_1, transforming growth factor-β_1; LIF, leukemia inhibitory factor, bFGF, basic fibroblast growth factor; GSK-3, glycogen synthase kinase 3; SCF, stem cell factor; Flt-3L, fetal liver tyrosine kinase-3 ligand; MEF ECM, mouse embryonic fibroblasts extracellular matrix; LiCl, lithium chloride; GABA, γ-aminobutyric acid

TeSR1 containing all five factors (bFGF, LiCl, GABA, pipecolic acid and TGF-β) is sufficient to support feeder-independent hESC derivation and culture, as well as or better than fibroblast-conditioned medium, as these factors do not overlap with the factors that sustain mouse ESCs in defined conditions.[60] Unlike previous hESC culture media, which included proprietary, poorly defined serum components with undisclosed formulations, all TeSR1 components are disclosed, and should therefore serve as a starting point for further optimization. Nevertheless, an aspect that needs improvement is the matrix, as the components of the purified human matrix are expensive and may provide a potential route of contamination by human pathogens. In this context, HSA should be marked as the only component of the TeSR1 medium that is not fully defined, and it is possible that components that bind to it have an influence on hESCs. HSA is routinely used for embryo culture, so its inclusion in TeSR1 does not qualitatively increase the risk of introducing pathogens to the hESC; nevertheless, the replacement of this component with cloned materials will be desirable in the near future.[17]

Finally, a significant fact is that when established hESC lines previously derived and expanded on MEFs (H1 and H9 lines) were transferred to this human matrix in the presence of TeSR1 medium, the animal products were eliminated, and the non-human sialic acid, Neu5Gc, previously positive in these two hESC lines completely disappeared,[17] thus enhancing its importance for future applications.

CONCLUSIONS

To enable their eventual application to cell replacement therapy, hESCs should be established and maintained under stable xeno-free culture conditions. Many researchers have attempted to eliminate animal cells/products/contaminants for the establishment and culture of hESCs. However, the definitive xeno-free culture condition is yet to be developed, as animal materials continue to be used in the process of ICM isolation, feeder cell culture and hESC culture. Even the use of SR cannot be considered as a complete xeno-free system because of the specific albumin fraction that it contains, which is purified from animal serum.

Until now, many sources of human fibroblast feeders have been demonstrated to support the growth of hESC lines in an undifferentiated stage. However, not all human feeders seem to function to the same degree, and availability is also a restricting factor. In this context, human foreskin, placental fibroblasts and autogeneic feeders have been shown to meet the best requirements, both for derivation and propagation in the presence of SR[12–14,30,32] and as a source of conditioned medium. All three seem to have advantages: foreskin fibroblasts are commercially available;[30] human placental feeders aim to recreate the hESCs niche in vitro;[12,13] and autogeneic feeders protect against the transfer of pathogens.[14,32] However, the derivation and propagation conditions do not completely eliminate exposure to animal products and/or pathogens transfer.

Nowadays, feeder-free derivation and expansion of hESCs are feasible in animal-derived ECM and in human ECM. Much progress has been made in animal ECM expansion since conditioned medium is not needed when SR is supplemented with defined factors such as noggin or bFGF. Human ECM obtained from HS supports growth and expansion in the presence of conditioned media from autogeneic feeders. Klimanskaya and co-workers[16] made a great accomplishment when they achieved the first derivation of an hESC line in feeder-free conditions using ECM extracted from MEF and non-conditioned medium containing SR.

Another important breakthrough was made by Ludwig and colleagues[17] when they reported the first derivation in defined medium, using TeSR1 as culture medium. This medium is completely defined except for HSA, which is also used in human embryo culture. The main components of TeSR1 are vitamins, antioxidants, trace minerals, specific lipids and five cloned growth factors supposed to participate in stemness, which are bFGF, LiCl, GABA, pipecolic acid and TGF-β. Two lines, WA15 and WA16, were derived under these conditions, and both display typical hESC undifferentiation characteristics. Unfortunately, WA15 eventually converted to trisomy in chromosome 12 and WA16 was shown to be XXY.

Despite the enormous accumulative efforts in this field, further studies are required to overcome significant backdraws in present culture conditions such as the genetic instability of new hESCs. The appearance of aneuploidy changes due to chromosomal gain have been detected during prolonged periods in feeder and feeder-free conditions.[61–63] As mentioned above, WA15 and WA16 present chromosomal anomalies.[17] The emergence of abnormal karyotype 12 in hESCs has been reported,[43] and is usually associated with clonal events that are probably a result of enzymatic passaging,[17] thus highlighting the need for further definition of stress culture conditions.

Great advances have been made in the development of an hESC derivation and propagation process of clinical grade, as shown in Table 14.2 and Figure 14.2. Progress in this area has been amazingly rapid, with significant results emerging almost daily, and representing important steps towards the clinical application of hESCs.[15] However, there still remain important challenges: the need to avoid immune reactions in transplantation, to prevent chromosomal, epigenetic, and genetic changes during long-term culture, and to control the differentiation of the cells, underline the importance of future research.[54]

All of the hESCs currently approved for federal funding in the USA were derived on mouse feeder layers and were exposed to a variety of other poorly defined animal products. Derivation and culture in serum-free, animal product-free feeder-independent conditions suggest that new hESC lines are qualitatively different from the original lines, and thus makes current public policy in the USA increasingly inadequate. FDA regulations highlight the necessity of obtaining xeno-free hESC lines for therapeutic lines. European directives are quite strict in following GMP conditions for hESC derivation and propagation: a new European directive that applies to all tissue and cell donors for transplantation was implemented in 2006.

REFERENCES

1. Thomson JA, Itskovitz-Eldor J, Shapiro SS et al. Embryonic stem cell lines derived from human blastocysts. Science 1998; 282: 1145–7.

2. Zwaka TP, Thomson JA. Homologous recombination in human embryonic stem cells. Nat Biotechnol 2003; 21: 319–21.
3. Schuldiner M, Yanuka O, Itskovitz-Eldor J et al. Effects of eight growth factors on the differentiation of cells derived from human embryonic stem cells. Proc Natl Acad Sci USA 2000; 97: 11307–12.
4. Henderson JK, Draper JS, Baillie HS et al. Preimplantation human embryos and embryonic stem cells show comparable expression of stage-specific embryonic antigens. Stem Cells 2002; 20: 329–37.
5. Hanna LA, Foreman RK, Tarasenko IA, Kessler DS, Labosky PA. Requirement for Foxd3 in maintaining pluripotent cells of the early mouse embryo. Genes Dev 2002; 16: 2650–61.
6. Brivanlou AH, Gage FH, Jaenisch R et al. Stem cells. Setting standards for human embryonic stem cells. Science 2003; 300: 913–16.
7. Hart AH, Hartley L, Ibrahim M, Robb L. Identification, cloning and expression analysis of the pluripotency promoting Nanog genes in mouse and human. Dev Dyn 2004; 230: 187–98.
8. Reubinoff BE, Pera MF, Fong CY, Trounson A, Bongso A. Embryonic stem cell lines from human blastocysts: somatic differentiation in vitro. Nat Biotechnol 2000; 18: 399–404.
9. Martin MJ, Muotri A, Gage F, Varki A. Human embryonic stem cells express an immunogenic nonhuman sialic acid. Nat Med 2005; 11: 228–32.
10. Galán A, Escobedo C, Valbuena D, Berna A, Simón C. In: Animal free to feeder free conditions: the desired derivation process. Embryonic Stem Cell Research. Hauppauge NY, Nova Publishers, 2006.
11. Richards M, Fong CY, Chan WK, Wong PC, Bongso A. Human feeders support prolonged undifferentiated growth of human inner cell masses and embryonic stem cells. Nat Biotechnol 2002; 20: 933–6.
12. Genbacev O, Krtolica A, Zdravkovic T et al. Serum-free derivation of human embryonic stem cell lines on human placental fibroblast feeders. Fertil Steril 2005; 83: 1517–29.
13. Simon C, Escobedo C, Valbuena D et al. First derivation in Spain of human embryonic stem cell lines: use of long-term cryopreserved embryos and animal-free conditions. Fertil Steril 2005; 83: 246–9.
14. Stojkovic P, Lako M, Stewart R et al. An autogeneic feeder cell system that efficiently supports growth of undifferentiated human embryonic stem cells. Stem Cells 2005; 23: 306–14.
15. Rodríguez CI, Galan A, Valbuena D, Simon C. Derivation of clinical-grade human embryonic stem cells. Reprod Biomed Online 2006; 12: 112–18.
16. Klimanskaya I, Chung Y, Meisner L et al. Human embryonic stem cells derived without feeder cells. Lancet 2005; 365: 1601–3.
17. Ludwig TE, Levenstein ME, Jones JM et al. Derivation of human embryonic stem cells in defined conditions. Nat Biotechnol 2006; 24: 185–7.
18. Cowan CA, Klimanskaya I, McMahonet J et al. Derivation of embryonic stem-cell lines from human blastocysts. N Engl J Med 2004; 350: 1353–6.
19. Richards M, Tan S, Fong CY et al. Comparative evaluation of various human feeders for prolonged undifferentiated growth of human embryonic stem cells. Stem Cells 2003; 21: 546–56.
20. Rodríguez CI, Simón C. Human embryonic stem cell derivation: from the IVF perspective to therapeutic applications. Regenerative Med 2006; 1: 103–9.
21. Mercader A, García-Velasco JA, Escudero E et al. Clinical experience and perinatal outcome of blastocyst transfer coculture of human embryos on human endometrial epithelial cells: a 5-year follow up study. Fertil Steril 2003; 80: 1162–8.
22. Simon C, Mercader A, Garcia-Velasco J, Remohí J, Pellicer A. Co-culture of human embryos with autologous human endometrial epithelial cells in patients with repeated implantation failures. J Clin Endocrinol Metab 1999; 84: 2638–46.
23. Domínguez F, Yáñez-Mó M, Sanchez-Madrid F, Simón C. Embryonic implantation and leukocyte transendothelial migration: different processes with similar players? FASEB J 2005; 19: 1056–60.
24. Lee JB, Song JM, Lee JE et al. Available human feeder cells for the maintenance of human embryonic stem cells. Reproduction 2004; 128: 727–35.
25. Lee JB, Lee JE, Park JH et al. Establishment and maintenance of human embryonic stem cell lines on human feeder cells derived from uterine endometrium under serum-free condition. Biol Reprod 2005; 72: 42–9.
26. Amit M, Itskovitz-Eldor J. Derivation and spontaneous differentiation of human embryonic stem cells. J Anat 2002; 200: 225–32.
27. Amit M, Margulets V, Segev H et al. Human feeder layers for human embryonic stem cells. Biol Reprod 2003; 68: 2150–6.
28. Hovatta O, Mikkola M, Gertow K et al. A culture system using human foreskin fibroblasts as feeder cells allows production of human embryonic stem cells. Hum Reprod 2003; 18: 1404–9.
29. Choo AB, Padmanabhan J, Chin AC, Oh SK. Expansion of pluripotent human embryonic stem cells on human feeders. Biotechnol Bioeng 2004; 88: 321–31.
30. Inzunza J, Gertow K, Stromberg, MA et al. Derivation of human embryonic stem cell lines in serum replacement medium using postnatal human fibroblasts as feeder cells. Stem Cells 2005; 23: 544–9.
31. Gearhart J. New human embryonic stem cell lines – more is better. N Engl J Med 2004; 350: 1275–6.

32. Wang Q, Fang Z, Jin F et al. Derivation and growing human embryonic stem cells on feeders derived from themselves. Stem Cells 2005; 23: 1221–7.

33. Ponsaerts P, Van der Sar S, Van Tenedlo VF et al. Highly efficient mRNA-based gene transfer in feeder-free cultured H9 human embryonic stem cells. Cloning Stem Cells 2004; 6: 211–16.

34. Mecham RP. Extracellular matrix. In: Galán A, Escobedo C, Valbuena D eds. Animal Free to feeder free conditions: The desired derivation process. Embryonic Stem Cell Research. Hauppauge NY: Nova Publishers: 2006: Current Protocols in Cell Biology. 1998; 1–14.

35. Kleinman HK. Extracellular matrix. In: Advances in Molecular and Cellular Biology, Vol. 6. Greenwich, Conn. JAI Press, 1993.

36. Bornstain P. Diversity of function is inherent in matricellular proteins: an appraisal of thrombospondin 1. J Cell Biol 1995; 130: 503–56.

37. Xu C, Inokuma MS, Denham J et al. Feeder-free growth of undifferentiated human embryonic stem cells. Nat Biotechnol 2001; 19: 971–4.

38. Brimble SN, Zeng X, Weiler DA et al. Karyotypic stability, genotyping, differentiation, feeder-free maintenance, and gene expression sampling in three human embryonic stem cell lines derived prior to August 9, 2001. Stem Cells Dev 2004; 13: 585–97.

39. Rosler ES, Fisk GJ, Ares X et al. Long-term culture of human embryonic stem cells in feeder-free conditions. Dev Dyn 2004; 229: 259–74.

40. Wang G, Zhang H, Zhao Y et al. Noggin and bFGF cooperate to maintain the pluripotency of human embryonic stem cells in the absence of feeder layers. Biochem Biophys Res Commun 2005; 330: 934–42.

41. Xu C, Rosler E, Jiang J et al. Basic fibroblast growth factor supports undifferentiated human embryonic stem cell growth without conditioned medium. Stem Cells 2005; 23: 315–23.

42. Xu RH, Peck RM, Li DS et al. Basic FGF and suppression of BMP signaling sustain undifferentiated proliferation of human ES cells. Nat Methods 2005; 2: 185–90.

43. Sato N, Meijer L, Skaltsounis L, Greengard P, Brivanlou AH. Maintenance of pluripotency in human and mouse embryonic stem cells through activation of Wnt signaling by a pharmacological GSK-3-specific inhibitor. Nat Med 2004; 10: 55–63.

44. Smith AG, Heath JK, Donaldson DD et al. Inhibition of pluripotential embryonic stem cell differentiation by purified polypeptides. Nature 1988; 336: 688–90.

45. Williams RL, Hilton DJ, Pease S et al. Myeloid leukaemia inhibitory factor maintains the developmental potential of embryonic stem cells. Nature 1988; 336: 684–7.

46. Pera MF, Filipczyk AA, Hawes SM, Laslett AL. Isolation, characterization, and differentiation of human embryonic stem cells. Methods Enzymol 2003; 365: 429–46.

47. Sato N, Sanjuan IM, Heke M et al. Molecular signature of human embryonic stem cells and its comparison with the mouse. Dev Biol 2003; 260: 404–13.

48. Meijer L, Skaltsounis AL, Magiatis P et al. GSK-3-selective inhibitors derived from Tyrian purple indirubins. Chem Biol 2003; 10: 1255–66.

49. Pera MF, Trounson AO. Human embryonic stem cells: prospects for development. Development 2004; 131: 5515–25.

50. Vallier L, Reynolds D, Pedersen RA. Nodal inhibits differentiation of human embryonic stem cells along the neuroectodermal default pathway. Dev Biol 2004; 275: 403–21.

51. Amit M, Shariki C, Margulets V, Itskovitz-Eldor J. Feeder layer- and serum-free culture of human embryonic stem cells. Biol Reprod 2004; 70: 837–45.

52. Stojkovic P, Lako M, Przyborski S et al. Human-serum matrix supports undifferentiated growth of human embryonic stem cells. Stem Cells 2005; 23: 895–902

53. Carpenter MK, Rosler ES, Fisk GJ et al. Properties of four human embryonic stem cell lines maintained in a feeder-free culture system. Dev Dyn 2004; 229: 243–58.

54. Hovatta O, Skottman H. Feeder-free derivation of human embryonic stem-cell lines. Lancet 2005; 365: 1601–3.

55. Hedman M, Kurkinen M, Alitalo K et al. Isolation of the pericellular matrix of human fibroblast cultures. J Cell Biol 1979; 81: 83–91.

56. Gordon MY, Riley GP, Watt SM, Greaves MF. Compartmentalization of a haematopoietic growth factor (GM-CSF) by glycosaminoglycans in the bone marrow microenvironment. Nature 1987; 326: 376–8.

57. Roberts R, Gallagher J, Spooncer E et al. Heparan sulfate bound growth factors: a mechanism for stromal cell mediated haemopoiesis. Nature 1988; 332: 376–8.

58. Pera MF. Stem cell culture, one step at a time. Nat Methods 2005; 2: 164–5.

59. Amit M, Carpenter MK, Inokuma MS et al. Clonally derived human embryonic stem cell lines maintain pluripotency and proliferative potential for prolonged periods of culture. Dev Biol 2000; 227: 271–8.

60. Ying QL, Nichols J, Chambers I, Smith A. BMP induction of Id proteins suppresses differentiation and sustains embryonic stem cell self-renewal in collaboration with STAT3. Cell 2003; 115: 281–92.

61. Buzzard JJ, Gough NM, Crook JM, Colman A. Karyotype of human ES cells during extended culture. Nat Biotechnol 2004; 22: 381–2.

62. Draper JS, Smith K, Gokhale P et al. Recurrent gain of chromosomes 17q and 12 in cultured human embryonic stem cells. Nat Biotechnol 2004; 22: 53–4.

63. Mitalipova MM, Rao RR, Hoyer DM et al. Preserving the genetic integrity of human embryonic stem cells. Nat Biotechnol 2005; 23: 19–20.

CHAPTER 15

Cell polarity, pluripotency and differentiation

Ana Krtolica and Olga Genbacev

CELL POLARITY, TIGHT JUNCTIONS AND THEIR FUNCTIONS

Cell polarity is defined by asymmetric distribution of structural and other macromolecules (proteins, lipids and carbohydrates) within the cell. Epithelial cell polarity is based on compartmentalization of the cell and its membrane into two major domains: apical, facing an open space or lumen; basolateral, taking part in cell–cell and cell–matrix interactions. At the boundary between these two domains, called the subapical zone, epithelial cells form tight junctions that seal the membranes of adjacent cells together to prevent the admixing of apical and basolateral membrane proteins and free diffusion through the intercellular space (Figure 15.1). Tight junctions are complex multiprotein structures that, apart from the described function in mediating selective diffusion across the epithelial sheet, also play an important role in regulating cell polarity, proliferation and differentiation. The role of tight junctions in epithelial polarity has recently been extensively reviewed.[1,2] We will focus here on just a few key issues pertinent to our discussion of the establishment of polarity in mammalian embryo and the role of the polarized phenotype in human embryonic stem cells (hESCs).

Tight junction components

In tight junctions, integral membrane proteins mediate direct contact between cells to make a tight seal. There are three major families of transmembrane proteins that are found in tight junctions: occludin, claudins and junctional adhesion molecules (JAMs). While both claudins and occludin span plasma membrane four times and form intermembrane strands, claudins are the main proteins important for tight junction strand formation and critical for its barrier function. Occludin seems to play an important role in tight junction assembly, and its extracellular domains are involved in cell–cell adhesion. Unlike occludin and claudins, JAMs have a single transmembrane domain and are members of the immunoglobulin superfamily. JAM-1/JAM-A and JAM-3/JAM-C localize to tight junctions in epithelial cells and are implicated in the formation of tight junctions and regulation of the pericellular barrier.

All three groups of transmembrane proteins interact through their cytoplasmic domains with an array of peripheral membrane proteins. These act as adaptors in linking integral membrane proteins to the actin cytoskeleton and thus stabilizing the tight junction structure and/or as scaffolds that recruit other proteins into the tight junction plaque and initiate signal transduction cascades. The most prominent group of peripheral tight junction proteins are zonula occludens (ZO) proteins. They belong to the membrane-associated guanylate kinase (MAGUK) family of proteins which do not have catalytic activity and instead act as molecular scaffolds. They contain guanylate kinase (GUK), postsynaptic density/zonula occludens (PDZ) and Src homology 3 (SH3) domains that mediate their multiple protein–protein interactions. ZO-1 localizes to the tight junctions of epithelial and endothelial

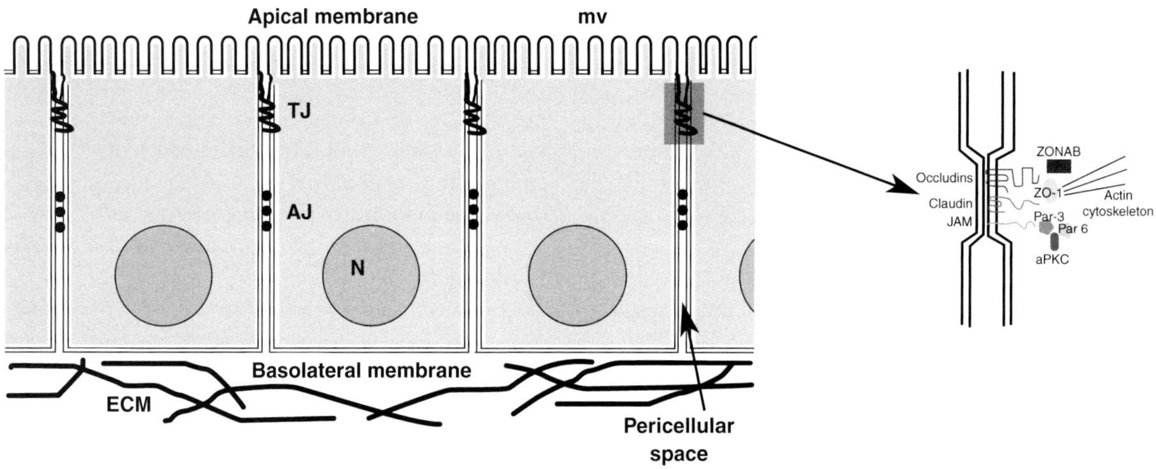

Figure 15.1 The polarized epithelial cells and the tight junction complex. The positions of the tight (TJ) and adherens (AJ) junctions, nuclei (N), the extracellular matrix (ECM), and the basolateral and apical membranes with microvilli (mv) are indicated. Enlarged areas of the TJ, with the main protein components, is depicted on the right

cells and is also present in non-epithelial cells such as fibroblasts and astrocytes. It localizes to the nucleus during the maturation of the epithelial monolayer and regulates proliferation by interacting with a Y-box transcription factor, ZO-1-associated nucleic acid-binding protein (ZONAB).[3] Moreover, ZO-1 plays an important role in the assembly and function of tight junctions. It has been implicated in the development of tight junctions during mouse blastocyst formation, and epithelial cells derived from ZO-1 knockout mice show delayed tight junction formation following a calcium-switch assay.[4] As mentioned above, ZO proteins act as scaffolding proteins and interact with many binding partners at the tight junction, including transmembrane proteins and proteins of actin cytoskeleton. In non-polarized cells in which tight junctions have not formed, ZO proteins form a complex with adherens junction proteins such as E-cadherin and catenins, but, upon polarization, they can separate from the adherens junction and concentrate in the tight junction, where they interact with tight junction proteins such as claudins and occludin.[5]

Establishment and maintenance of tight junctions

Structural proteins such as claudins play an important role as a fence preventing the mixing of apical and basolateral membranes. In this manner they act to reinforce polarity, but it appears unlikely that this fence function initiates polarity. The establishment and maintenance of epithelial cell polarity is a function of the two evolutionarily conserved polarization complexes that are localized at the tight junction: CRB and Par protein complexes. Their presence determines the apical domain of epithelial cells by excluding a lateral determinant, the Scrib complex, from the apical domain. Similarly, the Scrib complex antagonizes CRB and Par complexes at the lateral membrane. This mutual exclusion between polarity complexes leads to the establishment and maintenance of apico–basal polarity in epithelia. Most likely, the polarity complexes function to determine the site of the tight junction in the process of cell polarization. An emerging concept is that polarity complexes define the apico–basal polarity and create the landmark where the tight junction will form. This leads to a close interdependence between polarity complexes and tight junction structural components. Polarity complexes target proteins to the tight junction, and the formation of the tight junction then serves to reinforce polarity by preventing admixing of apical and basolateral membrane proteins.[1,2]

ESTABLISHMENT OF CELL POLARITY IN EARLY EMBRYO

The first differentiation event in mammalian development occurs during blastocyst formation of the preimplantation embryo. Depending on their position following the mitotic division, blastomeres at the morula stage are predetermined to become either inner cell mass (ICM) cells, which will give rise to the embryo proper, or an epithelial-like layer of trophectoderm (TE) cells that will develop into extraembryonic tissues such as placenta.

Numerous studies have suggested that TE differentiation requires cell polarity to be established in the outer cells of the morula (reviewed in Reference 6). Such apical–basal cell polarity develops progressively, as indicated by the distribution of a variety of cellular markers, including endocytotic vesicles,[7,8] β-catenin[9] and ezrin,[10] and the localization of microvilli to outer apical surfaces.[11] The cell–cell adhesion molecule E-cadherin is also first uniformly distributed on all cell surfaces until the early 8-cell stage. Then, after the process known as compaction, E-cadherin becomes restricted to regions of cell–cell contact.[12]

In mouse embryo, polarization of blastomeres occurs at the 8-cell stage. When the mouse embryo develops past the 8-cell stage, two types of cell division occur. Symmetric divisions, with the cleavage plane approximately perpendicular to the surface of the embryo, result in both progeny inheriting apical and basal regions of cytoplasm. Thus, both daughter cells are polar and retain an outer apical surface. By contrast, division planes, aligned approximately tangential to the surface of the embryo, are asymmetric and result in two types of daughter cell: one cell inheriting all of the apical surface and some inner surfaces and one cell inheriting only inner surfaces. Consequently, one daughter cell retains an apical outer surface and is polar, whereas the other remains internal and is non-polar. As outer cells of morula mature to functional TE epithelial cells, they initiate Na^+/K^+-channel-mediated active transport (reviewed in Reference 12), which causes internal fluid accumulation and formation of the blastocyst cavity.

The establishment of cellular polarity during cell division is regulated by the Par (partitioning defective) complex that consists of molecules Par3 and Par6 in complex with atypical protein kinase C (aPKC) (reviewed in Reference 12). Cell polarity is believed to play an important role in orienting cell divisions and therefore in establishing the ICM and TE lineages. Concomitant with the establishment of trophectoderm polarity, there is an assembly of tight junctions. It is a multistep process, which starts with E-cadherin adhesion at compaction, that is crucial for polarized membrane recruitment of tight junction proteins. Indeed in mouse embryo, tight junction constituents localize with the adherens junction until the 32-cell stage. The two junctions only become molecularly distinct once occludin and specific claudins assemble as a final event in tight junction construction, apparently mediated by late transcription of the cytoplasmic binding partner ZO-1a+ isoform.[4] Thus, formation of functional tight junctions is intimately connected with the establishment of functional TE and formation of the blastocoele cavity. In the context of early morphogenesis, tight junction biogenesis provides the means to control the microenvironment of the ICM via TE transport pathways for ions, amino acids, energy substrates, growth factors and other metabolites.

An ultrastructural analysis of blastocyst-stage human embryos suggests a similar link between polarization and cell fate in human embryos. Our unpublished data obtained by electron and confocal microscopy show that, similar to mouse embryo, TE cells of the human blastocyst form a polarized unilaminar epithelium which encapsulates non-polar cells of epiblast (Figure 15.2). The only cells exhibiting polarized phenotype within the ICM were cells of hypoblast, a single layer of cells on the border of the

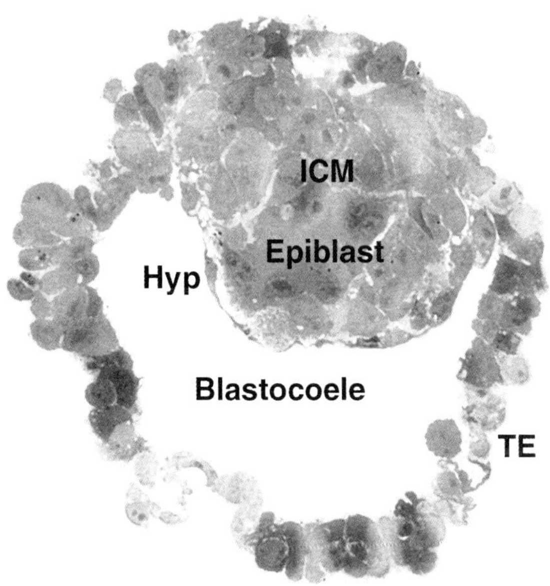

Figure 15.2 Semifine section of the human blastocyst. The inner cell mass (ICM) with prominent epiblast and hypoblast (Hyp) is surrounded by a trophectoderm layer (TE) and a blastocoele cavity (Courtesy of Dr Carlos Simon and Dr Carman Escobedo).

ICM that is facing the blastocoele cavity in mature blastocyst. Indeed, whereas TE cells that formed the outer surface of the embryo exhibited tight junctions at the cell–cell contacts, epiblast cells of the ICM lacked these specializations.

HUMAN EMBRYONIC STEM CELL DERIVATION AND ESTABLISHMENT OF POLARITY

ESCs are derived in culture from the ICM of the blastocyst. Like the ICM cells from which they are derived, ESCs are pluripotent, have very little heterochromatin, and large nuclei with a high nucleus to cytoplasm ratio, indicative of the short cell division cycle.[13–15] Interestingly, although they arise from the non-polar cells of the ICM, hESCs acquire a polarized phenotype during the derivation process (Krtolica, Genbacev and Fisher, unpublished work). Indeed, we have noticed that very early during the derivation process, at the time that the outgrowth of the first colony is formed and cells start appearing morphologically homogeneous, they acquire the morphology of the epithelial-like polarization. This polarized phenotype is maintained throughout the passaging process and may be the reason why the majority of hESCs differentiate if they are separated into single cell suspension: when kept in small clumps, they can still maintain their tight junctions and, thus, may reinforce their polarized phenotype.

If indeed, polarization is necessary for the long-term maintenance of the pluripotent phenotype, it is not surprising that the presence and type of extracellular matrix (ECM) are crucial for the derivation of hESCs from the ICM. After zona pellucida removal by spontaneous or assisted hatching, human embryos are capable of attaching to a variety of surfaces, including culture-treated plastic. However, empirical evidence suggests that the successful hESC derivation requires a specific matrix – containing either a mixture of basement membrane components or the one produced by the feeder cells, typically fibroblasts. This implies that in order to proliferate in culture, apart from the adequate supply of basic nutrients and survival, growth and differentiation inhibiting signals, ICM cells need to initiate interactions with appropriate matrix component which may enable them to establish and/or maintain the polarized phenotype. Our unpublished data suggest that the established hESCs produce, secrete and organize on the extracellular side of their basal membrane, several matrix components, including fibronectin. Moreover, fibronectin production was increased when cells were grown on a matrix that did not contain significant amounts of this ECM protein such as Matrigel.

Unlike cells of the mouse embryo, which can survive in a state of embryonic diapause, a condition of delayed implantation in mammals in which blastocyst growth is very slow, with minimal or no cell division,[16] human embryos exist in a blastocyst stage for only a very limited time – between 24 and 48 hours. Therefore, one can hypothesize that ICM cells of these two species have a very different capacity for extended survival in a pluripotent state: in humans, their presence is only transient, whereas in mice they must have developed some mechanisms for sustaining their undifferentiated state during dormancy. Interestingly, it has been suggested that the LIF– JAK–STAT3 pathway, which is present only in mouse cells, is an adaptation for sustaining self-renewal during embryonic diapause.[17] We hypothesize that during ESC derivation, human (more than mouse) ICM cells need to undergo extensive epigenetic changes to obtain the ability for long-term self-renewal and maintenance of pluripotency, and that this process is catalyzed by their development of a polarized phenotype. This establishment of an epithelial-like polarity in ICM-derived cells may be due to the partial activation of the gene expression characteristic for the cells of the primitive ectoderm, a pluripotent stem cell population which develops from epiblast at the time of implantation. Interestingly, in mouse embryo, development of the primitive ectoderm is characterized by cell polarization and reorganization of the pluripotent cells into a pseudostratified epithelial sheet, features that are present in hESCs in culture. Moreover, pluripotent cells of the primitive ectoderm retain expression of pluripotency genes such as Oct 3/4 at the levels that are indistinguishable from those in ESCs and, as ESCs, give rise to all three germ layers.[18]

For obvious ethical reasons we do not have such an in-depth knowledge of the early development in humans. How close hESCs may resemble the pluripotent cells of the primitive ectoderm remains to be seen. What is clear is that human ICM cells had to undergo profound changes in their phenotype in order to adjust themselves to perpetual undifferentiated growth in culture and that these changes appear inseparable from the establishment of the epithelial-like polarized phenotype.

ROLE OF CELL POLARITY IN DIFFERENTIATION

During ESC differentiation in culture, as well as ESC differentiation in vivo, regions of heterochromatin that are formed within the nucleus selectively suppress gene expression, resulting in a loss of expression of pluripotency-associated transcription factors such as Oct 3/4, Nanog and Sox2, and leading to diminishment of cell pluripotent potential.[19] Like mESCs, human ESCs are capable of differentiating into all three germ layers and, therefore, hold a therapeutic potential of creating cell replacement therapy for almost any type of tissue in the human body. As discussed earlier, epithelial polarization is often intimately linked with differentiation into the particular cell types and is necessary for the appropriate function of numerous epithelia within our body such as epidermis of the skin, lining of the intestines, respiratory and gland ducts, to name just a few. It is also the initial differentiation event in mammalian development that excludes TE cells from the pluripotent cell population of the embryo. However, our data (Krtolica, Genbacev and Fisher, unpublished work) strongly suggest that hESCs form functional tight junctions and express major morphological characteristics of the polarized phenotype while retaining pluripotent potential.

This seemingly puzzling finding may be easier to grasp if we think of it in the context of the other pluripotent cell populations that are polarized, such as cells of primitive ectoderm or germ stem cells.[20,21] Interestingly, hESC polarized phenotype retains extraordinary responsiveness to the external signals and the ability to be reverted to the non-polarized state (Krtolica, Genbacev and Fisher, unpublished work). It appears that during the derivation process, hESCs assume the reversible polarized state, which allows them long-term self-renewal and potentially brings their phenotype closer to the pluripotent cells of polarized primitive ectoderm. While still pluripotent, these cells possess altered developmental potential.[18] Indeed, when depolarized hESCs were subjected to in-vitro differentiation into embryoid bodies, we observed a distinct change in their differentiation capacity relative to the polarized controls. In the depolarized group, our immunocytochemical analysis revealed a prominent prevalence of cells of mesodermal origin, and a significant decrease in the expression of early endodermal and ectodermal markers (Krtolica, Genbacev and Fisher, unpublished work). Like cells from the ICM and primitive ectoderm, both control and depolarized hESCs had potential to differentiate into cells of all three germ layers, but the efficacy and the timing for acquiring the particular cell fates varied significantly between the two groups.

POTENTIAL IMPLICATIONS

Although we still lack an understanding of all the intricate molecular mechanisms involved in the establishment and maintenance of cell polarity, its critical importance for mammalian development is beyond any doubt. Our findings that hESCs express a polarized phenotype that appears to be associated with their long-term pluripotent potential may have implications in designing the optimal hESC derivation and maintenance protocols. For example, it suggests that conditions that promote establishment of polarity, such as the presence of an adequate ECM, may increase the efficiency of the derivation process. In addition, our results showing that depolarization of hESCs promotes mesodermal differentiation may provide an alternative approach for obtaining differentiated cells that can be used in future therapeutic applications.

Acknowledgments

The image of the human blastocyst (Figure 15.2) was kindly provided by Dr Carlos Simon and Dr Carmen Escobedo. The authors are indebted to Dr Susan Fisher for the insightful scientific discussions and support. This work was supported in part by grants from the UC Discovery Grant program (bio02-10302) and the California Breast Cancer Research Program (8KB-0100).

REFERENCES

1. Shin K, Fogg VC, Margolis B. Tight junctions and cell polarity. Annu Rev Cell Dev Biol 2006; Jan 13, [Epub ahead of print].
2. Munro EM. PAR proteins and the cytoskeleton: a marriage of equals. Curr Opin Cell Biol 2006; 18(1): 86–94.

3. Mostov K, Su T, ter Beest M. Polarized epithelial membrane traffic: conservation and plasticity. Nat Cell Biol 2003; 5(4): 287–93.

4. Sheth B, Fesenko I, Collins JE et al. Tight junction assembly during mouse blastocyst formation is regulated by late expression of ZO-1 alpha+ isoform. Development 1997; 124(10): 2027–37.

5. Muller SL, Portwich M, Schmidt A et al. The tight junction protein occludin and the adherens junction protein alpha-catenin share a common interaction mechanism with ZO-1. J Biol Chem 2005; 280(5): 3747–56.

6. Johnson MH, McConnell JM. Lineage allocation and cell polarity during mouse embryogenesis. Semin Cell Dev Biol 2004; 15(5): 583–97.

7. Fleming TP, Pickering SJ. Maturation and polarization of the endocytotic system in outside blastomeres during mouse preimplantation development. J Embryol Exp Morphol 1985; 89: 175–208.

8. Maro B, Johnson MH, Pickering SJ, Louvard D. Changes in the distribution of membranous organelles during mouse early development. J Embryol Exp Morphol 1985; 90: 287–309.

9. Goval JJ, Van Cauwenberge A, Alexandre H. Respective roles of protein tyrosine kinases and protein kinases C in the upregulation of beta-catenin distribution, and compaction in mouse preimplantation embryos: a pharmacological approach. Biol Cell 2000; 92(7): 513–26.

10. Louvet S, Aghion J, Santa-Maria A, Mangeat P, Maro B. Ezrin becomes restricted to outer cells following asymmetrical division in the preimplantation mouse embryo. Dev Biol 1996; 177(2): 568–79.

11. Johnson MH, Ziomek CA. Cell interactions influence the fate of mouse blastomeres undergoing the transition from the 16- to the 32-cell stage. Dev Biol 1983; 95(1): 211–18.

12. Vestweber D, Gossler A, Boller K, Kemler R. Expression and distribution of cell adhesion molecule uvomorulin in mouse preimplantation embryos. Dev Biol 1987; 124(2): 451–6.

13. Draper JS, Fox V. Human embryonic stem cells: multilineage differentiation and mechanisms of self-renewal. Arch Med Res 2003; 34(6): 558–64.

14. Amit M, Carpenter MK, Inokuma MS et al. Clonally derived human embryonic stem cell lines maintain pluripotency and proliferative potential for prolonged periods of culture. Dev Biol 2000; 227(2): 271–8.

15. Krtolica A. Stem cell: balancing aging and cancer. Int J Biochem Cell Biol 2005; 37(5): 935–41.

16. Hamatani T, Daikoku T, Wang H et al. Global gene expression analysis identifies molecular pathways distinguishing blastocyst dormancy and activation. Proc Natl Acad Sci USA 2004; 101(28): 10326–31.

17. Kristensen DM, Kalisz M, Nielsen JH. Cytokine signalling in embryonic stem cells. APMIS 2005; 113(11–12): 756–72.

18. Pelton TA, Sharma S, Schulz TC, Rathjen J, Rathjen PD. Transient pluripotent cell populations during primitive ectoderm formation: correlation of in vivo and in vitro pluripotent cell development. J Cell Sci 2002; 115(2): 329–39.

19. Rasmussen TP. Embryonic stem cell differentiation: a chromatin perspective. Reprod Biol Endocrinol 2003; 1(1): 100.

20. Okamura D, Kimura T, Nakano T, Matsui Y. Cadherin-mediated cell interaction regulates germ cell determination in mice. Development 2003; 130(26): 6423–30.

21. Li L, Arman E, Ekblom P et al. Distinct GATA6- and laminin-dependent mechanisms regulate endodermal and ectodermal embryonic stem cell fates. Development 2004; 131(21): 5277–86.

CHAPTER 16

Role of oxygen in early development and embryonic stem cell derivation

Olga Genbacev, Paolo F Rinaudo and Emin Maltepe

INTRODUCTION

Human embryonic stem cells (hESCs) are derived from the inner cell mass (ICM) of the blastocyst produced by in-vitro fertilization (IVF) techniques. They share with ICM the ability to self-renew and the pluripotent capacity.[1] In addition, their morphological characteristics are similar to ICM cells:[2] large nuclei with a high nucleus-to-cytoplasm ratio, characteristic for the short cell cycle; prominent nucleoli and very little heterochromatin, indicative of open chromatin structure, a feature of pluripotent cells; expression of markers of pluripotency. We can anticipate that in-vitro manipulations to maintain their unlimited self-renewal and the artificially created microenvironment (stem cell niche) induce epigenetic changes to adjust to cell culture conditions. This is the reason why ESCs can be considered as culture 'artifacts' in the sense that their properties and fate are to some extent different from those of the ICM cells of the blastocyst. In spite of these limitations, hESCs can be used to model early human development that is, for ethical reasons, impossible to study directly. The other application of hESCs is to 'tailor' them to meet our needs by acquiring sometimes therapeutically useful, unphysiological properties that are not exhibited in a blastocyst. As the most important characteristic of hESCs is their pluripotency, the ability to generate every cell type of a body, it is important to ensure that hESCs remain capable of generating functionally normal cells. We hypothesize that to retain this ability the in-vitro conditions for hESC derivation and propagation in the undifferentiated state should mirror to some extent the in-vivo environment. What do we know about the transitional microenvironment of the ICM cells? Can we use some of the available information to produce optimal culture systems that will provide the environment for the most accurate gene replication, activation and epigenetic modifications? Here, we are going to address the role of oxygen tension and present evidence to support derivation and propagation of hESCs in low oxygen.

OXYGEN AND MAMMALIAN DEVELOPMENT

Since biological organisms can be characterized as open systems, continuously interacting with and dependent on their environments, environment–organism interactions are perpetually operating to influence development. Thus, even the most basic metabolic substrates have the potential to influence developmental states. An important example of this is oxygen.

Oxygen is critical for aerobic respiration. As the terminal electron acceptor of the mitochondrial electron transport chain, its reduction enables the conversion of ADP to ATP – the metabolic currency of the cell.[3] As such, oxygen is essential for the maintenance of a multicellular existence. However, the exact amount of oxygen needed is unclear. Mammalian cells and tissues are exposed to a fairly large range of oxygen tensions. However, limiting conditions for electron transport occur only under extremely low oxygen concentrations. This is because the K_m of cytochrome c oxidase is less than 1 μmol/l.[4] Thus, mitochondria have the capacity to generate maximal ATP throughout the entire physiological range of oxygen tensions.[5,6] At a partial pressure of ~3 mmHg (torr), or ~0.5% (as compared with atmospheric oxygen, i.e. 21%), mitochondrial electron transport of cultured cells is inhibited and apoptotic death is initiated.[7,8] Above this level, although still well below atmospheric conditions, cells are able to grow for extended periods. In mouse embryonic fibroblasts, prolonged culture under 'hypoxic' (3% O_2) conditions even prevents cell senescence.[9] Thus, a range of oxygen tensions considered hypoxic in relation to the 'normoxic' atmosphere of the air we breathe is perfectly compatible with cellular existence. This 'physiological hypoxia' (1–10% O_2), as opposed to 'pathological hypoxia' (<1% O_2) during which metabolism becomes compromised, represents the natural environment for most mammalian tissues. In the context of development, the role of physiological hypoxia becomes even more pronounced.

Insight into the role of oxygen tension during development came from investigators attempting to improve the culture conditions for growing mammalian embryos in vitro. They found the optimum oxygen concentration for mammalian embryonic development to be about 5%.[10–17] Furthermore, the oviducts and uterine horns of mammals also have been found to exhibit oxygen tensions in this range.[18–23] Additionally, in humans, follicular fluid aspirates exhibit oxygen tensions in the hypoxic range, varying from <1 to 5.5%.[24] Also, the first 10–12 weeks of human pregnancy transpires without significant maternal blood flow to the conceptus. Cytotrophoblasts, human placental cells cultured under hypoxic conditions (2% oxygen), that mimic the environment near the uterine surface before 10 weeks of gestation, continued proliferating and differentiated poorly. When cultured in 20% oxygen, mimicking the environment near uterine arterioles, the cells stopped proliferating and differentiated normally. Thus, oxygen tension determines whether placental cells proliferate or invade, thereby regulating placental growth and cellular architecture.[25,26] At this point the placental bed becomes perfused with maternal blood in a pulsatile fashion.[27,28] Thus, the entire process of organogenesis unfolds under hypoxic conditions. Direct measurements of fetal blood oxygen partial pressure (pO_2) following establishment of the maternal–fetal circulation indicate a continued hypoxemia throughout the remainder of human gestation. Whereas human maternal arterial pO_2 is normally ~90 mmHg and venous pO_2 is ~70 mmHg (~13 to ~10% O_2, respectively), fetal arterial and venous pO_2 values rarely exceed ~30 mmHg (~4–5% O_2).[29] Thus, even after access to the relatively oxygen-rich maternal vasculature, the fetal circulation provides developing tissues with hypoxic levels of oxygen that are nonetheless physiological.

OXYGEN AND CULTURE OF PREIMPLANTATION EMBRYOS

Assisted reproductive techniques (ART) require that preimplantation embryos are manipulated and maintained in vitro for different lengths of time (from 3 to 5 days) and then transferred to the uterus. It is known from animal systems that embryo culture conditions affect both metabolism[30] and gene expression.[31] Multiple IVF programs achieve good success rate by using 20% O_2 to culture human embryos for up to 3 days. However, there are reports[17] suggesting that culture in 20% oxygen is associated with a decrease in the implantation and pregnancy rates. As culture of the embryos is getting more and frequently extended from 3 to 6 days to reach the blastocyst stage, the role of oxygen tension has appeared to be critical. It has been shown that prolonged exposure to 20% oxygen from day 3 to the blastocyst stage is associated with a reduction in the cell number in the blastocyst and a lower morphology score.[32,33] Ample animal evidence supports the protective role of the low oxygen tension in preimplantation embryo development, as opposed to high oxygen concentration, which is associated with abnormal preimplantation development.[34]

Moreover, comet assays, which detect DNA damage, revealed that atmospheric oxygen compromises the genomic integrity of the mouse embryos developed in vitro.[35] Such damage is likely to be associated with increased production of the reactive oxygen species (ROS) in these embryos;[36] ROS can damage proteins, lipids and DNA (Figure 16.1). The results reported by Katz-Jaffe et al[37] provided further

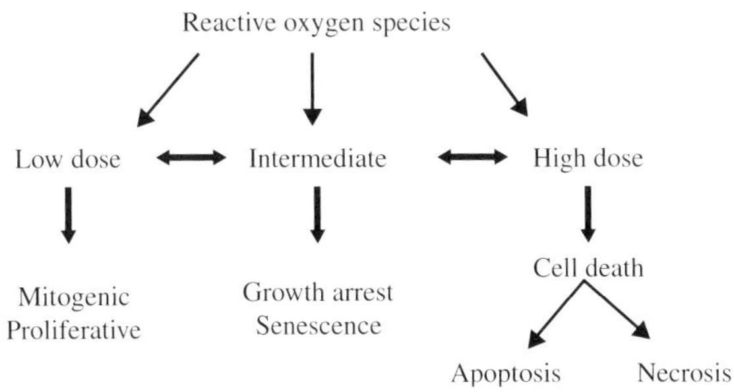

Figure 16.1 Dose-dependent effects of reactive oxygen species (ROS). Reactive oxygen species induce an array of cell effects that are highly dependent on the amount of ROS produced

support in favor of the use of low oxygen for embryo cultures. These authors showed by a proteomic approach that the protein profiles of embryos cultured in 5% oxygen were much more similar to in-vivo developed embryos than those from embryos cultured in 20% oxygen.

More recently, the phenotype and genotype of the preimplantation mouse embryos cultured in vitro to the blastocyst stage under 5% and 20% oxygen were compared with their in-vivo counterparts – the blastocyst-stage embryos flushed from the fallopian tubes.[38] Embryos cultured in 5% oxygen produced more blastocysts and had higher number of cells than embryos cultured in 20% oxygen. The global pattern of gene expression showed that, compared with in-vivo controls, more genes were misregulated in embryos cultured in 20% than in 6% oxygen. Particular attention was paid to genes that are regulated by the hypoxic condition (genes containing the hypoxia response element [HRE]) and to genes that are regulated by high oxygen concentration (antioxidant response element [ARE]). None of these genes were differentially expressed following the culture in 5% oxygen when compared with embryos that developed in vivo. This is consistent with the fact that 5% oxygen is a physiological and not a hypoxic condition. Harvey et al[39] showed that the expression of hypoxia-inducible factor-1α (HIF-1α) in the blastocysts was not up-regulated in embryos cultured in 5% oxygen and that the expression of Slc2a1 (another hypoxia response gene) did not change in embryos cultured in 7% and 20% O_2 but was up-regulated in cultures maintained in 2% oxygen (a true hypoxic condition).

OXYGEN AND STEM CELLS

What role does oxygen play during derivation and propagation of the hESCs? As oxygen concentration to which naturally conceived embryos are exposed is between 1.5 and 6%, we may reason that, at least for derivation, oxygen concentration should be within this range. In order to prove that this is correct, it is necessary to determine the range of oxygen concentration that is 'normoxic' and to define the 'hypoxic' range for these cells. As we manipulate these cells by creating their 'niche' in vitro, it is in our hands to make the best product that would fulfill our needs. The knowledge of the role of oxygen, the molecular mechanisms of oxygen sensing and gene activation is rapidly growing and many excellent reviews are available (see Hirota and Semenza[40] and Lahiri et al,[41] and references within). In this chapter we are going to summarize only some of the most relevant data.

Hypoxia-inducible factor and the transcriptional response to hypoxia

A widely accepted mechanism of oxygen tension-mediated regulation of cellular physiology is the activation of the transcriptional factor HIF-1α, which in turn regulates the transcription of a number of downstream target genes.[42,43] Under normoxic conditions, HIF-1α is constitutively transcribed, translated and hydroxylated at multiple proline residues by a set of prolyl-4-hydroxylase (PHD1, -2 and -3) enzymes.[44–46] These enzymes hydroxylate HIF-1α at highly conserved proline residues via a reaction that utilizes iron, oxygen, 2-oxoglutarate and ascorbate. The hydroxylated prolines are then recognized by the Von Hippel-Lindau (pVHL) E3 ubiquitin ligase complex, which targets HIF-1α for proteosomal degradation, thus explaining the ability to induce HIF-1α protein with iron chelators or anoxic conditions. This system is exquisitely sensitive to oxygen, such that following as little as 5 minutes of reoxygenation, most stabilized HIF-1α is degraded. In contrast, non-hydroxylated HIF-1α translocates to the nucleus, heterodimerizes with ARNT (arylhydrocarbon receptor nuclear translocator) and binds to HREs within the promoters or enhancers of hypoxia-induced genes (Figure 16.2). The related HIF-2α is regulated in a similar fashion. In addition, other post-translational modifications are also important for regulating HIF transcriptional activity.

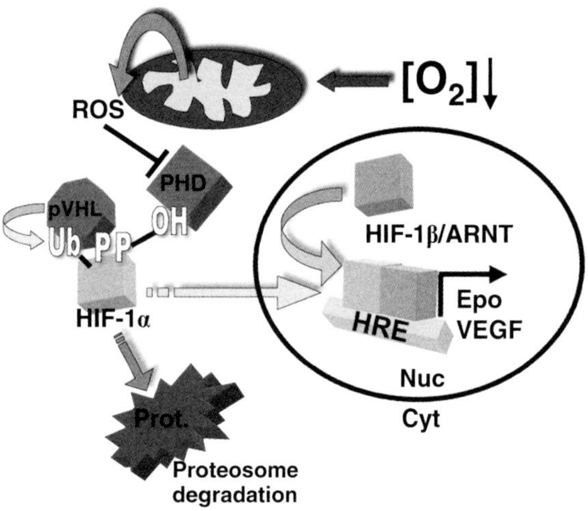

Figure 16.2 Mechanism of HIF induction in low oxygen. See detailed explanation in the text. ROS, reactive oxygen species; PHD, prolyl 4-hydroxylase; pVHL, Von Hippel–Lindau E3 ubiquitin ligase complex; HIF-1, hypoxia-inducible factor 1; ARNT, aryl-hydrocarbon receptor nuclear translocator; VEGF, vascular endothelial growth factor; HRE, hypoxia response element; P, proline residue; Ub, ubiquitine; Nuc, nucleus; Cyt, cytoplasm; Prot, proteosome; Epo, erythropoietin

The carboxyl terminus of the protein contains asparagine residues that can be hydroxylated by the factor inhibiting HIF-1 (FIH-1). As the name implies, this modification results in the transcriptional inactivation of this protein by preventing its interaction with the p300 histone acetyl transferase necessary for its transcriptional activity.[47] Finally, protein acetylation is also involved in regulating HIF activity. Mouse ARD1, an acetyltransferase that shares 57% identity with its homolog in *Saccharomyces cerevisiae*, was recently found to acetylate HIF-1α, promoting its interaction with pVHL, thereby augmenting its destruction.[48] This acetylation is reversible, however, being mediated by the interaction of HIF-1α with histone deacetylase 1 (HDAC1) and the metastasis tumor associated protein 1 (MTA1).[49] Finally, the extracellular regulated kinases are also activated by hypoxia, leading to HIF-1α phosphorylation.[50] Thus, the response to hypoxia involves complex modifications of HIF-1α by multiple pathways.

Whereas the identity of the oxygen sensor remains an intensely debated topic in the field, a leading model proposes that, under hypoxic conditions, mitochondrially generated ROS inhibit HIF-1α prolyl hydroxylation and degradation.[51–54] An alternative model proposes that the PHD (prolyl 4-hydroxylase) proteins are themselves the oxygen sensors, as they require oxygen to catalyze the hydroxylation of HIF-1α proline residues. However, recombinant prolyl hydroxylases have a K_m of ambient air (21%) in vitro indicating that the PHDs are decreasing their catalytic activity beginning above the physiological range of oxygen tension encountered by normal tissues.[55] Thus, one would expect to see HIF-1α stabilization beginning at 21% O_2, whereas it is only activated beginning around 5%,[56] largely discounting the ability of the PHDs to act as physiological oxygen sensors. Major evidence that mitochondria act as oxygen sensors came from studies in which cells were depleted of mitochondrial DNA and hence mitochondrial DNA-derived electron transport chain components.[57] These cells are unable to induce HIF-1α under physiological hypoxia[51] but do so under anoxia.[58] According to this model, ROS are generated at mitochondria as a function of decreasing oxygen tension, beginning at around 6% oxygen.[51,59–61] Consistent with this, free radical scavengers are able to also inhibit HIF-1α accumulation in this range of oxygen tensions.[62] Also, total protein carbonylation is increased during oxygen deprivation in yeast. This oxidant-induced protein modification was due to ROS generated by the mitochondrial electron transport chain.[63] More recently, mitochondrially targeted antioxidants have been shown to inhibit HIF-1α accumulation during hypoxia,[64] providing yet further evidence for a role for this pathway in cellular oxygen sensing.

Hypoxia-inducible factors and development

The first indication that hypoxia-induced gene expression pathways were critical regulators of mammalian development followed the genetic inactivation of the murine *Arnt (Hif-1β)* locus.[65,66] These animals exhibited midgestational embryonic lethality due to impaired hypoxia-induced *Vegf* expression and angiogenesis. Subsequently, multiple groups produced knockouts at the murine *Hif-1α* locus that largely recapitulated the findings of *Arnt*-null embryos.[67,68] VHL deficiency also resulted in embryonic lethality due to vascular defects in the placenta,[69] indicating that constitutively active HIF is just as detrimental as its absence. These studies strongly suggest that the environment of the developing mammalian embryo plays an informative role during organogenesis and that oxygen should be considered a developmental morphogen. Furthermore, this is a dynamic process that depends on the ability to modulate HIF activity with varying environmental conditions. Additional analyses with these genetically manipulated embryos and ESCs revealed roles for this pathway in organ systems other than the vasculature. The proliferation of hematopoietic stem cells was shown to be dependent on hypoxic HIF activity, as embryoid bodies derived from *Arnt*-null ESCs produced fewer hematopoietic precursors across multiple lineages when cultured under physiological hypoxia.[70] *Arnt*-null yolk sacs also contained fewer hematopoietic precursors as assessed by methylcellulose-based colony formation assays, indicating that the hypoxic environment in vivo was promoting hematopoietic stem cell proliferation. Consistent with the ability of oxygen tension to regulate human placental development,[25] the placentas of these mice were severely defective.[65,71] Beyond impaired vascularization, these placentas displayed gross disorganization of structure, indicated by the inappropriate differentiation and maintenance of trophoblast precursors. Derivation of trophoblast stem (TS) cells from *Arnt*-null blastocysts indicated that HIF activity determines cell fate decisions in the placenta.[71,72] This was largely due to the ability of the HIFs to interact with and modulate chromatin remodeling complexes associated with HDAC activity. In fact, pharmacological HDAC inhibition in wild-type TS cell lines was able to reproduce the differentiation defect in wild-type TS cells. This ability to intersect with epigenetic regulatory pathways significantly broadens the repertoire of HIF functions during development.

The related HIF-2α is also required for proper embryonic development. Multiple groups have produced knockouts of HIF-2α with varying phenotypes largely due to differences in genetic background. McKnight's laboratory described a requirement for HIF-2α in maintaining catecholamine homeostasis during embryonic development.[73] The expression of Hif-2α in developing adrenergic tissues such as the sympathetic chain and organ of Zuckerkandl, along with the decreased production of dopaminergic agents, was consistent with this. These embryos thus expired in utero due to impaired hypoxia-induced catecholamine production and depressed cardiac output. Carmeliet's group also witnessed an embryonic lethality in their Hif-2α-null embryos. However, a significant fraction of them survived to term, only to succumb to a condition highly reminiscent of respiratory distress syndrome (RDS) associated with preterm birth in humans.[74] In this case, impaired hypoxia-induced *Vegf* production in the lung prevented proper maturation of the alveolar epithelium, resulting in reduced surfactant production and subsequent perinatal demise due to respiratory distress. Together, these results highlight the pleiotropic roles played by oxygen in the developing and early postnatal mammalian embryo.

Whereas global inactivation of hypoxia-induced transcriptional pathways has revealed a great deal regarding the role of oxygen in development, targeted inactivation in individual organ systems has provided yet more evidence of the importance of this pathway during embryogenesis. Inactivation of *Hif-1α* gene expression in chondrocytes indicated that the developing mammalian growth plate is significantly hypoxic and that HIF activity is necessary for proper chondrocyte *Vegf* production, proliferation, extracellular matrix deposition and maturation.[75–78] Similarly, VHL deletion in these tissues also resulted in impaired endochondral bone formation. In addition to endochondral bone development, hypoxic HIF activity is required for proper tracheal development. Deficient HIF-1α expression in chondrocytes results in perinatal lethality due to airway malformations reminiscent of tracheomalacia in humans. Mammary epithelial differentiation is also dependent on hypoxic HIF activity. Targeted inactivation of HIF-1α in this tissue results in impaired secretory differentiation and activation of the mammary gland.[79]

The combined results from these experiments strongly argue for a vital role for physiological hypoxia-induced HIF activity during mammalian development. These effects are probably operative as early as fertilization and certainly are relevant for ESC biology.

Derivation and propagation of human embryonic stem cells in low oxygen

In collaboration with the Geron Corporation we have used low oxygen to derive ESCs (unpublished data). We have derived 5 ESC lines (that are not yet fully characterized) from discarded embryos in 6% oxygen with an efficiency of derivation that increased from 33% of attached blastocysts in 20% oxygen [80] to 50% in 6% oxygen (unpublished data). All the cell lines derived, in both 20% and 6% oxygen, showed normal karyotype and expressed markers of stemness. Because of the small number of total blastocysts used, these results are considered as preliminary, and more experiments are required to confirm the statistical significance of these results.

The beneficial effect of low oxygen on ESC propagation has been recently reported.[81] The authors have shown that the ESC colonies maintained at 5% oxygen grew better and showed less spontaneous differentiation than colonies cultured at 20% oxygen. Cells maintained under low oxygen were capable of forming embryoid bodies (EBs) and the number formed was significantly higher than in controls. In addition, the hypoxic EBs showed better attachment to the substrate and developed the outgrowths and cystic structures more readily than EBs cultured in 20% oxygen.

We have cultured two cell lines (H9 and H1) on placental fibroblasts as a feeder at both 6% and 20% oxygen. In spite of the differences in feeders (placental fibroblasts vs mouse embryonic fibroblasts [MEFs]), the results obtained were the same as reported by Ezashi et al.[81] Both cell lines proliferated more readily and exhibited less spontaneous differentiation in 6% than in 20% oxygen (Figure 16.3). Our preliminary results from cell cycle analysis did not show any significant differences in the number of cells detected at any phase of the cell cycle at either 6% or 21% oxygen, suggesting that oxygen tension has no effect on the progression of ESCs through the cell cycle. In addition, we did not detect any significant effect of low pO_2 on the rate of apoptosis. These results suggest that, compared with air, ESCs are able to progress faster through a normal cell cycle at low pO_2 (see Figure 16.3a) by reducing their average doubling time from 36 hours (at 20% oxygen) to 20–24 hours at 6% oxygen. In this experiment both feeder cells and ESCs were exposed to low oxygen. In order to exclude the effect of low oxygen on feeder cells, we cultured H9 cells on Matrigel in MEF conditioned medium that was produced under atmospheric oxygen. The same effects were observed in the absence of feeders (see Figure 16.3b), suggesting that low oxygen has a direct effect on ESCs. In addition, to prove that 6% oxygen is not an hypoxic environment for ESCs, we measured the expression of hypoxia-induced factors

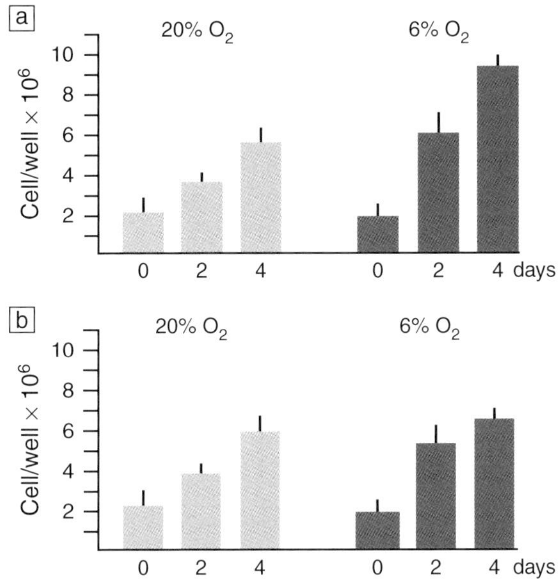

Figure 16.3 Effect of oxygen on hESC proliferation. H9 cells were cultured on placental fibroblasts (a) and on Matrigel in MEF-conditioned medium (b) for 4 days

(HIF-1 and HIF-2α) in ESCs cultured in both 6% and 1.5% oxygen. Neither of the two factors was up-regulated in 6% oxygen, indicating that this oxygen concentration is not hypoxic for these cells. In contrast, in cells cultured in 1.5% oxygen, HIF-1α was significantly up-regulated (unpublished data). We hypothesize that oxygen concentration within the range of 3–6% regulates self-renewal vs differentiation in hESCs through the induction of specific growth factors and cytokines and their respective receptors. It is known that low oxygen stimulates the production of vascular endothelial growth factor (VEGF) and platelet-derived growth factor-B (PDGF-B) in endothelial cells.[82] Furthermore, the receptor of hepatocyte growth factor (HGF) is also up-regulated by low oxygen.[83] Experiments designed to examine the production of growth factors and their receptors in hESCs cultured in low oxygen are in progress. Data supporting the use of low oxygen to culture ESCs are also coming from the somatic stem cell field. For example, in a recently published paper, D'Ippolito et al[84] examined the role of pO_2 in regulating the capacity of the unique subpopulation of human stromal cell from bone marrow to self-renew and maintain their pluripotency or to progress toward osteoblastic differentiation. The proliferation rate of cells exposed to 3% oxygen was three times higher than of cells exposed to air. Compared with controls, cells cultured at low oxygen (3–5%) upregulated at mRNA level markers of stemness: OCT-3/4, REX-1, telomerase reverse transcriptase and SSEA-4. It appears that low oxygen is essential to maintain the stem cell fate. The 'niche' model elaborated initially by Schofield,[85] and recently discussed by D'Ippolito et al,[84] suggests that stem cells in vivo are located within a specific area characterized by a unique microenvironment, which is, among other specific characteristics, low in oxygen, which contributes to maintenance of their limitless self-renewing potential (to proliferate without differentiation). This niche provides a sheltering environment that protects stem cells from differentiation, apoptotis and any other stimuli that would challenge them.[86] If we accept this concept, borrowed from the somatic stem cell niche, we may consider the derivation and propagation of undifferentiated ESCs in low oxygen as the best approach. Manipulation of oxygen tensions to closely approximate in-vivo conditions thus represents more than just an academic enterprise. For example, the ability of the HIFs to interact with and manipulate epigenetic regulatory pathways suggests that in-vitro culture conditions could produce heritable alterations in cell lines with potential long-term implications.

Much less is known on how to create the niche for targeted differentiation of ESCs. Low oxygen can inhibit, slow down or delay differentiation of several cell types such as, for example, human placental trophoblasts[25] and osteoblasts.[84,87,88] One of the most urgent tasks is therefore to determine how to manipulate oxygen concentration to create the optimal niche for differentiation of specific cell types. Studies of mammalian embryogenesis in the 1970s showed that successful development of the neural fold is highly sensitive to oxygenation levels. Interestingly, these studies[89] also showed that switching from a hypoxic to a normoxic condition and ultimately to a hyperoxic state is essential for the successful formation and closure of the neural fold of mammalian embryos, at least under in-vitro conditions. This embryonic oxygenation shift has never been well characterized, a task that should be accomplished if we are going to use stem cells to generate populations of various types of differentiated cells.

SUMMARY

Published data and our results support the use of a more physiological, low oxygen atmosphere to derive and propagate ESCs. As stem cells exist in a physicological environment of organic and inorganic components, a thorough understanding of the effects that changes in these components have on stem cell function is important to achieve therapeutic goals. Therefore, establishing cell culture conditions based on such an understanding is critical. A lot of work remains to be done to define specific niches for targeted differentiation of stem cells.

Acknowledgment

This work was supported in part by a grant from the UC Discovery Grant program (bio 02-10302).

REFERENCES

1. Amit M, Carpenter MK, Inokuma MS et al. Clonally derived human embryonic stem cell lines maintain pluripotency and proliferative potential for prolonged periods of culture. Dev Biol 2000; 22(6): 271–8.
2. Krtolica A. Stem cell-balancing aging and cancer. Int J Biochem Cell Biol 2005; 37: 935–41.
3. Chance B. Electron transfer: pathways, mechanisms, and controls. Annu Rev Biochem 1997; 46: 967–80.
4. Chandel NS, Budinger GR, Schumacker PT. Molecular oxygen modulates cytochrome c oxidase function. J Biol Chem 1996; 271(31): 18672–7.
5. Aw TY, Jones DP. Secondary bioenergetic hypoxia. Inhibition of sulfation and glucuronidation reactions in isolated hepatocytes at low O_2 concentration. J Biol Chem 1982; 257(15): 8997–9004.
6. Wilson DF, Rumsey WL, Green TJ, Vanderkooi JM. The oxygen dependence of mitochondrial oxidative phosphorylation measured by a new optical method for measuring oxygen concentration. J Biol Chem 1988; 263(6): 2712–18.
7. Graeber TG, Osmanian C, Jacks T et al. Hypoxia-mediated selection of cells with diminished apoptotic potential in solid tumours. Nature 1996; 379(6560): 88–91.
8. Brunelle JK, Chandel NS. Oxygen deprivation induced cell death: an update. Apoptosis 2002; 7(6): 475–82.
9. Parrinello S, Samper E, Krtolica A et al. Oxygen sensitivity severely limits the replicative lifespan of murine fibroblasts. Nat Cell Biol 2003; 5(8): 741–7.

10. Quinn P, Harlow GM. The effect of oxygen on the development of preimplantation mouse embryos in vitro. J Exp Zool 1978; 206(1): 73–80.

11. Pabon JE Jr, Findley WE, Gibbons WE. The toxic effect of short exposures to the atmospheric oxygen concentration on early mouse embryonic development. Fertil Steril 1989; 51(5): 896–900.

12. Thompson JG, Simpson AC, Pugh PA, Donnelly PE, Tervit HR. Effect of oxygen concentration on in-vitro development of preimplantation sheep and cattle embryos. J Reprod Fertil 1990; 89(2): 573–8.

13. Umaoka Y, Noda Y, Narimoto K, Mori T. Effects of oxygen toxicity on early development of mouse embryos. Mol Reprod Dev 1992; 31(1): 28–33.

14. Li J, Foote RH. Culture of rabbit zygotes into blastocysts in protein-free medium with one to twenty per cent oxygen. J Reprod Fertil 1993; 98(1): 163–7.

15. Eppig JJ, Wigglesworth K. Factors affecting the developmental competence of mouse oocytes grown in vitro: oxygen concentration. Mol Reprod Dev 1995; 42(4): 447–56.

16. Bernardi ML, Flechon JE, Delouis C. Influence of culture system and oxygen tension on the development of ovine zygotes matured and fertilized in vitro. J Reprod Fertil 1996; 106(2): 161–7.

17. Catt JW, Henman M. Toxic effects of oxygen on human embryo development. Hum Reprod 2000; 15 (Suppl 2): 199–206.

18. Mitchell JA, Yochim JM. Intrauterine oxygen tension during the estrous cycle in the rat: its relation to uterine respiration and vascular activity. Endocrinology 1968; 83(4): 701–5.

19. Mitchell JA, Yochim JM. Measurement of intrauterine oxygen tension in the rat and its regulation by ovarian steroid hormones. Endocrinology 1968; 83(4): 691–700.

20. Yochim JM, Mitchell JA. Intrauterine oxygen tension in the rat during progestation: its possible relation to carbohydrate metabolism and the regulation of nidation. Endocrinology 1968; 83(4): 706–13.

21. Rodesch F, Simon P, Donner C, Jauniaux E. Oxygen measurements in endometrial and trophoblastic tissues during early pregnancy. Obstet Gynecol 1992; 80(2): 283–5.

22. Fischer B, Bavister BD. Oxygen tension in the oviduct and uterus of rhesus monkeys, hamsters and rabbits. J Reprod Fertil 1993; 99(2): 673–9.

23. Kaufman DL, Mitchell JA. Intrauterine oxygen tension during the oestrous cycle in the hamster: patterns of change. Comp Biochem Physiol Comp Physiol 1994; 107(4): 673–8.

24. Van Blerkom J, Antczak M, Schrader R. The developmental potential of the human oocyte is related to the dissolved oxygen content of follicular fluid: association with vascular endothelial growth factor levels and perifollicular blood flow characteristics. Hum Reprod 1997; 12(5): 1047–55.

25. Genbacev O, Zhou Y, Ludlow JW, Fisher SJ. Regulation of human placental development by oxygen tension. Science 1997; 277(5332): 1669–72.

26. Genbacev O, Krtolica A, Kaelin W, Fisher SJ. Human cytotrophoblast expression of the von Hippel–Lindau protein is downregulated during uterine invasion in situ and upregulated by hypoxia in vitro. Dev Biol 2001; 233(2): 526–36.

27. Jaffe R, Jauniaux E, Hustin J. Maternal circulation in the first-trimester human placenta – myth or reality? Am J Obstet Gynecol 1997; 176(3): 695–705.

28. Burton GJ, Jauniaux E, Watson AL. Maternal arterial connections to the placental intervillous space during the first trimester of human pregnancy: the Boyd collection revisited. Am J Obstet Gynecol 1999; 181(3): 718–24.

29. Emmanouilides G, Allen H, Riemenschneider T, Gutgesell H. Moss and Adams' Heart Disease in Infants, Children, and Adolescents, 5th edn. Baltimore: Williams & Wilkins, 1995.

30. Gardner DK. Changes in requirements and utilization of nutrients during mammalian preimplantation embryo development and their significance in embryo culture. Theriogenology 1998; 49: 83–102.

31. Rinaudo P, Schultz RM. Effects of embryo culture on global pattern of gene expression in preimplantation mouse embryos. Reproduction 2004; 128: 301–11.

32. Dumoulin JC, Meijers CJ, Bras M et al. Effect of oxygen concentration on human in-vitro fertilization and embryo culture. Hum Reprod 1999; 14: 465–9.

33. Gardner DK, Schoolcraft WB. Culture and transfer of human blastocysts. Curr Opin Obstet Gynecol 1999; 11: 307–11.

34. Karagenc L, Sertkaya Z, Ciray N, Ulug U, Bahceci M. Impact of oxygen concentration on embryonic development of mouse zygotes. Reprod Biomed online 2004; 9: 409–17.

35. Takahashi M, Keicho K, Takahashi H et al. Effect of oxidative stress on development and DNA damage in in-vitro cultured bovine embryos by Comet assay. Theriogenology 2000; 54: 137–45.

36. Kitagawa Y, Suzuki K, Yoneda A, Watanabe T. Effects of oxygen concentration and antioxidants on the in vitro developmental ability, production of reactive oxygen species (ROS), and DNA fragmentation in porcine embryos. Theriogenology 2004; 62: 1186–97.

37. Katz-Jaffe MG, Linck DW, Schoolcraft WB, Gardner DK. A proteomic analysis of mammalian preimplantation embryonic development. Reproduction 2005; 130: 899–905.

38. Rinaudo P, Giritharan G, Dobson AT, Schultz RM. Effects of oxygen tension on gene expression in preimplantation mouse embryos. Fertil Steril 2006.

39. Harvey AJ, Kind KL, Pantaleon M, Armstrong DT, Thompson JG. Oxygen-regulated gene expression in bovine blastocysts. Biol Reprod 2004; 71(4): 1108–19.

40. Hirota K, Semenza GL. Regulation of hypoxia-inducible factor 1 by prolyl and asparaginyl hydroxylases. Biochem Biophys Res Commun 2005; 9; 338(1): 610–16.

41. Lahiri S, Roy A, Baby SM et al. Oxygen sensing in the body. Prog Biophys Mol Biol. 2006; 91(3): 249–86.

42. Semenza GL. Hypoxia-inducible factor 1: master regulator of O_2 homeostasis. Curr Opin Genet Dev 1998; 8(5): 588–94.

43. Semenza GL. HIF-1, O(2), and the 3 PHDs: how animal cells signal hypoxia to the nucleus. Cell 2001; (5)107(1): 1–3.

44. Bruick RK, McKnight SL. A conserved family of prolyl-4-hydroxylases that modify HIF. Science 2001; 294(5545): 1337–40.

45. Epstein AC, Gleadle JM, McNeill LA et al. *C. elegans* EGL-9 and mammalian homologs define a family of dioxygenases that regulate HIF by prolyl hydroxylation. Cell 2001; 107(1): 43–54.

46. Ivan M, Kondo K, Yang H et al. HIFalpha targeted for VHL-mediated destruction by proline hydroxylation: implications for O_2 sensing. Science 2001; 292(5516): 464–8.

47. Mahon PC, Hirota K, Semenza GL. FIH-1: a novel protein that interacts with HIF-1alpha and VHL to mediate repression of HIF-1 transcriptional activity. Genes Dev 2001; 15(20): 2675–86.

48. Jeong JW, Bae MK, Ahn MY et al. Regulation and destabilization of HIF-1alpha by ARD1-mediated acetylation. Cell 2002; 111(5): 709–20.

49. Yoo YG, Kong G, Lee MO. Metastasis-associated protein 1 enhances stability of hypoxia-inducible factor-1alpha protein by recruiting histone deacetylase 1. Embo J 2006; 25(6): 1231–41.

50. Minet E, Arnould T, Michel G et al. ERK activation upon hypoxia: involvement in HIF-1 activation. FEBS Lett 2000; 468(1): 53–8.

51. Chandel NS, Maltepe E, Goldwasser et al. Mitochondrial reactive oxygen species trigger hypoxia-induced transcription. Proc Natl Acad Sci USA 1998; 95(20): 11715–20.

52. Brunelle JK, Bell EL, Quesada NM et al. Oxygen sensing requires mitochondrial ROS but not oxidative phosphorylation. Cell Metab 2005; 1(6): 409–14.

53. Guzy RD, Hoyos B, Robin E et al. Mitochondrial complex III is required for hypoxia-induced ROS production and cellular oxygen sensing. Cell Metab 2005; 1(6): 401–8.

54. Mansfield KD, Guzy RD, Pan Y et al. Mitochondrial dysfunction resulting from loss of cytochrome c impairs cellular oxygen sensing and hypoxic HIF-alpha activation. Cell Metab 2005; 1(6): 393–9.

55. Hirsila M, Koivunen P, Gunzler V, Kivirikko KI, Myllyharju J. Characterization of the human prolyl 4-hydroxylases that modify the hypoxia-inducible factor. J Biol Chem 2003; 278(33): 30772–80.

56. Jiang BH, Semenza GL, Bauer C, Marti HH. Hypoxia-inducible factor 1 levels vary exponentially over a physiologically relevant range of O_2 tension. Am J Physiol 1996; 271(4 Pt 1): C1172–80.

57. King MP, Attardi G. Injection of mitochondria into human cells leads to a rapid replacement of the endogenous mitochondrial DNA. Cell 1988; 52(6): 811–19.

58. Schroedl C, McClintock DS, Budinger GR, Chandel NS. Hypoxic but not anoxic stabilization of HIF-1alpha requires mitochondrial reactive oxygen species. Am J Physiol Lung Cell Mol Physiol 2002; 283(5): L922–31.

59. Duranteau J, Chandel NS, Kulisz A, Shao Z, Schumacker PT. Intracellular signaling by reactive oxygen species during hypoxia in cardiomyocytes. J Biol Chem 1998; 273(19): 11619–24.

60. Wood JG, Johnson JS, Mattioli LF, Gonzalez NC. Systemic hypoxia promotes leukocyte-endothelial adherence via reactive oxidant generation. J Appl Physiol 1999; 87(5): 1734–40.

61. Killilea DW, Hester R, Balczon R, Babal P, Gillespie MN. Free radical production in hypoxic pulmonary artery smooth muscle cells. Am J Physiol Lung Cell Mol Physiol 2000; 279(2): L408–12.

62. Bell EL, Emerling BM, Chandel NS. Mitochondrial regulation of oxygen sensing. Mitochondrion 2005; 5(5): 322–32.

63. Dirmeier R, O'Brien KM, Engle M et al. Exposure of yeast cells to anoxia induces transient oxidative stress. Implications for the induction of hypoxic genes. J Biol Chem 2002; 277(38): 34773–84.

64. Sanjuan-Pla A, Cervera AM, Apostolova N et al. A targeted antioxidant reveals the importance of mitochondrial reactive oxygen species in the hypoxic signaling of HIF-1alpha. FEBS Lett 2005; 579(12): 2669–74.

65. Kozak KR, Abbott B, Hankinson O. ARNT-deficient mice and placental differentiation. Dev Biol 1997; 191(2): 297–305.

66. Maltepe E, Schmidt JV, Baunoch D, Bradfield CA, Simon MC. Abnormal angiogenesis and responses to glucose and oxygen deprivation in mice lacking the protein ARNT. Nature 1997; 386(6623): 403–7.

67. Iyer NV, Kotch LE, Agani F et al. Cellular and developmental control of O_2 homeostasis by hypoxia-inducible factor 1 alpha. Genes Dev 1998; 12(2): 149–62.

68. Ryan HE, Lo J, Johnson RS. HIF-1 alpha is required for solid tumor formation and embryonic vascularization. EMBO J 1998; 17(11): 3005–15.

69. Gnarra JR, Ward JM, Porter FD et al. Defective placental vasculogenesis causes embryonic lethality in VHL-deficient mice. Proc Natl Acad Sci USA 1997; 94(17): 9102–7.

70. Adelman DM, Maltepe E, Simon MC. Multilineage embryonic hematopoiesis requires hypoxic ARNT activity. Genes Dev 1999; 13(19): 2478–83.

71. Adelman DM, Gertsenstein M, Nagy A, Simon MC, Maltepe E. Placental cell fates are regulated in vivo by HIF-mediated hypoxia responses. Genes Dev 2000; 14(24): 3191–203.

72. Maltepe E, Krampitz GW, Okazaki KM et al. Hypoxia-inducible factor-dependent histone deacetylase activity determines stem cell fate in the placenta. Development 2005; 132(15): 3393–403.

73. Tian H, Hammer RE, Matsumoto AM, Russell DW, McKnight SL. The hypoxia-responsive transcription factor EPAS1 is essential for catecholamine homeostasis and protection against heart failure during embryonic development. Genes Dev 1998; 12(21): 3320–4.

74. Compernolle V, Brusselmans K, Acker T et al. Loss of HIF-2alpha and inhibition of VEGF impair fetal lung maturation, whereas treatment with VEGF prevents fatal respiratory distress in premature mice. Nat Med 2002; 8(7): 702–10.

75. Schipani E, Ryan HE, Didrickson S et al. Hypoxia in cartilage: HIF-1alpha is essential for chondrocyte growth arrest and survival. Genes Dev 2001; 15(21): 2865–76.

76. Pfander D, Cramer T, Schipani E, Johnson RS. HIF-1alpha controls extracellular matrix synthesis by epiphyseal chondrocytes. J Cell Sci 2003; 116(Pt 9): 1819–26.

77. Pfander D, Kobayashi T, Knight MC et al. Deletion of Vhlh in chondrocytes reduces cell proliferation and increases matrix deposition during growth plate development. Development 2004; 131(10): 2497–508.

78. Zelzer E, Mamluk R, Ferrara N et al. VEGFA is necessary for chondrocyte survival during bone development. Development 2004; 131(9): 2161–71.

79. Seagroves TN, Hadsell D, McManaman J et al. HIF1-alpha is a critical regulator of secretory differentiation and activation, but not vascular expansion, in the mouse mammary gland. Development 2003; 130(8): 1713–24.

80. Genbacev O, Krtolica A, Zdravkovic T et al. Serum free derivation of human embryonic stem cell lines on human placental fibroblast feeders. Fertil Steril 2005; 85(5): 1517–29.

81. Ezashi T, Das P, Roberts RM. Low oxygen tensions and the prevention of differentiation of hES cells. Proc Natl Acad Sci USA 2005; 102: 4783–8.

82. Namiki A, Brogi E, Kearney M et al. Hypoxia induces vascular endothelial growth factor in cultured human endothelial cells. J Biol Chem 1995; 270: 31189–95.

83. Pennacchietti S, Michieli P, Galluzzo M et al. Hypoxia promotes invasive growth by transcriptional activation of the met protooncogene. Cancer Cell 2003; 3: 347–61.

84. D'Ippolito G, Diabira S, Howard GA, Roos BA, Schiller PC. Low oxygen tension inhibits osteogenic differentiation and enhances stemness of human MIAMI cells. Bone 2006 Apr 6; [Epub ahead of print].

85. Schofield R. The relationship between the spleen colony-forming cell and the haemapoietic stem cell. Blood Cells 1978; 4: 7–25.

86. Moore KA, Lemischka IR. Stem cells and their niches. Science 2006; 311: 1880–5.

87. Brighton CT, Schaffer JL, Shapiro DB, Tang JJ, Clark CC. Proliferation and macromolecular synthesis by rat calvarial bone cells grown in various oxygen tensions. J Orthop Res 1991; 9: 847–54.

88. Park JH, Park BH, Kim HK, Park TS, Back HS. Hypoxia decreases Runx2/Cbfa1 expression in human osteoblast-like cells. Mol Cell Endocrinol 2002; 192: 197–203.

89. Morriss GM, New DA. Effect of oxygen concentration on morphogenesis of cranial neural folds and neural crest in cultured rat embryos. J Embryol Exp Morphol 1979; 54: 17–35.

CHAPTER 17

Nuclear reprogramming

Keith HS Campbell

INTRODUCTION

The technique of nuclear transfer (NT) involves the transfer of a nucleus from a donor cell (karyoplast) into an enucleated oocyte or zygote from which the nuclear genetic material has been removed (cytoplast). The term 'nuclear reprogramming' has been used to describe the changes in gene expression which are induced in the donor nucleus following NT, or more generally the changes that are induced experimentally by introducing nuclei into a new cytoplasmic environment.[1] NT was proposed by Spemann[2] as a technique to study cell differentiation and commitment; by transferring nuclei from progressively later stages of development, the point at which the nucleus became fixed (committed), or lost the ability to control all development, could be determined. We now know that nuclear instructions are in the form of DNA and that the majority of nuclei within an adult contain two complete copies of the genome derived from the maternal and paternal germ cells at the point of fertilization. In 1996 the birth of 'Dolly', a sheep produced by nuclear transfer from an adult-derived somatic cell[3] demonstrated that the oocyte was able to reprogram nuclear DNA from a differentiated cell and recapitulate the temporal and spatial pattern of gene expression associated with development to produce offspring which developed to adulthood and were reproductively normal. Thus, NT provides a route to the dedifferentiation and redifferentiation of somatic nuclei, thereby producing the entire range of cell types associated with normal development and, in particular, providing a method for the derivation of autologous multipotential embryonic stem cells for human therapeutics. It is now accepted that nuclear reprogramming following NT is controlled by epigenetic mechanisms and not by rearrangement of DNA sequences. However, it should be remembered that nuclear reprogramming is not restricted to NT embryos and that nuclear programming by epigenetic mechanisms is an ongoing event throughout development and differentiation and has also been implicated in the disease process.

EPIGENETICS IN DEVELOPMENT AND DIFFERENTIATION

Eukaryotic DNA is assembled into chromatin and chromosomes by association with histones. Briefly, the DNA helix is wrapped around core histones to form a simple bead-like structure (nucleosome) that is then folded into higher-order chromatin. Higher-order chromatin contains other proteins that are required for a range of functions, including assembly and maintenance of structure, DNA replication, repair, transcription and recombination. By means of nucleosomal DNA, the genome is organized into functional regions that are transcriptionally active or transcriptionally repressive. However, the transcriptional state is not fixed and the covalent modification of nucleosomal DNA or the core histones is important in the control of many biological processes, including transcription and DNA replication. Such mechanisms, which are heritable through mitosis but do not involve alterations in DNA sequence, are termed 'epigenetic' and include modifications at the DNA level, i.e. DNA methylation, chromatin structure, modification of histones and modifications of nuclear structure (for reviews see References 4 and 5).

DNA methylation

Methylation of genomic DNA at CpG repeats is an important mechanism regulating gene expression. Methylation of the promoter regions of specific genes can regulate gene expression in an allele-specific manner and is involved in the phenomenon of parental genetic imprinting (reviewed in Reference 6), allowing regulated gene expression during early development and in particular during fetal growth. In fact, incorrect patterns of DNA methylation are involved in a number of so-called 'imprinted' developmental abnormalities such as Beckwith–Wiedemann syndrome and Prader–Willi syndrome (reviewed in Reference 7). Two major periods of alterations in methylation status occur during development: the first period occurs during development of the germ cells when genome-wide demethylation of the primordial germ cells is followed by mitotic (male) or meiotic (female) arrest. Sex-specific remethylation then occurs in the prospermatogonia or during oocyte growth, the resultant gametes being highly methylated. A second major period of reprogramming of methylation state occurs during early embryonic development. During the first cell cycle of the fertilized zygote, rapid demethylation of the sperm DNA occurs by an active mechanism immediately after fertilization. On formation of the pronuclei, both paternal and maternal DNA are then demethylated by a passive mechanism that continues through development, erasing methylation on all but the imprinted genes by the blastocyst stage. Following implantation, remethylation of specific genes occurs in a lineage-specific manner. In different species, the timing of the reprogramming of DNA methylation patterns during early development varies: in cattle, for instance, demethylation of both maternal and paternal genomes occurs between the 2- and 4-cell stage followed by de-novo methylation at the 8-cell stage onwards, with a characteristic hypermethylation of the inner cell mass (ICM) at the blastocyst stage;[8] in sheep, demethylation occurs slowly up to the 8-cell stage and then remains almost constant.[9] Although the role of demethylation in development is unknown, it appears that imprinted marks are maintained, suggesting that demethylation is not genome-wide and is not random (for review see Reference 10).

Histone modification

The modifications of the core histones have been implicated in a range of cellular processes, including both transcriptional activation and repression, cell cycle progression, chromatin condensation and chromosome organization. Modifications that occur at the amino termini of histones include acetylation, phosphorylation, methylation, ubiquitination and ADP ribosylation (for review see Reference 11). The roles of histone modification in development and differentiation are slowly being elucidated and have been reviewed elsewhere.[12] In this article, I briefly mention only those modifications for which there is some evidence also gathered from NT embryos.

Acetylation and deacetylation of specific lysine residues are achieved by histone acetyl transferases (HATs) and histone deacetylases (HDACs).[13] Histone acetylation has been reported to have major roles in cell function, including repression or activation of transcription,[14–16] control of cell cycle progression,[17] inheritance of epigenetic information (reviewed in Reference 18), DNA repair and apoptosis,[19] and is also important in the remodeling of the embryonic genome during normal development.[20] Studies in early embryos have shown that, in the mouse, both maternal and paternal gametes are unacetylated. Following fertilization, the paternal chromatin becomes rapidly hyperacetylated; this is followed by a slower acetylation of the female chromatin. However, both pronuclei become acetylated, which may correlate with the onset of zygotic transcription, which occurs at the 1–2 cell stage.[21] In our studies in cattle, we also found that both parental gametes are unacetylated. During the 1st cell cycle of the fertilized zygote, both pronuclei become transiently hyperacetylated. A decrease in the level of acetylation was then observed until the 8–16-cell stage, after which a gradual increase occurred. This correlates with the onset of zygotic transcription in cattle embryos. Following the onset of transcription, it appears that differential acetylation occurs and, by the blastocyst stage, the ICM is less acetylated than the trophectoderm (TE) cells. In particular, ICM cells are hypoacetylated on lysine residues 5 and 12.[22]

NUCLEAR TRANSFER

Methodology

The term nuclear transfer can refer to the transplantation of a nucleus between any cell types; however, in general, it is understood to refer to the creation of a new embryo by transplantation of a donor nucleus into an enucleated oocyte, zygote or early embryo. The production of embryos and offspring by NT or so-called cloning is a multistep process requiring production of a suitable recipient cell, enucleation, transfer of the donor nucleus, activation, culture and, if required, transfer to a suitable surrogate recipient. Historically, oocytes arrested at metaphase of the second meiotic division (MII), pronuclear zygotes and 2-cell embryos have all been used as recipient cells for NT, however, the recipient of choice based on development is presently the MII oocyte.[23] MII oocytes obtained following in-vivo or in-vitro maturation are physically enucleated by aspirating the maternal chromosomes using a fine glass pipette (for reviews see References 23–25). Following enucleation, the donor nucleus is transferred into the cytoplasm of the recipient cell (cytoplast). In general, this is achieved by cell fusion induced by a DC electric pulse; however, both viral and chemically induced fusion have been reported, as well as injection of either the whole cell or the nucleus and some associated cytoplasm (reviewed in Reference 26). Following reconstruction, the reconstructed oocyte is activated and then cultured to a stage suitable for transfer to a surrogate recipient. In general, for many species, embryos are cultured in vitro; however, embryos can be transferred to a recipient immediately after reconstruction and allowed to develop to term, as in pigs,[27] or transferred to a temporary recipient, recovered and assessed prior to final transfer.[28] The improvement in culture techniques has superseded the use of temporary recipients in many species.

Each of the stages involved in the reconstruction process can affect the success of NT via both physical as well as biological mechanisms. In particular, the culture conditions have been shown to be involved in producing fetal overgrowth through epigenetic mechanisms.[29,30] However, it is considered that the most important factors involved in obtaining successful development are the stage and quality of the recipient cytoplast, the differentiated status of the donor cell, the coordination of nuclear and cytoplasmic phases between donor and recipient and the method of activation.

Coordination of donor nucleus and recipient cytoplasm

The process of oocyte maturation involves both nuclear and cytoplasmic events. The immature or germinal vesicle (GV) stage oocyte is arrested at prophase of the first meiotic division (MI); on resumption of meiosis, two cytoplasmic kinase activities, maturation promoting factor (MPF) and mitogen-activated protein kinase (MAPK), increase and induce germinal vesicle breakdown (GVBD) and chromosome condensation. MPF activity peaks at metaphase of the MI, and then transiently declines, reaching maximum activity again at MII. MAPK activity remains elevated throughout maturation to prevent nuclear reformation and DNA synthesis. When a donor nucleus is transferred into an MII cytoplasmic environment, the levels of MPF and MAPK are high and induce nuclear envelope breakdown (NEBD) and premature chromosome condensation (PCC). The effects of NEBD and PCC on the donor nucleus are dependent upon the cell cycle stage at the time of transfer and have been extensively reviewed elsewhere.[31,32] Briefly, diploid or mitotic nuclei are suitable for transfer into MII cytoplasm, S-phase nuclei undergo DNA damage due to PCC and this is followed by uncoordinated DNA replication resulting in aneuploid embryos, G_2 phase nuclei undergo DNA rereplication resulting in tetraploid embryos.[33] In contrast, if enucleated oocytes have low kinase activities or are activated prior to NT, which causes a decline in kinase activities, then NEBD and PCC do not occur and regulated DNA replication occurs in donor nuclei which are in G_1, S or G_2 phases of the cell cycle. The use of activated oocytes as recipients with low levels of kinase activity can be used to advantage when cloning from embryonic blastomeres[34] (see below).

The donor cell

The first successful report of NT in mammals involved the transfer of pronuclei between mouse zygotes,[35] demonstrating that the manipulations required did not prevent development. However, in subsequent experiments when embryonic blastomeres were used as nuclear donors, no development was reported.[36] In similar experiments in farm animals, the use of enucleated zygotes as cytoplast recipients also resulted in a lack of development.[37,38] In contrast, when MII oocytes were used as cytoplast recipients, live lambs were obtained using donor nuclei from embryos at the 8–16-cell stage.[39] These experiments demonstrated that the mature oocyte had a greater ability to reprogram blastomere nuclei than did enucleated zygotes; however, this may be due to removal of factors localized within the pronuclei (see below). Even when MII oocytes were used as recipients, there still appeared to be a species-specific maximum developmental stage which could result in development; furthermore, this appeared to be related to the timing of the onset of zygotic transcription. In a comparison of species, it appeared that the later the onset of zygotic transcription the later in development nuclear donors could result in development: at the two extremes were the mouse, which initiates transcription at the 1–2-cell stage, and *Xenopus laevis*, which initiates transcription at the 4000-cell stage. Two explanations emerged to explain this apparent block; first, following the onset of transcription, the embryonic nuclei becomes progressively committed to a particular lineage and is less able to be reprogrammed and, secondly, in species where transcription is initiated later, the transferred nucleus has more time to be reprogrammed.[23,40] In truth, both of these concepts are probably involved in the reprogramming process; however, it is now apparent that the differentiated status of the donor cell can profoundly affect the frequency of early embryonic development.

During early embryonic cell cycles, S phase (or the period of DNA replication) is the predominant cell cycle stage at any one time. Transfer of S-phase nuclei into an MII cytoplasmic environment results in DNA damage and incorrect ploidy in the reconstructed embryo.[33] In contrast, transfer of S-phase nuclei into an interphase cytoplasmic environment avoids this damage and significantly improved development of ovine embryos reconstructed using 16-cell blastomeres as nuclear donors.[34] In mammals, the time required to complete DNA synthesis in embryonic cell cycles and in many somatic cell types is very similar, and therefore simply coordinating nuclear and cytoplasmic events may avoid problems of aneuploidy; however, there are many reports of abnormal ploidies in cloned embryos.[41–44] Whether these result from incomplete or uncoordinated DNA replication or faulty chromosome segregation is unknown.[44] In amphibians, differences in replication timing have much more serious consequences. Embryonic replication occurs much more rapidly than in somatic cells, the onset of mitosis during early embryonic cycles is not affected by replication status and chromosomal abnormalities have been reported as a consequence of incomplete DNA synthesis.[45,46] However, complete DNA replication of somatic nuclei can occur in the correct time frame in a *Xenopus* cytoplasmic extract following sufficient time for remodeling of nuclear/chromatin structure.[47] These observations suggest that preconditioning of the somatic nucleus may result in correct replication following transplantation.

Although the use of interphase cytoplasts increased embryo development when using embryonic blastomeres,[34] or early passage ICM cells as nuclear donors when more differentiated cells were used, there appeared to be a reduction in developmental competence.[28] However, when MII cytoplasts and quiescent (G_0) donor cells were used, an apparent increase in development was observed.[48] Therefore, it appeared that the cell cycle stage of the recipient cytoplast, the donor cell type and the donor cell cycle stage all contributed to increasing development. The production of live offspring from cultured embryonic cells,[28] followed by the birth of animals from fetal- and adult-derived cells,[3] heralded the development of somatic cell nuclear transfer (SCNT) techniques. Subsequently, SCNT has been reported in a range of species (Table 17.1), with a range of cell types derived from embryonic, fetal and adult tissues. Although a comparison of development between species and cell types is difficult, owing to differences in methodology between species and between laboratories, it is now generally accepted that differences in development exist between cell types, with development decreasing from embryonic to fetal to adult cell types (reviewed in Reference 49).

The recipient oocyte

The recipient oocyte is essential to the development of NT embryos; however, it has been demonstrated that many factors can influence oocyte quality and subsequent development. In sheep, the use of superovulation has been shown to decrease the frequency of development to both blastocyst and term of fertilized embryos and also to reduce the birth weight of the offspring. In mice, similar studies have demonstrated an altered pattern of DNA methylation

Table 17.1 Major milestones in somatic cell animal cloning

Date	*Species*	*Cell donor comments*	*Reference*
1995	Sheep	Embryo-derived cultured cells	28
1996	Sheep (Dolly)	Embryo-; fetal- and adult-derived cells	3
1997	Sheep	Embryo. 1st transgenic animal for pharmaceutical	138
1997	Cattle	Transgenic, fetal	139
1998	Mice	Uncultured cumulus cells	74
1999	Goats	Transgenic, fetal	61
2000	Pigs	Adult	27
2000	Sheep	Fetal. 1st gene targeted farm animal	140
2000	Gaur	Adult. Interspecies	111
2001	Mouflon	Postmortem adult cell, ovine oocyte	112
2002	Cat	Adult cell	141
2003	Deer	Adult	142
2003	Rabbit	Adult cell	143
2003	Rat		144
2003	Mule	Fetal	145
2003	Horse	Adult. Dam twin as surrogate	146
2005	Dog	Adult	147
2006	Ferret	Adult	148

[Q1]

in the zygotes. Preparation of the oocyte for NT requires removal of the maternal chromosomes. This process also removes a proportion of the cytoplasm, and it has been suggested that this may remove specific proteins localized around the meiotic spindle that are essential for subsequent development.[42] The age of the oocyte, in terms of hours after onset of maturation, and also the age of the oocyte donor, may also affect development. Both of these factors can impact on the levels of MPF and MAPK present in the oocyte; oocytes from prepubertal sheep have reduced kinase activities[50] and MII oocyte kinase activities can decline rapidly on aging, i.e in rats.[51] MPF and MAPK activities may be important in NT; indeed, in the majority of species cloned so far, MII oocytes were used as cytoplast recipients. The roles of MPF and MAPK in nuclear reprogramming are unclear. Studies carried out in mice[52] and cattle[53–56] have directly compared the efficiency of development of SCNT embryos produced in both high and low MPF activity cytoplasts. Development is greatest when high MPF activity cytoplasts are used, indicating that reprogramming activity is present in young matured oocytes. When somatic cells are transferred into low MPF cytoplasts with active MAPK activity, development to blastocysts is reduced, suggesting that MAPK activity is not involved in nuclear reprogramming.[54] Although this evidence strongly suggests that MPF and MAPK are not reprogramming molecules acting by themselves, the possibility exists that they are involved in nuclear reprogramming through other mechanisms. A simple explanation is that the occurrence of NEBD and PCC in the donor nucleus following NT first allows greater access of oocyte components to the donor chromatin, facilitating changes in nuclear and chromatin architecture; furthermore, the condensation of the donor chromatin may aid this remodeling process by removing chromatin-bound transcription factors due to torsional stress[57] and the abortion of nascent somatic transcripts.[58] Although the potential roles of MPF and MAPK in reprogramming are unclear, the occurrence of NEBD and PCC are beneficial: this is supported by an apparent increase in development when cells containing condensed chromatin are used as nuclear donors.[59]

In contrast to these studies, other reports in sheep,[60] goats[61] and cattle[62–65] show that embryos can also develop and give offspring when preactivated recipients (with low MPF activity) are used for SCNT. The discrepancy between studies is difficult to interpret; however, considering the variations in the manipulation protocols used and the assessment of the oocyte status as well as the remodeling of the transferred nuclei in the different studies makes it difficult to draw a final conclusion. Determination of a high or low MPF activity in the recipient oocyte is used as the main indicator of a preactivated or non-activated state. However, it is also well known that MAPK activity undergoes dephosphorylation after oocyte activation, and its inactivation is correlated with pronuclear formation, although this occurs at a much slower rate than the MPF inactivation.[66–69] It has also been shown that MPF and MAPK activities have no influence in chromatin condensation, since condensed chromosomes are observed prior to GVBD in butyrolactone I-arrested oocytes, which have no active MPF or MAPK.[70]

The role of quiescence

The use of quiescent or G_0 cells as nuclear donors in the first instance provides a convenient method for the coordination of the donor nucleus with the MII oocyte cytoplasmic environment, allowing NEBD and PCC to occur but reducing possible DNA damage and maintaining ploidy.[32] However, the use of such cell cycle-arrested donor cells may also have further benefits. Following quiescence, cells undergo a variety of changes, which include a reduction in transcription and condensation of the chromatin. As discussed previously, little transcription occurs in early embryos until the zygotic genome is activated. In NT embryos, transcription of the donor nucleus must be halted and then reprogrammed to replicate the spatial and temporal pattern observed in early embryos. Therefore, reducing transcription in the nuclear donor cell prior to transfer may be beneficial. In addition, the condensation of the nuclear DNA may displace certain transcription factors, allowing greater access of oocyte factors and thus aiding the potential beneficial effects of PCC induced by MPF (see above). Although few studies have adequately compared development of different donor/recipient cell cycle combinations, a single report in cattle suggests that the use of G_0 donor cells results in greater viability of embryos, which results in more live offspring.[71] When the donor cells were transgenic, it appeared that G_1-phase donors were superior; however, it cannot be ruled out that the location of the transgene may have altered reprogrammability of the donor nucleus. In a similar study carried out in sheep,[72] no differences were reported in the frequency of development or the occurrence of developmental abnormalities between quiescent and cycling fetal fibroblasts, which were used as nuclear donors. Although direct comparisons between development to term of cycling and quiescent donor cells have proved inconclusive, other studies suggest that quiescence in the nuclear donor may be beneficial. Quiescence can alter the epigenetic status of nuclear DNA. Studies in quiescent and cycling B lymphocytes showed a marked reduction in methylation of histone H3 at lysines 4 (H3K4), 9 (H3K9) and 27 (H3K27) and histone H4 at lysine 20 in quiescent cells. In addition, the quiescent cells also lacked heterochromatin-associated HP1β and Ikaros at pericentric chromatin and expressed low levels of Ezh2 and ESET histone methyltransferases (HMTases).[73] In these studies, the authors also demonstrated in NT-reconstructed embryos that quiescent donors were more developmentally competent than cells which had been stimulated to re-enter the cell cycle and in which HMTase expression, histone methylation and HP1β binding had been restored. Interestingly, freshly isolated cumulus cells which have been used in a number of studies are quiescent.[74] The method and duration of culture of the donor cell can also alter the epigenetic status of the nuclear DNA, and this may compromise development. In cultured bovine cumulus and fetal fibroblast cells, acetylation of histones H1, H3 and H4 increased with cell passage. In addition, cell cycle differences occur: for instance, acetylation was lower in cells in the

G_0/G_1-stage than in those in the S or G_2 phases.[75] In a study using adult fibroblasts as nuclear donors,[76] the authors noted that development was greater with cells which had been cultured for longer, suggesting that changes occurring during culture may be beneficial for development.

EPIGENETICS IN NUCLEAR TRANSFER-DERIVED EMBRYOS

Epigenetic modifications to the donor nucleus in NT embryos have primarily been studied by measuring gene expression levels or by assessing individual epigenetic markers by immunofluorescence techniques. A number of studies have shown aberrant gene expression patterns in bovine blastocysts produced by NT, including changes in the relative abundance of a number of genes involved in early development.[77] Interestingly, the cytoplast recipient used for embryo reconstruction and the method of culture of bovine embryos can both alter expression levels.[77,78] It has also been reported in NT-derived bovine blastocysts that Acrogranin, Cdx2 and ERR2 genes, which are critical for early placental and preimplantation development, are down-regulated.[79] However, in a separate study where global gene expression patterns were studied, the expression profiles of NT-derived bovine blastocysts closely resembled that of naturally fertilized controls, but differed significantly from the nuclear donor cells, demonstrating that significant reprogramming of gene expression had occurred.[80] In mice, abnormal gene expression patterns have been reported in the placenta of cloned fetuses[81] and in blastocyst-stage embryos; in particular, reactivation of Oct4 is found to be incomplete, resulting in misregulation of a number of Oct4-regulated genes.[82] Taken together, these studies suggest that, at least by the blastocyst stage, many genes have correct expression and that the lack of development may either be due to incomplete reprogramming of a few key genes or that errors in reprogramming occur later in development. Such errors may be related to incomplete erasure of epigenetic marks or some form of epigenetic memory.

Although the birth of live offspring shows that complete reprogramming of the nuclear genome can occur, many studies of individual markers of epigenetic programming, including both nuclear and chromatin structure and DNA status, have reported incomplete or incorrect reprogramming and add evidence to the phenomenon of epigenetic memory. In immunofluorescence studies of NT bovine embryos, transient demethylation of the donor genome occurs during early cell cycles; this is followed by remethylation, resulting in hypermethylation of trophectodermal cells at the blastocyst stage.[8,83] Interestingly, the pattern of methylation observed in individual nuclei closely resembled that seen in the donor cells,[84] possibly reflecting incomplete erasure of this epigenetic marker or some form of epigenetic memory that was not erased prior to remethylation. In contrast to global methylation patterns, when methylation of specific DNA sequences was examined by bisulfite sequencing in porcine NT embryos, normal patterns were observed.[85] Changes in histone composition, acetylation and methylation of histone tails, X-chromosome inactivation and nuclear structure have all been reported following NT. Interestingly, the rate of occurrence and extent of each of these changes vary with the cell cycle stage of the donor cytoplasm and recipient nucleus at the time of NT; in addition, the presence of the maternal chromosomes and the method of activation can further influence the outcome (for review see Reference 32).

SUMMARY OF REPROGRAMMING IN NUCLEAR TRANSFER EMBRYOS AND POTENTIAL ROUTES TO IMPROVEMENT

Although many factors, including the method of reconstruction, activation protocol and culture conditions, are involved in the development of embryos reconstructed by NT, in this Chapter I wish to discuss only two of these variables in terms of improving NT – the recipient oocyte and the donor cell. As discussed above, cell cycle regulation of the donor and recipient cell is essential to prevent DNA damage and maintain correct ploidy; however, it is also apparent that different cell cycle combinations result in differing levels of development. It is now generally accepted that the use of MII oocytes as cytoplast recipients and the occurrence of NEBD and PCC is optimal for subsequent development. However, the occurrence and extent of NEBD and PCC varies between individual oocytes and is dependent upon donor age and time of maturation. Although MPF and MAPK activities are maximal at MII, these activities do not remain constant but decline with time spent at

MII (i.e. ovine[86]). In addition, MPF and MAPK activities may be lower in oocytes from young donors rather than older donors (i.e. ovine[50]). In studies in our laboratory we have quantified MPF and MAPK activities in in-vitro matured ovine oocytes before and after enucleation and correlated this with the occurrence of NEBD and PCC. Our experiments demonstrated that enucleation did not affect the activities of these kinases; however, the occurrence of NEBD and PCC in the donor nucleus was extremely low. By treating MII oocytes with caffeine, a phosphatase inhibitor, the levels of MPF and MAPK could be increased by up to 50%. This resulted in a significant increase in the occurrence of NEBD and PCC (86.2 vs 11.1); furthermore, when these oocytes were used as cytoplast recipients for SCNT, an increase in cell number at the blastocyst stage[86] and an increase in pregnancy rates were observed.[87] To extend these observations we have examined expression levels of a range of developmentally regulated genes in blastocyst-stage ovine NT embryos using semiquantitative polymerase chain reaction (PCR). In control NT embryos, aberrant gene expression patterns were observed for Oct-4 and a number of genes regulated by Oct-4 (H2A.Z, IF-tau, FGF-4, and Sox-2). Oct-4, H2AZ, FGF-4 and Sox-2 were down-regulated and IF-tau was up-regulated. In contrast, the expression patterns of NT embryos reconstructed using caffeine-treated oocytes as cytoplast recipients, resembled that of control in-vitro fertilization (IVF) embryos. Oct-4, FGF-4 and H2A.Z were up-regulated, whereas IF-tau was down-regulated.[88] The mechanisms behind this alteration in cell number and gene expression profiles are unknown but may reflect a number of pathways. Increased cell number may simply reflect an increase in cell division, which may be due to accelerated DNA synthesis. Changes in gene expression may reflect increased reprogramming, which may occur as a result of the physical displacement and exclusion of somatic transcription factors from the condensed chromatin due to the extent and duration of PCC, as has been reported to occur during mitosis.[57] Alternatively, it may also reflect an active process by oocyte components which is time dependent prior to the initiation of embryo development. In particular, MAPK has been implicated in a number of pathways that regulate the epigenetic state of the donor nucleus such as phosphorylation of HDACs and disruption of corepressor interactions inducing transcriptional repression,[89] modulation of transcription by phosphorylation of histone H3 and coupling of phosphorylation to acetylation[90] and alteration of DNA methylation patterns, which are dependent upon histone acetylation.[91,92]

Attempts to increase reprogramming based on the donor cell have addressed donor cell type, culture conditions and cell cycle stage, as previously described. In addition, attempts have been made to erase some of the donor epigenetic marks prior to NT using chemical and biological means. Treatment of donor cells with 5-aza-cytidine prior to NT causes demethylation of the donor DNA but resulted in a decrease in the frequency of development of bovine NT embryos. In contrast, treatment with trichostatin A, which increases histone acetylation, resulted in an increase in embryo development.[93] Chemical modification of the epigenetic state has also been reported following embryo reconstruction. In the mouse, treatment with trichostatin A during the first 10 hours of culture following NT increased development 2–5 fold, dependent upon donor cell type. Interestingly, there was no effect on development when embryonic stem (ES) cells were used as nuclear donors.[94]

Attempts to improve the outcome of SCNT have demonstrated that alteration of epigenetic state may be crucial to nuclear reprogramming. A range of biological approaches have also been taken to alter epigenetic status and reverse or alter the differentiated state of somatic cells, and these are discussed below.

ISOLATION OF EMBRYONIC STEM CELLS FROM SOMATIC CELL NUCLEAR TRANSFER-DERIVED EMBRYOS

To date, proven ES cells have only been obtained from mice, humans and primates, and only in the mouse from SCNT embryos.[95–98] In the mouse, although the majority of SCNT-derived blastocysts do not produce live offspring, the frequency of isolation of ES cells is equal to that derived from fertilized controls. Such ntES (nuclear transfer embryonic stem) cells have been derived from a variety of donor cell types, including cumulus cells,[95] tail tip fibroblasts[96] and neuronal cells,[99] and can differentiate into a range of cell types. In addition, the transcriptional profile of ntES cells is indistinguishable from ES cells derived from fertilized controls, suggesting that selection for epigenetic erasure occurs.[100] However, when EC (embryonal carcinoma) cells were used as nuclear donors, the resultant ES lines had characteristics of their nuclear donors.[101] The role of epigenetic status is also a determinant in the ability to isolate ES cells from murine embryos. The transcription factor Oct-4 is a key determinant of pluripotency. During development, the level of Oct-4 varies with the differentiated state of different cell populations, being lost on differentiation. In SCNT murine embryos, Oct-4 expression in the inner cell mass is variable and correlates with the ability to form outgrowths and ntES cells.[102] Furthermore, unlike fertilized controls, the distribution and expression of Oct-4 was dependent upon the culture environment.[103] These authors concluded that, although ntES cells can be isolated, development to the blastocyst stage is not equivalent to full reprogramming and that ES and ICM cells are not functionally equivalent. The loss of Oct-4 expression also varies with genetic background and may be why some mouse strains are more refractory to ES cell isolation. However, treatment with PD98059, a MAPK inhibitor which suppresses activation of the MAPKs Erk1 and Erk2, results in an increased persistence of Oct-4-expressing cells. When PD98059 treatment of isolated ICM cells was combined with ovariectomy to delay implantation, ES cells were isolated from the normally refractory CBA strain of mice,[104] providing further support that modification of epigenetic status can be achieved by alterations in cellular physiology.

In the mouse, the frequency of development to term of blastocyst-stage NT embryos reconstructed with ES cell nuclei is increased 3–10-fold compared with somatic nuclei.[105] Thus, the ability to derive ntES cells provides an additional route to the generation of live offspring by NT by first producing an ntES line, and then using this as nuclear donors for the production of live offspring. Interestingly, the success of this method does not differ from SCNT.[106] Although the use of NT technologies for the production of autologous ntES cells is limited in humans, not only by the availability of recipient cytoplasts but also by moral, legal and ethical objections to the creation of potentially viable cloned human embryos, it is generally accepted that, from an immunological point of view, this approach would be advantageous. An alternative would be the generation of human ntES cells from non-viable embryos. Such an approach has been reported in the mouse; ntES cells were derived using donor cells in which Cdx2 expression was restricted. Cdx2 is essential for trophoblast formation, and therefore the resultant embryos would not implant and would be non-viable. This approach yielded functional ntES cells and has been termed altered nuclear transfer (ANT).[107]

OTHER APPROACHES TO NUCLEAR REPROGRAMMING

The technical difficulties associated with SCNT, coupled with the low frequency of development to term, has stimulated significant research effort into developing alternative strategies for nuclear reprogramming. On the whole these strategies seek to dedifferentiate or transdifferentiate somatic cells into stem cell-like cells or their derivatives. Such techniques would offer numerous possibilities in reprogramming cells prior to use to improve the outcome of NT, developing cells with high rates of homologous recombination for use in transgenesis or in providing autologous cells for human cell therapies without the need for the production of viable embryos. NT transfer studies in amphibians[108–110] and mammals[3,60] demonstrated the ability of the oocyte to reprogram gene expression in somatic nuclei and produce all cell types required for development. A number of alternative biological approaches to achieving reprogramming using oocytes or oocyte cytoplasm from other species or a range of undifferentiated cell types have been reported, and these are discussed below.

Inter- and trans-species nuclear transfer in mammals

The lack of availability of oocytes from rare or endangered species prompted the use of oocytes from closely related species (inter) and from different species (trans) as cytoplasts for NT. When using interspecies oocytes, development has been relatively successful with the production of a live gaur calf using bovine oocytes[111] and a mouflon using ovine oocytes.[112] In trans-species, NT results have been more mixed. Bovine oocytes have been shown to support early embryonic development up to the blastocyst stage using donor somatic nuclei from cattle, sheep, pigs, monkeys and rats.[113] In addition, rabbit oocytes not only supported early development of human nuclei but also permitted isolation of ES cells that were capable of self-renewal and differentiation into all three germ layers.[114]

Trans-species reprogramming using amphibian oocytes and cytoplasmic extracts

If reprogramming activity is conserved across species, then amphibian oocytes and eggs could provide a valuable supply of reprogramming components. Oocytes from *Xenopus laevis* are approximately 1000 × the volume of mammalian eggs and contain sufficient components to assemble 4000 embryonic nuclei. Two approaches to the use of amphibian (primarily *Xenopus*) oocytes have been reported:

- direct injection of isolated nuclei or permeabilized cells into GV- and MII-stage oocytes
- the use of cytoplasmic extracts from oocytes, activated eggs and early development stage embryos.

Early studies which injected isolated somatic nuclei into oocyte cytoplasm demonstrated that cytoplasmic factors could alter nuclear and chromatin structure.[115] Injected HeLa cell nuclei continue to synthesize RNA;[116] however, gene expression patterns are altered, with the majority of somatic genes being switched off.[117] In further studies, when *Xenopus* somatic nuclei were injected into oocytes of the newt *Pleurodeles waltlii*, in addition to suppression of somatic gene expression patterns, oocyte specific genes were activated.[118] More recently nuclei of adult mouse thymocytes and of adult human blood lymphocytes were reported to reactivate Oct4 expression when injected into the GV of *Xenopus* oocytes.[119] Moreover, this reactivation was dependent upon the demethylation of the proximal region of the Oct4 promotor,[120] demonstrating demethylation activity in *Xenopus* GV oocytes. This ability to alter nuclear and chromatin structure, and suppress and reactivate gene expression, is not restricted to intact oocytes but has also been reported in extracts prepared from different stages of oocyte and embryo development. The properties of such extracts also closely mimic the differences between different developmental stages. In our laboratory we have characterized extracts produced from GV-stage oocytes (oocyte extract) and activated MII-stage oocytes (egg extracts). Egg extracts are able to support DNA replication, whereas oocyte extracts are not; however, DNA replication is dependent upon remodeling of the nuclear lamina and, specifically, the incorporation of *Xenopus*-specific lamin Liii into the somatic nucleus.[121] Both extracts can remodel the nuclear lamina, removing somatic lamin A/C in an active process that requires permeable nuclear pores. This process is lamin A/C specific, since B-type lamins are not changed, and it is not dependent on the incorporation of *Xenopus* lamin III. In egg extracts, lamin Liii is incorporated into the somatic nucleus; however, this does not occur in oocyte extracts, which do not contain lamin Liii. Other differences include differential regulation of transcriptional activity; both Pol I and II transcriptions are maintained in oocyte extracts but are abolished in egg extracts[122] and in demethylation of DNA. Both oocyte and egg extracts are able to demethylate mammalian somatic DNA; however, in egg extracts DNA replication is required, suggesting differences in the mechanisms of demethylation.[123] In other studies, extracts produced from *Xenopus* eggs and early embryos were reported to reactivate Oct4 gene expression in human leukocytes; this requires the chromatin remodeling factor BRG1.[124]

Reprogramming by cell fusion to produce heterokaryons

Decades of research using cell fusion to produce heterokaryons has provided a raft of evidence that the terminally differentiated state of a cell could be altered, silent genes could be reactivated and active genes silenced (for reviews see References 125 and 126). The production of heterokaryons by fusion of a differentiated cell to undifferentiated cell populations may therefore be expected to induce reprogramming of the somatic nucleus to an undifferentiated state. Such undifferentiated populations may include ES, EG (embryonic germ) and EC cells. Early experiments with EC cells demonstrated reactivation of the inactive X chromosome.[127] Similarly, fusion of murine lymphocytes or thymocytes to murine EG cells demonstrated alterations in the epigenetic/imprinted state of the somatic nucleus, including reactivation of the inactive X-chromosome, differential demethylation of imprinted genes and reactivation of silent genes.[128,129] Fusion to ES cells has now been reported from a number of laboratories, demonstrating their reprogramming activity. In stable tetraploids, generated by fusion of human fibroblasts with human ES (hES) cells, genome-wide reprogramming to an embryonic state occurs;[130] however, differences in reprogramming activity between ES and EG cells have been described, in particular the absence of demethylation of imprinted genes in ES cells, thymocyte fusions.[131] Problems associated with the use of cell fusion as a reprogramming strategy include the generation of tetraploid or aneuploid embryos;[130] consequently, several groups have tried to develop strategies whereby only stable diploid cells are produced containing only the reprogrammed genome. The use of enucleated ES cells has been suggested as one route;[132] however, studies in murine ES fusions have demonstrated that the presence of a nucleus is required for reactivation of Oct4.[133] Whether it is the continued presence of an ES nucleus or whether it is the release of nuclear factors required for reprogramming is currently unclear; one possibility is that the small number of reprogrammed cybrids reported by Strelchenko et al[132] may reflect the small number of ES cells in mitosis at the time of enucleation when nuclear contents are released into the cytoplasm. A further adaptation of the technique is the creation of stable tetraploid ES cell lines that have an increased cell volume.[134] This method not only has the advantage of a greater cell volume to achieve fusion and possible reprogramming but also the presence of the tetraploid nucleus provides an opportunity for differential enucleation to leave only the diploid donor nucleus.

These studies have demonstrated the reprogramming capacity of ES and other cell types, but so far there is no reported involvement of the cell cycle. As in NT studies, inappropriate coordination of nuclear and cytoplasmic cell cycle stages may cause DNA damage and result in aneuploidy. Although certain cell cycle stages of donor and/or recipient may facilitate improved reprogramming, control of the cell cycle in ES cells is difficult to achieve.

Reprogramming with heterologous cell extracts

An alternative to cell fusion is the treatment of permeabilized cells with extract from other cell types in order to alter the differentiated state. Treatment of 293T and skin fibroblasts with lymphocyte extracts induced epigenetic modifications of the treated cell nuclei, which led to changes in phenotype and gene expression that could be maintained for long periods in culture.[135,136] In similar experiments, treatment of NIH3T3 and 293 cells with extracts from ES and EC cells resulted in the formation of ES cell-like colonies.[137] These changes in morphology were associated with genome-wide reprogramming of gene expression, including down-regulation of somatic genes associated with differentiation such as Lamin A and up-regulation of embryonic and stem cell-associated genes, including OCT4, SOX2, NANOG, and Oct4-responsive genes. These cells were able to differentiate toward neurogenic, adipogenic, osteogenic and endothelial lineages and, furthermore, retinoic acid treatment resulted in down-regulation of Oct4.

CONCLUSIONS

During development and differentiation, the phenotype and gene expression patterns of differentiated cells become more difficult to alter; however, NT experiments proved that the differentiated state could be reversed. This chapter has described some of the major events associated with nuclear reprogramming and some of the approaches to achieving control of the differentiated state. The ability to control cellular potency has numerous applications, particularly in human and animal therapeutic medicine, disease research, toxicology testing and animal biotechnology. Research to date demonstrates that reversal and reprogramming of the differentiated state is a multistage process that involves numerous biological processes. An initial erasure of epigenetic status provides a template upon which epigenetic marks can be reprogrammed, but, as demonstrated by the low frequency of development in NT embryos, the processes involved are subject to error. Alteration of current protocols or the combination of a range of reprogramming strategies may improve animal development. However, the reprogramming requirements to achieve cell therapies may not be as stringent as those required for the generation of live offspring. Many studies have demonstrated that numerous factors can influence the epigenetic state: by achieving a greater understanding of the mechanisms that regulate epigenetic status, we will be more able to control the differentiated state.

REFERENCES

1. Gurdon JB, Byrne JA, Simonsson S. Nuclear reprogramming and stem cell creation. Proc Natl Acad Sci USA 2003; 100 (Suppl 1): 11819–22.
2. Spemann H. Embryonic Development and Induction. New Haven, CT: Yale University Press, 1938: 210–11. Reprinted New York: Hafner, 1967.

3. Wilmut I, Schnieke AE, McWhir J, Kind AJ, Campbell KHS. Viable offspring derived from fetal and adult mammalian cells. Nature 1997; 385: 810–13.
4. Roloff TC, Nuber UA. Chromatin, epigenetics and stem cells. Eur J Cell Biol 2005; 84: 123–35.
5. Cheung P, Lau P. Epigenetic regulation by histone methylation and histone variants. Mol Endocrinol 2005; 19: 563–73.
6. Kelly TL, Trasler JM. Reproductive epigenetics. Clin Genet 2004; 65: 247–60.
7. Deal CL. Parental genomic imprinting. Curr Opin Pediatr 1995; 7: 445–58.
8. Dean W, Santos F, Stojkovic M et al. Conservation of methylation reprogramming in mammalian development: aberrant reprogramming in cloned embryos. Proc Natl Acad Sci USA 2001; 98: 13734–8.
9. Beaujean N, Taylor JE, McGarry M et al. The effect of interspecific oocytes on demethylation of sperm DNA. Proc Natl Acad Sci USA 2004; 101: 7636–40.
10. Young LE, Beaujean N. DNA methylation in the preimplantation embryo: the differing stories of the mouse and sheep. Anim Reprod Sci 2004; 82–83: 61–78.
11. Lachner M, O'Sullivan RJ, Jenuwein T. An epigenetic road map for histone lysine methylation. J Cell Sci 2003; 116: 2117–24.
12. Lin W, Dent SY. Functions of histone-modifying enzymes in development. Curr Opin Genet Dev 2006; 16: 137–42.
13. Wolffe AP. Histone deacetylase: a regulator of transcription. Science 1996; 272: 371–2.
14. Wolffe AP, Matzke MA. Epigenetics: regulation through repression. Science 1999; 286: 481–6.
15. Allfrey VG, Faulkner R, Mirsky AE. Acetylation and methylation of histones and their possible role in the regulation of RNA synthesis. Proc Natl Acad Sci USA 1964; 51: 786–94.
16. Tse C, Sera T, Wolffe AP, Hansen JC. Disruption of higher-order folding by core histone acetylation dramatically enhances transcription of nucleosomal arrays by RNA polymerase III. Mol Cell Biol 1998; 18: 4629–38.
17. Aoki E, Schultz RM. DNA replication in the 1-cell mouse embryo: stimulatory effect of histone acetylation. Zygote 1999; 7: 165–72.
18. Turner BM. Histone acetylation and an epigenetic code. Bioessays 2000; 22: 836–45.
19. Carrozza MJ, Utley RT, Workman JL, Cote J. The diverse functions of histone acetyltransferase complexes. Trends Genet 2003; 19: 321–9.
20. Xu RH, Peng Y, Fan J et al. Histone acetylation is a checkpoint in FGF-stimulated mesoderm induction. Dev Dyn 2000; 218: 628–35.
21. Kim JM, Liu H, Tazaki M, Nagata M, Aoki F. Changes in histone acetylation during mouse oocyte meiosis. J Cell Biol 2003; 162: 37–46.
22. Maalouf WE, Alberio R, Campbell KHS. Acetylation of histone H4 lysine-5 and lysine-8 during development of in-vitro produced bovine embryos. Reprod Fertil Dev 2004; 16: 125.
23. Campbell KHS, Wilmut I. Nuclear transfer. In: Clark AJ, ed., Animal Breeding: Technology for the 21st Century. Amsterdam: Harwood Academic Publishers, 1998: 47–62.
24. Campbell KHS, Alberio R, Denning C, Lee J-H. Somatic cell nuclear transplantation. In: Celis JE, ed., Cell Biology: A Laboratory Handbook, 3rd edn. New York: Academic Press, 2006: 45–51.
25. Li GP, White KL, Bunch TD. Review of enucleation methods and procedures used in animal cloning: state of the art. Cloning Stem Cells 2004; 6: 5–13.
26. Campbell KHS, Alberio R, Choi I et al. Cloning: eight years after Dolly. Reprod Domest Anim 2005; 40: 265–8.
27. Polejaeva IA, Chen SH, Vaught TD et al. Cloned pigs produced by nuclear transfer from adult somatic cells. Nature 2000; 407: 86–90.
28. Campbell KHS, McWhir J, Ritchie WA, Wilmut I. Sheep cloned by nuclear transfer from a cultured cell line [see comments]. Nature 1996; 380: 64–6.
29. Young LE, Sinclair KD, Wilmut I. Large offspring syndrome in cattle and sheep. Rev Reprod 1998; 3: 155–63.
30. Young LE, Fernandes K, McEvoy TG et al. Epigenetic change in IGF2R is associated with fetal overgrowth after sheep embryo culture. Nat Genet 2001; 27: 153–4.
31. Campbell KHS, Loi P, Otaegui PJ, Wilmut I. Cell cycle co-ordination in embryo cloning by nuclear transfer. Rev Reprod 1996; 1: 40–6.
32. Campbell KHS, Alberio R. Reprogramming the genome: role of the cell cycle. Reprod Suppl 2003; 61: 477–94.
33. Campbell KHS, Ritchie WA, Wilmut I. Nuclear–cytoplasmic interactions during the first cell cycle of nuclear transfer reconstructed bovine embryos: implications for deoxyribonucleic acid replication and development. Biol Reprod 1993; 49: 933–42.
34. Campbell KHS, Loi P, Cappai P, Wilmut I. Improved development to blastocyst of ovine nuclear transfer embryos reconstructed during the presumptive S-phase of enucleated activated oocytes. Biol Reprod 1994; 50: 1385–93.
35. McGrath J, Solter D. Nuclear transplantation in the mouse embryo by microsurgery and cell fusion. Science 1983; 220: 1300–2.
36. McGrath J, Solter D. Inability of mouse blastomere nuclei transferred to enucleated zygotes to support development in vitro. Science 1984; 226: 1317–19.

37. Prather RS, Sims MM, First NL. Nuclear transplantation in early pig embryos. Biol Reprod 1989; 41: 414–18.

38. Robl JM, Prather R, Barnes F et al. Nuclear transplantation in bovine embryos. J Anim Sci 1987; 64: 642–7.

39. Willadsen SM. Nuclear transplantation in sheep embryos. Nature 1986; 320: 63–5.

40. Campbell KHS, Wilmut I. Recent advances on in vitro culture and cloning of ungulate embryos. Vth World Congress on Genetics as Applied to Livestock 1994; 20: 180–7.

41. Shi W, Dirim F, Wolf E, Zakhartchenko V, Haaf T. Methylation reprogramming and chromosomal aneuploidy in in vivo fertilized and cloned rabbit preimplantation embryos. Biol Reprod 2004; 71: 340–7.

42. Simerly C, Dominko T, Navara C et al. Molecular correlates of primate nuclear transfer failures. Science 2003; 300: 297.

43. Booth PJ, Viuff D, Tan S et al. Numerical chromosome errors in day 7 somatic nuclear transfer bovine blastocysts. Biol Reprod 2003; 68: 922–8.

44. Bureau WS, Bordignon V, Leveillee C, Smith LC, King WA. Assessment of chromosomal abnormalities in bovine nuclear transfer embryos and in their donor cells. Cloning Stem Cells 2003; 5: 123–32.

45. Di Berardino MA, Hoffner N. Development and chromosomal constitution of nuclear-transplants derived from male germ cells. J Exp Zool 1971; 176: 61–72.

46. Di Berardino MA, Hoffner N. Origin of chromosomal abnormalities in nuclear transplants – a reevaluation of nuclear differentiation and nuclear equivalence in amphibians. Dev Biol 1970; 23: 185–209.

47. Kill IR, Bridger JM, Campbell KHS, Maldonado-Codina G, Hutchison CJ. The timing of the formation and usage of replicase clusters in S-phase nuclei of human diploid fibroblasts. J Cell Sci 1991; 100(Pt 4): 869–76.

48. Campbell KHS, Ritchie WA, McWhir J, Wilmut I. Live lambs by nuclear transfer from an established cultured cell line. Theriogenology 1996; 45: 287.

49. Shi W, Zakhartchenko V, Wolf E. Epigenetic reprogramming in mammalian nuclear transfer. Differentiation 2003; 71: 91–113.

50. Ledda S, Bogliolo L, Leoni G, Naitana S. Cell coupling and maturation-promoting factor activity in in vitro-matured prepubertal and adult sheep oocytes. Biol Reprod 2001; 65: 247–52.

51. Goren S, Piontkewitz Y, Dekel N. Meiotic arrest in incompetent rat oocytes is not regulated by cAMP. Dev Biol 1994; 166: 11–17.

52. Kim JM, Ogura A, Nagata M, Aoki F. Analysis of the mechanism for chromatin remodeling in embryos reconstructed by somatic nuclear transfer. Biol Reprod 2002; 67: 760–6.

53. Tani T, Kato Y, Tsunoda Y. Direct exposure of chromosomes to nonactivated ovum cytoplasm is effective for bovine somatic cell nucleus reprogramming. Biol Reprod 2001; 64: 324–30.

54. Tani T, Kato Y, Tsunoda Y. Reprogramming of bovine somatic cell nuclei is not directly regulated by maturation promoting factor or mitogen-activated protein kinase activity. Biol Reprod 2003; 69: 1890–4.

55. Du F, Sung LY, Tian XC, Yang X. Differential cytoplast requirement for embryonic and somatic cell nuclear transfer in cattle. Mol Reprod Dev 2002; 63: 183–91.

56. Shin MR, Park SW, Shim H, Kim NH. Nuclear and microtubule reorganization in nuclear-transferred bovine embryos. Mol Reprod Dev 2002; 62: 74–82.

57. Martinez-Balbas MA, Dey A, Rabindran SK, Ozato K, Wu C. Displacement of sequence-specific transcription factors from mitotic chromatin. Cell 1995; 83: 29–38.

58. Schermoen AW, O'Farrell PH. Progression of the cell cycle through mitosis leads to abortion of nascent transcripts. Cell 1991; 67: 303–10.

59. Sullivan EJ, Kasinathan S, Kasinathan P, Robl JM, Collas P. Cloned calves from chromatin remodeled in vitro. Biol Reprod 2004; 70: 146–53.

60. Campbell KHS, Ritchie WA, McWhir J, Wilmut I. Sheep cloned by nuclear transfer from a cultured cell line. Nature 1996; 380: 64–6.

61. Baguisi A, Behboodi E, Melican DT et al. Production of goats by somatic cell nuclear transfer. Nat Biotechnol 1999; 17: 456–61.

62. Liu JL, Wang MK, Sun QY, Xu Z, Chen DY. Effect of telophase enucleation on bovine somatic nuclear transfer. Theriogenology 2000; 54: 989–98.

63. Bordignon V, Keyston R, Lazaris A et al. Transgene expression of green fluorescent protein and germ line transmission in cloned calves derived from in vitro-transfected somatic cells. Biol Reprod 2003; 68: 2013–23.

64. Kurosaka S, Nagao Y, Minami N, Yamada M, Imai H. Dependence of DNA synthesis and in vitro development of bovine nuclear transfer embryos on the stage of the cell cycle of donor cells and recipient cytoplasts. Biol Reprod 2002; 67: 643–7.

65. Vignon X, Chesne P, Le Bourhis D et al. Developmental potential of bovine embryos reconstructed from enucleated matured oocytes fused with cultured somatic cells. C R Acad Sci III 1998; 321: 735–45.

66. Liu L, Yang X. Interplay of maturation-promoting factor and mitogen-activated protein kinase inactivation during metaphase-to-interphase transition of activated bovine oocytes. Biol Reprod 1999; 61: 1–7.

67. Alberio R, Kubelka M, Zakhartchenko V et al. Activation of bovine oocytes by specific inhibition of

cyclin-dependent kinases. Mol Reprod Dev 2000; 55: 422–32.

68. Liu L, Ju JC, Yang X. Parthenogenetic development and protein patterns of newly matured bovine oocytes after chemical activation. Mol Reprod Dev 1998; 49: 298–307.

69. Liu L, Ju JC, Yang X. Differential inactivation of maturation-promoting factor and mitogen-activated protein kinase following parthenogenetic activation of bovine oocytes. Biol Reprod 1998; 59: 537–45.

70. Kubelka M, Motlik J, Schultz RM, Pavlok A. Butyrolactone I reversibly inhibits meiotic maturation of bovine oocytes, without influencing chromosome condensation activity. Biol Reprod 2000; 62: 292–302.

71. Wells DN, Laible G, Tucker FC et al. Coordination between donor cell type and cell cycle stage improves nuclear cloning efficiency in cattle. Theriogenology 2003; 59: 45–59.

72. Peura TT, Hartwich KM, Hamilton HM, Walker SK. No differences in sheep somatic cell nuclear transfer outcomes using serum-starved or actively growing donor granulosa cells. Reprod Fertil Dev 2003; 15: 157–65.

73. Baxter J, Sauer S, Peters A et al. Histone hypomethylation is an indicator of epigenetic plasticity in quiescent lymphocytes. EMBO J 2004; 23: 4462–72.

74. Wakayama T, Perry AC, Zuccotti M, Johnson KR, Yanagimachi R. Full-term development of mice from enucleated oocytes injected with cumulus cell nuclei. Nature 1998; 394: 369–74.

75. Enright BP, Jeong BS, Yang X, Tian XC. Epigenetic characteristics of bovine donor cells for nuclear transfer: levels of histone acetylation. Biol Reprod 2003; 69: 1525–30.

76. Kubota C, Yamakuchi H, Todoroki J et al. Six cloned calves produced from adult fibroblast cells after long-term culture. Proc Natl Acad Sci USA 2000; 97: 990–5.

77. Wrenzycki C, Wells D, Herrmann D et al. Nuclear transfer protocol affects messenger RNA expression patterns in cloned bovine blastocysts. Biol Reprod 2001; 65: 309–17.

78. Wrenzycki C, Herrmann D, Carnwath JW, Niemann H. Alterations in the relative abundance of gene transcripts in preimplantation bovine embryos cultured in medium supplemented with either serum or PVA. Mol Reprod Dev 1999; 53: 8–18.

79. Hall VJ, Ruddock NT, French AJ. Expression profiling of genes crucial for placental and preimplantation development in bovine in vivo, in vitro, and nuclear transfer blastocysts. Mol Reprod Dev 2005; 72: 16–24.

80. Smith SL, Everts RE, Tian XC et al. Global gene expression profiles reveal significant nuclear reprogramming by the blastocyst stage after cloning. Proc Natl Acad Sci USA 2005; 102: 17582–7.

81. Humpherys D, Eggan K, Akutsu H et al. Abnormal gene expression in cloned mice derived from embryonic stem cell and cumulus cell nuclei. Dev Biol 2002; 99: 12889–94.

82. Bortvin A, Eggan K, Skaletsky H et al. Incomplete reactivation of Oct4-related genes in mouse embryos cloned from somatic nuclei. Development 2003; 130: 1673–80.

83. Bourc'his D, Le Bourhis D, Patin D et al. Delayed and incomplete reprogramming of chromosome methylation patterns in bovine cloned embryos. Curr Biol 2001; 11: 1542–6.

84. Santos F, Zakhartchenko V, Stojkovic M et al. Epigenetic marking correlates with developmental potential in cloned bovine preimplantation embryos. Curr Biol 2003; 13: 1116–21.

85. Kang YK, Koo DB, Park JS et al. Typical demethylation events in cloned pig embryos. Clues on species-specific differences in epigenetic reprogramming of a cloned donor genome. J Biol Chem 2001; 276: 39980–4.

86. Lee JH, Campbell KH. Effects of enucleation and caffeine on maturation-promoting factor (MPF) and mitogen-activated protein kinase (MAPK) activities in ovine oocytes used as recipient cytoplasts for nuclear transfer. Biol Reprod 2006; 74: 691–8.

87. Lee J-H, Marfil M, Panarce M, Medina M, Campbell KHS. Establishment of pregnancy by ovine nuclear transfer embryos reconstructed using caffeine-treated in vitro matured oocytes as cytoplast recipients. Reprod Fertil Dev 2006; 18(1): 135–6.

88. Choi I, Lee JH, Campbell K. Effect of treatment of ovine oocytes with caffeine on gene expression in nuclear transfer embryos. Reprod Fertil Dev 2006; 18(1): 122.

89. Galasinski SC, Resing KA, Goodrich JA, Ahn NG. Phosphatase inhibition leads to histone deacetylases 1 and 2 phosphorylation and disruption of corepressor interactions. J Biol Chem 2002; 277: 19618–26.

90. Clayton AL, Mahadevan LC. MAP kinase-mediated phosphoacetylation of histone H3 and inducible gene regulation. FEBS Lett 2003; 546: 51–8.

91. Gregory RI, Randall TE, Johnson CA et al. DNA methylation is linked to deacetylation of histone H3, but not H4, on the imprinted genes Snrpn and U2af1-rs1. Mol Cell Biol 2001; 21: 5426–36.

92. Gregory RI, O'Neill LP, Randall TE et al. Inhibition of histone deacetylases alters allelic chromatin conformation at the imprinted U2af1-rs1 locus in mouse embryonic stem cells. J Biol Chem 2002; 277: 11728–34.

93. Enright BP, Kubota C, Yang X, Tian XC. Epigenetic characteristics and development of embryos cloned from donor cells treated by trichostatin A or 5-aza-2'-deoxycytidine. Biol Reprod 2003; 69: 896–901.

94. Kishigami S, Mizutani E, Ohta H et al. Significant improvement of mouse cloning technique by treatment with trichostatin A after somatic nuclear transfer. Biochem Biophys Res Commun 2006; 340: 183–9.

95. Munsie MJ, Michalska AE, O'Brien CM et al. Isolation of pluripotent embryonic stem cells from reprogrammed adult mouse somatic cell nuclei Curr Biol 2000; 10: 989–92.

96. Wakayama T, Tabar V, Rodriguez I et al. Differentiation of embryonic stem cell lines generated from adult somatic cells by nuclear transfer. Science 2001; 292: 740–3.

97. Kishigami S, Wakayama S, van Thuan N, Wakayama T. Cloned mice and embryonic stem cell establishment from adult somatic cell. Hum Cell 2006; 19: 2–10.

98. Wakayama T. Cloned mice and embryonic stem cell lines generated from adult somatic cells by nuclear transfer. Oncol Res 2003; 13: 309–14.

99. Kawase E, Yamazaki Y, Yagi T, Yanagimachi R, Pedersen RA. Mouse embryonic stem (ES) cell lines established from neuronal cell-derived cloned blastocysts. Genesis 2000; 28: 156–63.

100. Brambrink T, Hochedlinger K, Bell G, Jaenisch R. ES cells derived from cloned and fertilized blastocysts are transcriptionally and functionally indistinguishable. Proc Natl Acad Sci USA 2006; 103: 933–8.

101. Blelloch RH, Hochedlinger K, Yamada Y et al. Nuclear cloning of embryonal carcinoma cells. Proc Natl Acad Sci USA 2004; 101: 13985–90.

102. Boiani M, Eckardt S, Scholer HR, McLaughlin KJ. Oct4 distribution and level in mouse clones: consequences for pluripotency. Genes Dev 2002; 16: 1209–19.

103. Boiani M, Gentile L, Gambles VV et al. Variable reprogramming of the pluripotent stem cell marker Oct4 in mouse clones: distinct developmental potentials in different culture environments. Stem Cells 2005; 23: 1089–104.

104. Buehr M, Smith A. Genesis of embryonic stem cells. Phil Trans R Soc Lond B 2003; 358: 1397–402.

105. Saito S, Liu B, Yokoyama K. Animal embryonic stem (ES) cells: self-renewal, pluripotency, transgenesis and nuclear transfer. Hum Cell 2004; 17: 107–15.

106. Wakayama S, Mizutani E, Kishigami S et al. Mice cloned by nuclear transfer from somatic and ntES cells derived from the same individuals. J Reprod Dev 2005; 51: 765–72.

107. Meissner A, Jaenisch R. Generation of nuclear transfer-derived pluripotent ES cells from cloned Cdx2-deficient blastocysts. Nature 2006; 439: 212–15.

108. Gurdon JB, Uehlinger V. "Fertile" intestine nuclei. Nature 1966; 210: 1240–1.

109. Gurdon JB. Genetic reprogramming following nuclear transplantation in Amphibia. Semin Cell Dev Biol 1999; 10: 239–43.

110. Gurdon JB. Multiple genetically identical frogs. J Hered 1962; 53: 5–9.

111. Lanza RP, Cibelli JB, Moraes CT et al. Cloning of an endangered species (*Bos gaurus*) using interspecies nuclear transfer. Cloning 2000; 2: 79–90.

112. Loi P, Ptak G, Barboni B et al. Genetic rescue of an endangered mammal by cross-species nuclear transfer using post-mortem somatic cells. Nat Biotechnol 2001; 19: 962–4.

113. Dominko T, Mitalipova M, Haley B et al. Bovine oocyte cytoplasm supports development of embryos produced by nuclear transfer of somatic cell nuclei from various mammalian species. Biol Reprod 1999; 60: 1496–502.

114. Chen Y, He ZX, Liu A et al. Embryonic stem cells generated by nuclear transfer of human somatic nuclei into rabbit oocytes. Cell Res 2003; 13: 251–63.

115. Gurdon JB. Injected nuclei in frog oocytes: fate, enlargement, and chromatin dispersal. J Embryol Exp Morphol 1976; 36: 523–40.

116. Gurdon JB, Partington GA, De Robertis EM. Injected nuclei in frog oocytes: RNA synthesis and protein exchange. J Embryol Exp Morphol 1976; 36: 541–53.

117. De Robertis EM, Partington GA, Longthorne RF, Gurdon JB. Somatic nuclei in amphibian oocytes: evidence for selective gene expression. J Embryol Exp Morphol 1977; 40: 199–214.

118. De Robertis EM, Gurdon JB. Gene activation in somatic nuclei after injection into amphibian oocytes. Proc Natl Acad Sci USA 1977; 74: 2470–4.

119. Byrne JA, Simonsson S, Western PS, Gurdon JB. Nuclei of adult mammalian somatic cells are directly reprogrammed to oct-4 stem cell gene expression by amphibian oocytes. Curr Biol 2003; 13: 1206–13.

120. Simonsson S, Gurdon J. DNA demethylation is necessary for the epigenetic reprogramming of somatic cell nuclei. Nat Cell Biol 2004; 6: 984–90.

121. Alberio R, Fisher P, Campbell KHS. DNA replication of bovine fetal fibroblasts in Xenopus egg extracts is dependent on lamin B3 incorporation. Chromatin and Epigenetics abstracts book (Chromatin and Epigenetics Workshop, 19–22 June 2003, EMBL, Germany), 2003; 33.

122. Alberio R, Johnson AD, Stick R, Campbell KH. Differential nuclear remodeling of mammalian somatic cells by *Xenopus laevis* oocyte and egg cytoplasm. Exp Cell Res 2005; 307: 131–41.

123. Bian Y, Alberio R, Johnson A, Campbell K. Demethylation of mammalian somatic DNA by Xenopus egg and oocyte extracts. Reprod Fertil Dev 2006; 18(1): 169.

124. Hansis C, Barreto G, Maltry N, Niehrs C. Nuclear reprogramming of human somatic cells by Xenopus

egg extract requires BRG1. Curr Biol 2004; 14: 1475–80.

125. Blau HM. How fixed is the differentiated state? Lessons from heterokaryons. Trends Genet 1989; 5: 268–72.

126. Blau HM, Blakely BT. Plasticity of cell fate: insights from heterokaryons. Semin Cell Dev Biol 1999; 10: 267–72.

127. Takagi N, Yoshida MA, Sugawara O, Sasaki M. Reversal of X-inactivation in female mouse somatic cells hybridized with murine teratocarcinoma stem cells in vitro. Cell 1983; 34: 1053–62.

128. Surani MA. Reprogramming a somatic nucleus by trans-modification activity in germ cells. Semin Cell Dev Biol 1999; 10: 273–7.

129. Tada M, Tada T, Lefebvre L, Barton SC, Surani MA. Embryonic germ cells induce epigenetic reprogramming of somatic nucleus in hybrid cells. EMBO J 1997; 16: 6510–20.

130. Cowan CA, Atienza J, Melton DA, Eggan K. Nuclear reprogramming of somatic cells after fusion with human embryonic stem cells. Science 2005; 309: 1369–73.

131. Tada M, Takahama Y, Abe K, Nakatsuji N, Tada T. Nuclear reprogramming of somatic cells by in vitro hybridization with ES cells. Curr Biol 2001; 11: 1553–8.

132. Strelchenko N, Kukharenko V, Shkumatov A et al. Reprogramming of human somatic cells by embryonic stem cell cytoplast. Reprod Biomed Online 2006; 12: 107–11.

133. Do JT, Scholer HR. Nuclei of embryonic stem cells reprogram somatic cells. Stem Cells 2004; 22: 941–9.

134. Pralong D, Mrozik K, Occhiodoro F et al. A novel method for somatic cell nuclear transfer to mouse embryonic stem cells. Cloning Stem Cells 2005; 7: 265–71.

135. Hakelien AM, Landsverk HB, Robl JM, Skalhegg BS, Collas P. Reprogramming fibroblasts to express T-cell functions using cell extracts. Nat Biotechnol 2002; 20: 460–6.

136. Hakelien AM, Gaustad KG, Taranger CK et al. Long-term in vitro, cell-type-specific genome-wide reprogramming of gene expression. Exp Cell Res 2005; 309: 32–47.

137. Taranger CK, Noer A, Sorensen AL et al. Induction of dedifferentiation, genomewide transcriptional programming, and epigenetic reprogramming by extracts of carcinoma and embryonic stem cells. Mol Biol Cell 2005; 16: 5719–35.

138. Schnieke AE, Kind AJ, Ritchie WA et al. Human factor IX transgenic sheep produced by transfer of nuclei from transfected fetal fibroblasts. Science 1997; 278: 2130–3.

139. Cibelli JB, Stice SL, Golueke PJ et al. Cloned transgenic calves produced from nonquiescent fetal fibroblasts. Science 1998; 280: 1256–8.

140. McCreath KJ, Howcroft J, Campbell KHS et al. Production of gene-targeted sheep by nuclear transfer from cultured somatic cells. Nature 2000; 405: 1066–9.

141. Shin T, Kraemer D, Pryor J et al. A cat cloned by nuclear transplantation. Nature 2002; 415: 859.

142. Cloned Deer. 2006. [Q

143. Chesne P, Adenot PG, Viglietta C et al. Cloned rabbits produced by nuclear transfer from adult somatic cells. Nat Biotechnol 2002; 20: 366–9.

144. Zhou Q, Renard JP, Le Friec G et al. Generation of fertile cloned rats by regulating oocyte activation. Science 2003; 302: 1179.

145. Woods GL, White KL, Vanderwall DK et al. A mule cloned from fetal cells by nuclear transfer. Science 2003; 301: 1063.

146. Galli C, Lagutina I, Crotti G et al. Pregnancy: a cloned horse born to its dam twin. Nature 2003; 424: 635.

147. Lee BC, Kim MK, Jang G et al. Dogs cloned from adult somatic cells. Nature 2005; 436: 641.

148. Li Z, Sun X, Chen J et al. Cloned ferrets produced by somatic cell nuclear transfer. Dev Biol 2006; 293: 439–48.

CHAPTER 18

Nuclear transfer and its applications in regenerative medicine

Vanessa Jane Hall and Miodrag Stojkovic

AN HISTORICAL PERSPECTIVE

The first attempt to create identical individuals ex vivo was performed by embryo splitting at the turn of the 19th century. The earliest study was published in 1885 by Hans Dreisch, which involved shaking a sea urchin embryo until it split apart, creating an identical second embryo. These embryos developed successfully into adult dwarf sea urchins. Seventeen years later, another German scientist, Hans Spemann, separated salamander embryo cells by tying a strand of baby hair between two embryonic blastomeres to separate them. Both cells were also able to grow into adult salamanders. Spemann eventually became a Nobel prize laureate in 1935. Shortly thereafter, in 1938, he proposed that it may be possible to transfer a single cell nucleus into an enucleated egg. This theory has now become the most fundamental method used today for the technique, of nuclear transfer (NT), otherwise known as cloning. It wasn't until 1962 that a British biologist, John Gurdon, was able to produce an adult organism using this method. In this study, Gurdon transferred the nucleus of a fully differentiated adult intestinal frog cell into an enucleated egg, or oocyte, to produce an NT South African frog, a genetic copy of the cell from which the cloned animal was derived.[1] The term 'clone' dates back to 1963, when JBS Haldane, another British biologist, used the word clone in a speech entitled: 'Biological possibilities for the human species of the next ten-thousand years.'

Cloning, or NT, is a complicated and fascinating process that reverts an adult differentiated genome into an embryonic-like genome. Interestingly, the term cloning is most widely used, and is easily used to distinguish between both 'therapeutic' and 'reproductive' cloning. However, cloning is considered an inappropriate label according to many in the scientific field. In 2004, the International Society for Stem Cell Research made a huge effort to re-educate both the scientific and non-scientific communities, recommending the use of the abbreviation NT rather than cloning. Nuclear transfer can be defined as the production of embryos following transfer of either embryonic, fetal or somatic cell/nuclei into enucleated eggs: ECNT (embryonic cell nuclear transfer) describes strictly nuclear transfer using embryonic cell nuclei and SCNT (somatic cell nuclear transfer), using somatic cell adult nuclei. In addition, pluripotent cells isolated from the inner cell mass of NT blastocysts should be described as nuclear transfer stem cells (NTSCs) but the term human embryonic stem cells (hESCs) should be used for cells derived from human preimplantation embryos, which are produced by in-vitro fertilization.

Little discussion was raised in regard to performing NT in humans prior to 1997. However, at that time, scientists from the Roslin Institute in Scotland revealed the first large animal to be produced by using SCNT. Dolly the sheep[2] was produced from a single adult mammary cell and was the only successfully surviving live born animal following the transfer of 29 blastocysts (an efficiency of 3.4%). Since then, many scientists have successfully used SCNT as a reproductive tool to create live offspring. The generation of many livestock animal species, including sheep,[2] cattle,[3] pigs[4] and a horse,[5] as well as domestic animals such as cats[6] and a dog,[7] can be added to the list of animals produced. Somatic cell nuclear transfer has been proposed as a technique that may help to improve the agricultural industry,[8] by improving livestock genetics and producing genetically superior animals.[8] Furthermore, SCNT may be used to preserve endangered animal breeds,[9,10] that are unable to reproduce in the wild as a result of species scarcity or failing fertility. In addition, genetic modification in combination with NT may become an important tool for the biotechnology and pharmaceutical industries in the future.[11] Genetically modified cows produced by NT may act as suitable 'biopharms' for producing bioactive proteins in their milk, like the spider silk protein.[12] Current research is focused on producing a supply of histocompatible pig organs that could circumvent the severe shortage of human organs for transplantation.[13] Similarly, genetic modification, coupled with NT in the primate, may help to find cures for neurodegenerative diseases.[14] Thus, the technique of NT may serve to deliver economic, agricultural and medicinal gains.

NUCLEAR TRANSFER AND NUCLEAR TRANSFER STEM CELLS IN ANIMALS

Animal SCNT is considered a reproductive tool that holds great promise for varying industries. It remains hampered by the low efficiencies[2] in producing large numbers of healthy offspring, despite the continued efforts of researchers to improve developmental efficiencies. Reasons for the unexplained inefficiencies may to be attributed to epigenetic and genetic defects in the resultant embryos. Epigenetic defects such as aberrant genomic imprinting and gene expression have been detected in many NT embryos and across a wide range of NT animals.[15–19] This is thought to lead to decreased levels of implantation, and developmental defects, which may, in turn, lead to fetal loss and death shortly following birth. This is primarily attributable to the lack of understanding of the molecular events that drive nuclear reprogramming and nuclear remodeling, both of which occur during the early stages following embryo reconstruction. Nevertheless, these defects don't appear to hamper early development until the preimplantation blastocyst stage and, morphologically, these embryos appear similar to their in-vitro produced counterparts.[18] Therefore, the successes in producing live offspring using NT in a wide range of species have been demonstrated to be partly due to improved techniques and embryo culture systems. However, the next barrier to overcome is to improve the developmental competence of the NT embryos and the feasibility of using this technique. This is likely to be achieved over the next few years, with increasing research focusing on the mechanisms that underlie the nuclear reprogramming process and determining which key reprogramming factors are involved in restoring genetic totipotency to the somatic cell nucleus.[15,16,19]

Studying the use and application of NT and NTSCs using animal models is critical in order to determine the potential of these cells for cell replacement therapies. To date, a number of NTSC lines have been derived in the mouse model.[20–22] In these studies, the generation of a number of different stem cell lines has been achieved. One study[22] investigated whether NTSCs could rescue a genetic phenotype by correcting the expression of *Rag2* following homologous recombination and then transplanting hematopoietic precursors derived from corrected NTSCs into double knockout *Rag2*, IL (interleukin) common cytokine γ-receptor null mice.[22] This syngenic approach may be one of the most prominent studies to date to investigate the effects of transplanting NTSCs in the rodent model. However, graft rejection was reported following transplantation of genetically modified NTSCs into *Rag2* null mice, which indicates an immunorejection response may have induced graft failure. One other useful study has reported the transplantation of NT fetal cells into the autologous host animal.[23] This study demonstrated that no T-cell response could be detected following transplantation of NT fetal cardiac, skeletal or renal cells into the host animal.[23] Even though the creation of NT fetal tissues is not an ethically feasible strategy to consider for the human, this study demonstrates the evident lack of immunorejection by using an autologous approach for cell replacement therapy. Further research is required to investigate the immunoresponse of transplanted NTSCs or differentiated cells derived from NTSCs back into the original host (from which the donor material was derived), before this NT strategy can be fully endorsed as a viable alternative for cell replacement therapies.

NUCLEAR TRANSFER: A ROLE FOR HUMAN MEDICINE?

The successful application of animal reproductive NT has brought the possibility of producing human NT embryos for therapeutic purposes much closer. Compared with the hundreds of reported articles on animal NT, few studies to date have performed human NT,[24–26] not including the retracted papers by Hwang et al in 2004 and 2005. Results from these human NT studies indicate that human NT is still a relatively inefficient technique and often results in poor embryonic development. In 2005, it was reported that one human NT blastocyst was produced, although an attempt to derive an NTSC line proved unsuccessful.[25] The question remains, however, as to why there is even a need to perform human NT and derivation of NTSC? This is based on the ethical dilemmas that arise from producing genetically cloned copies of living human beings. The primary response to the posed question is that NTSCs may deliver a histocompatible source of cells for cell transplantation therapies and the derivation of patient-specific embryonic stem cell (ESC) lines from NT embryos. This was proposed in the late 1990s as a concept to overcome the need to administer immunosuppressive drugs to patients following transplantation of human embryonic stem cell (hESC)-derived cells.[27] Patient-specific stem cell lines could be derived from NT embryos, which are initially produced by fusion of a single adult cell (obtained from the patient) into an enucleated human oocyte.[28–30] The first report to describe the derivation of human NT embryos was published by Cibelli et al.[24] The NT embryos did not develop to the blastocyst stage and arrested at the 6-cell stage. Whether this happened because of technical problems, oocyte quality, inefficient enucleation, inappropriate artificial activation or suboptimal in-vitro culture conditions is not clear. Further research in human NT has indicated that resultant embryos produced by using adult fibroblast nuclei, fused into failed-to-fertilize oocytes derived from infertile women, result in arrested development and failed to cleave, or arrested shortly following the first or second stage of embryonic cleavage.[25,26] Fluorescent in-situ hybridization, using varying chromosomal probes, indicates that most of these embryos are hyperdiploid and display chromosomal anomalies.[26] This may be primarily due to the suboptimal oocytes used in NT.[25,26] Obtaining high numbers of fresh oocytes from fertile women remains a huge obstacle for human NT (see below and in Problems in human nuclear transfer section).

From animal NT studies, it has been suggested that non-optimal oocyte enucleation or timing of oocyte enucleation may induce spindle defects in the resultant embryo, which occur as a direct consequence of centrosome and motor deficiencies.[31,32] Whether this may be the case for human oocyte enucleation is unknown and warrants further investigation. The source of oocytes used for human NT remains an unresolved, yet critical, issue. To overcome the limited availability of human oocytes, Chen et al[33] used rabbit oocytes as cytoplasts and human donor cells as karyoplasts. This research resulted in the production of hybrid-species NT embryos from which 14 NTSC lines were derived. The derivation of NTSCs appears independent of the age of the donor cells, which varied from 5 to 60 years. The NTSCs were maintained in an undifferentiated and proliferative state for up to 25 passages prior to cryopreservation and, upon differentiation, gave rise to different cell types, including neurons and muscle. Thus, NTSCs derived from human somatic cells fused into rabbit oocyte cytoplasts retain phenotypes similar to those of conventional hESCs, including the ability to undergo multilineage cellular differentiation. However, the analysis of human and rabbit mitochondrial DNA (mtDNA) shows that both human and rabbit mtDNA coexist in hybrid NTSC, which complicates the cell replacement strategy.[29] NTSCs produced strictly in the human system would also carry the nuclear genome of the patient (within a subpopulation of mitochondria inherited from the recipient oocyte), which has raised the question of whether histocompatibility may actually be negated between the donor and host tissues.[29] The in-vivo transplantation of bovine NT fetal tissues back into the original host suggests that there was no significant T-cell response in response to the grafted tissues, even though it is known that mitochondria bear at least two genes that could elicit a response from mtDNA-encoded minor histocompatibility antigens.[23] This study stands alone in evaluating whether histocompatibility may be overcome using NT-derived cells in cell transplantation. To date, no NTSCs have been transferred back into the animal from where the NTSCs were derived. Further research is clearly needed to address the unresolved issue of possible immunorejection.

What concerns should we also have for the epigenetic status of the human NT embryos and NTSC lines? Again, previous studies performed in animal models have shown that NT embryos harbor epigenetic defects.[18,19] In addition, does the epigenetic status of human NTSC lines affect the efficiency of targeted differentiation in hESCs and NTSCs[19] and may epigenetic defects, if present, impede on the proliferation of NTSCs? Preliminary studies in the mouse model are encouraging, confirming that NTSC lines derived from NT embryos, compared with lines derived from in-vitro fertilized embryos, have similar therapeutic potential.[34] In this study, the authors demonstrated that, in contrast to embryonic and fetal development of NT offspring, the process of NTSC derivation rigorously selects for immortal cells that have an erased epigenetic status and, thus, become functionally equivalent. Therefore, there is an increasing need to study and confirm this in the human model. In addition, examining the genetic profile of human NT embryos to examine whether they express key pluripotent markers such as *OCT4* will help to identify whether they may have a genetic cause for reduced potential to produce NTSC lines, which has previously been demonstrated in the mouse.[35]

Although much progress has been made in the animal field, the development of human NT remains a more scientific challenge that needs to be overcome if it is to be adapted as a tool for medical treatments. However, human NT and NTSCs could also be used for gene therapy treatments and as a model to study debilitating human diseases.[13,14,25,30] Specifically, pathogenesis of inherited diseases, toxicological effects and establishment of reliable screening systems could be investigated using such embryos and embryo-derived cell lines. It is important that new disease-specific stem cells could be derived from patients with neurodegenerative diseases, cancers and other conditions of unknown cause or multigenic origin.[36] The ability to re-establish NTSCs that can be differentiated under in-vitro conditions (see Potential of human embryonic stem cells and nuclear transfer stem cells section) and that will express the disease phenotype could be a very valuable source for screening for pathways and mechanisms involved in disease. Identifying these pathways and factors which may trigger disease will help to identify causes of diseases and enable the development of novel drugs and chemicals that may protect the tissue or treat the symptoms.[25,28–30,36] Therefore, further research is also needed to optimize the human NT techniques and culture methods currently used. There is also a need to continue this research in animal models in order to provide a proof of concept and to determine how pluripotent and useful NTSCs may be for future medicine.

POTENTIAL OF HUMAN EMBRYONIC STEM CELLS AND NUCLEAR TRANSFER STEM CELLS

A wide range of differentiating cell types can be derived from undifferentiated hESCs and theoretically from human NTSCs. Researchers have observed that hESCs have the potential to differentiate under in-vitro conditions into different cell types that are derived from ectodermal, mesodermal and endodermal tissues found in the developing fetus. Human embryonic stem cells may differentiate into neurons and oligodendrocytes following exogenous addition of varying growth factors, such as basic fibroblast growth factor (bFGF) and epidermal growth factor, and later by additional supplementation of all-trans retinoic acid.[37] These cells were shown to respond to neurotransmitters and are able to remylinate neurons in the shiver mouse model.[38] Dopaminergic or motor neurons can be formed from hESCs to cure spinal cord injury.[38,39] Mummery et al[40,41] showed that beating heart muscle cells derived from hESCs express cardiomyocyte markers, including α-myosin heavy chain, cardiac troponins and atrial natriuretic factor, as well as transcription factors typical of cardiomyocytes, e.g. Nkx2.5, MEF3, GATA4.[40–42] These cells respond to pharmacological drugs and were capable of integrating apparently normally when transplanted into rodent and porcine heart muscle, forming a functional network between the transplanted and recipient cells.[43–45]

Production of cell types from the endodermal lineage has been the most difficult, although continued interest remains for developing functional liver or β-islet cells because of their potential to treat diabetes. Differentiation of hESCs into liver-like cells has been observed following spontaneous differentiation of hESCs,[46] following treatment of embryoid bodies with sodium butyrate or following treatment of adherent hESCs with dimethyl sulfoxide, and later, sodium butyrate.[47] Pancreatic islet-like cells have been derived from protocols that elicit spontaneous differentiation of hESCs.[48] Embryoid bodies were produced in-vitro, following the removal of feeder cultures, grown for 7 days and then replated in insulin–transferrin–selenium–fibronectin medium. Disaggregated cells were grown in medium containing bFGF and later with nicotinamide and low glucose in suspension culture. A high percentage of insulin- and glucagon-expressing cells were observed. However, more research is required to improve the efficiency and functional capacity of hESCs derived β-cells, by optimizing differentiation protocols. This data suggest that the application of appropriate markers and optimized differentiation protocols may improve the differentiation of hESCs.[30,36]

Other obstacles that need to be solved, in order for differentiated hESCs to be suitable for cell transplantation therapy, include:

- the production of new lines that meet clinical grade regulations
- isolation of pure or homogeneous populations of differentiated cells[49]
- improvement in cell transplantation techniques.[50]

PROBLEMS IN HUMAN NUCLEAR TRANSFER

A number of dilemmas exist for human NT, including political pressures and non-flexible regulations; however, the biggest problem is most likely to be the lack of available viable oocytes.[25,30] Our recent findings indicate that human NT embryos can be derived following heterologous NT into enucleated human oocytes.[25] In this study, we evaluated different sources of human oocytes, using undifferentiated hESCs[51] (hES-NCL1 line) as a source of donor cells. Stem cells are better donor cells for human NT, since they have a lower level of genomic DNA methylation and the majority of the cell population is in the G_0/G_1 stage of the cell cycle.[17] This makes them an amenable source for ensuring complete nuclear reprogramming of the donor cell and allows us to identify the source and developmental potential of human oocytes after enucleation and the NT procedure.[25] Recently, it was reported that failed-to-fertilize oocytes obtained from women undergoing infertility treatment were a poor source of oocytes and were unable to support early development following NT.[25,26] This finding confirms that development was only obtained when fresh oocytes were used (following consent from a woman undergoing follicular reduction treatment) for NT.[25] However, the efficiencies of human SCNT remain low[51a] and the process for deriving patient-specific NTSC lines has been slow owing to non-flexible legislation and, most importantly, the lack of good-quality oocytes available for research.

There have been several proposals for overcoming the many hurdles that face human NT. For instance, Heng et al[52] have proposed that egg-sharing in return for subsidized fertility treatment may be a feasible strategy to obtain freshly superovulated oocytes from women undergoing infertility treatment. Recently, in the UK (July 2006), an egg sharing program has been approved by the HFEA for human NT research. In our studies, to overcome the shortage of donor oocytes for NT, we used human oocytes donated from women undergoing IVF. Either oocytes were recovered after follicle reduction[25] or women were asked to donate two of their superovulated oocytes if more than 12 oocytes were obtained following oocyte collection. Data suggest (Choudhary, pers comm) that pregnancy outcome is not impaired. The consent rates are high, with more than 80% of couples undergoing fertility treatment willing to participate and donate embryos or failed-to-fertilize oocytes for research,[53] although donation of fresh oocytes is much lower (Choudhary, pers comm). Assuming that appropriate and non-biased information is given during consent, this strategy may be acceptable as a means of obtaining the additional source of fresh and viable human oocytes.

Improving NT efficiency is crucial in order to minimize the number of oocytes required to use for the NT procedure. This can be performed by improving embryo manipulation techniques, by testing which donor cell types result in the most efficient outcomes and by improving embryo culture. Currently, the bovine NT system results in blastocyst formation fates of approximately 30–50%. This has been achieved following over a decade of technical and culture improvements. Simple translation of methods across to other species has proved detrimental, with many species-specific differences in terms of physiological, biochemical and environmental requirements. Therefore, the murine NT techniques and embryo culture differ significantly. Perhaps the primate model will prove to be the best system to improve NT methods and culture for the human system. To date, primate blastocysts have been produced, but at low efficiencies, and many of these harbor spindle defects that are thought to arise following enucleation.[31,32] Therefore, the method and timing of enucleation and superovulation may need careful optimization.

Legislative restraints have hampered the ability to perform human NT and, currently, only a few laboratories around the world can perform the technique. Human NT is being applied, for therapeutic purposes in only a handful of countries in Europe, including the UK, Belgium and Sweden. Many Asian countries, such as South Korea, China and Singapore, hold a permissive stance for conducting therapeutic NT. In the USA, NT may be performed, but may not be funded by the state. This stance is similarly upheld by the European Union. This is primarily the result of the moral and ethical issues that surround human NT. The slippery slope scaremongers suggest that if human NT becomes permissive, this may be a step towards endorsing reproductive NT legislation in the future which may endorse human reproductive NT. The legislation in permissive countries clearly state that reproductive NT is banned. Fierce fines and even jail terms are marked for those that may even contemplate abusing the privileges to perform human NT. However, with tight legislation, comes suboptimal working conditions, and the difficulty in obtaining fresh human oocytes is regarded as a continuing issue that needs to be resolved.

Therefore, hESCs and NTSCs are crucial tools for studying mechanisms that regulate early human development, gene expression, the role of mtDNA and epigenetics in artifact tissues derived from human embryos or their NT counterparts. Knowledge gained from studying these varying aspects of development may potentially be used for translation and applied research in medicine. The use of human material, if handled in an ethically acceptable manner, may accelerate modern science and could be useful for regenerative medicine.

REFERENCES

1. Gurdon J. Adult frogs derived from the nuclei of single somatic cells. Dev Biol 1962; 4: 256–73.
2. Wilmut I, Schnieke AE, McWhir J et al. Viable offspring derived from fetal and adult mammalian cells. Nature 1997; 385: 810–13.
3. Cibelli JB, Stice SL, Gouleke PJ et al. Cloned transgenic calves produced from nonquiescent fetal fibroblasts. Science 1998; 281: 1611.
4. Boquest AC, Grupen CG, Harrison SJ et al. Production of cloned pigs from cultured fetal fibroblast cells. Biol Reprod 2002; 66: 1283–7.
5. Galli C, Lagutina I, Crotti G et al. Pregnancy: a cloned horse born to its dam twin. Nature 2003; 424: 635.
6. Yin XJ, Lee HS, Lee YH et al. Cats cloned from fetal and adult somatic cells by nuclear transfer. Reproduction 2005; 129: 245–9.
7. Lee BC, Kim MK, Jang G et al. Dogs cloned from adult somatic cells. Nature 2005; 436: 641.
8. Vajta G, Gjerris M. Science and technology of farm animal cloning: state of the art. Anim Reprod Science 2006; 92: 211–30.
9. Wells DN. Cloning in livestock agriculture. Reprod Suppl 2003; 61: 131–50.
10. Lanza RP, Cibelli JB, Diaz F et al. Cloning of an endangered species (*Bos gaurus*) using interspecies nuclear transfer. Cloning 2000; 2: 79–90.
11. Denning C, Priddle H. New frontiers in gene targeting and cloning: success, application and challenges in domestic animals and human embryonic stem cells. Reproduction 2003; 126: 1–11.
12. Thomson AJ, McWhir J. Biomedical and agricultural applications of animal transgenesis. Mol Biotechnol 2004; 27: 231–44.
13. Harrison SJ, Guidolin A, Faast R et al. Efficient generation of alpha (1,3) galactosyltransferase knockout porcine fetal fibroblasts for nuclear transfer. Transgenic Res 2002; 11: 143–150.
14. Norgren RB Jr. Creation of non-human primate neurogenetic disease models by gene targeting and nuclear transfer. Reprod Biol Endocrinol 2004; 16: 40.
15. Dean W, Santos F, Stojkovic M et al. Conservation of methylation reprogramming in mammalian embryos: aberrant reprogramming in cloned embryos. Proc Natl Acad Sci USA 2001; 98: 13734–8.
16. Latham KE. Early and delayed aspects of nuclear reprogramming during cloning. Biol Cell 2005; 97: 119–32.
17. Morgan HD, Santos F, Green K et al. Epigenetic reprogramming in mammals. Hum Mol Genet 2005; 14: R47–58.
18. Wrenzycki C, Herrmann D, Lucas-Hahn A et al. Messenger RNA expression patterns in bovine embryos derived from in vitro procedures and their implications for development. Reprod Fertil Dev 2005; 17: 23–35.
19. Armstrong L, Lako M, Dean Stojkovic M. Epigenetic modification is central to genome reprogramming in somatic cell nuclear transfer. Stem Cells 2006; 24: 805–14.

20. Kawase E, Yamazaki Y, Yagi T et al. Mouse embryonic stem (ES) cell lines established from neuronal cell-derived cloned blastocysts. Genesis 2000; 28: 156–63.

21. Munsie MJ, Michalska AE, O'Brien CM et al. Isolation of pluripotent embryonic stem cells from reprogrammed adult mouse somatic cell nuclei. Curr Biol 2000; 10: 989–92.

22. Rideout WM 3rd, Hochedlinger K, Kyba M et al. Correction of a genetic defect by nuclear transplantation and combined cell and gene therapy. Cell 2002; 109: 17–27.

23. Lanza RP, Chung HY, Yoo JJ et al. Generation of histocompatible tissues using nuclear transplantation. Nat Biotechnol 2002; 20: 689–96.

24. Cibelli JB, Kiessling AA, Cunniff K et al. Somatic cell nuclear transfer in humans: pronuclear and early embryonic development. J Regen Med 2001; 2: 25–31.

25. Stojkovic M, Stojkovic P, Leary C et al. Derivation of a human blastocyst after heterologous nuclear transfer to donated oocytes. Reprod Biomed Online 2005; 11: 226–31 .

26. Lavoir MC, Weier J, Conaghan J et al. Poor development of human nuclear transfer embryos using failed fertilized oocytes. Reprod Biomed Online 2005; 11: 740–4.

27. Lanza RP, Cibelli JB, West MD. Prospects for the use of nuclear transfer in human transplantation. Nat Biotechnol 1999; 12: 1171–4.

28. Hochedlinger K, Jaenisch R. Monoclonal mice generated by nuclear transfer from mature B and T donor cells. Nature 2002; 415: 1035–8.

29. Stojkovic M, Lako L, Strachan T et al. Derivation and characterisation of human embryonic stem cells. Reproduction 2004; 128: 259–67.

30. Hall VJ, Stojkovic P, Stojkovic M. Using therapeutic cloning to fight human disease; a conundrum or reality? Stem Cells 2006; 24: 1628–37.

31. Simerly C, Dominko T, Navara C et al. Molecular correlates of primate nuclear transfer failures. Science 2003; 300: 297.

32. Simerly C, Navara C, Hyun SH et al. Embryogenesis and blastocyst development after somatic cell nuclear transfer in nonhuman primates: overcoming defects caused by meiotic spindle extraction. Dev Biol 2004; 276: 237–52.

33. Chen Y, He ZX, Liu A et al. Embryonic stem cells generated by nuclear transfer of human somatic nuclei into rabbit oocytes. Cell Res 2003; 13: 251–63.

34. Brambrink T, Hochedlinger K, Bell G, Jaenisch R. ES cells derived from cloned and fertilized blastocysts are transcriptionally and functionally indistinguishable. Proc Natl Acad Sci USA 2006; 103: 933–8.

35. Kishigami S, Hikichi T, Van Thuan N et al. Normal specification of the extraembryonic lineage after somatic nuclear transfer. FEBS Lett 2006; 580: 1801–6.

36. Trounson A. The production and directed differentiation of human embryonic stem cells. Endocr Rev 2006; 27: 208–19.

37. Carpenter MK, Inokuma MS, Denham J et al. Enrichment of neurons and neural precursors from human embryonic stem cells. Exp Neurol 2001; 172: 383–97.

38. Nistor GI, Totoiu MO, Haque N et al. Human embryonic stem cells differentiate into oligodendrocytes in high purity and myelinate after spinal cord transplantation. Glia 2005; 49: 385–96.

39. McDonald JW, Becker D, Holekamp TF et al. Repair of the injured spinal cord and the potential of embryonic stem cell transplantation. J Neurotrauma 2004; 21: 383–93.

40. Mummery C, Ward D, van den Brink CE et al. Cardiomyocyte differentiation of mouse and human embryonic stem cells. J Anat 2002; 200: 233–42.

41. Mummery C, Ward-van Oostwaard D, Doevendans P et al. Differentiation of human embryonic stem cells to cardiomyocytes: role of coculture with visceral endoderm-like cells. Circulation 2003; 107: 2733–40.

42. Xu C, Police S, Rao N et al. Characterization and production and directed diffentiation of hESCs enrichment of cardiomyocytes derived from human embryonic stem cells. Circ Res 2001; 91: 501–8.

43. Gertow K, Wolbank S, Rozell B et al. Organized development from human embryonic stem cells after injection into immunodeficient mice. Stem Cells Dev 2004; 13: 421–35.

44. Kehat I, Khimovich I, Caspi O et al. Electromechanical integration of cardiomyocytes derived from human embryonic stem cells. Nat Biotechnol 2004; 10: 1282–9.

45. Xue T, Cho HC, Akar FG et al. Functional integration of electrically active cardiac derivatives from genetically engineered human embryonic stem cells with quiescent recipient ventricular cardiomyocytes: insights into the development of cell-based pacemakers. Circulation 2005; 111: 11–20.

46. Stojkovic P, Lako M, Przyborski S et al. Human-serum matrix supports undifferentiated growth of undifferentiated human embryonic stem cells. Stem Cells 2005; 23: 895–902.

47. Rambhatla L, Chiu CP, Kundu P et al. Generation of hepatocyte-like cells from human embryonic stem cells. Cell Transplant 2003; 12: 1–11.

48. Segev H, Fishman B, Ziskind A, Shulman M, Itskovitz-Eldor J. Differentiation of human embryonic stem cells into insulin-producing clusters. Stem Cells 2004; 22: 265–74.

49. Conti L, Pollard SM, Gorba T et al. Niche-independent symmetrical self-renewal of a mammalian tissue stem cell. PLoS Biol 2005; 3: e283.

50. Park CH, Minn YK, Lee JY et al. In vitro and in vivo analyses of human embryonic stem cell-derived dopamine neurons. J Neurochem 2005; 92: 1265–76.

51. Stojkovic M, Lako M, Stojkovic P et al. Derivation of human embryonic stem cells from day-8 blastocysts recovered after three-step in vitro culture. Stem Cells 2004; 22: 790–7.

51a. Hall VJ, Compton D, Stojkovic P et al. Developmental competence of human in vitro oocytes as host cells for nuclear transfer. Hum Reprod 2006 Sept 6 [Epub ahead of print].

52. Heng BC, Tong GQ, Stojkovic M. The egg-sharing model for human therapeutic cloning: managing donor selection criteria, the proportion of shared oocytes allocated to research, and amount of financial subsidy given to the donor. Med Hypotheses 2006; 66: 1022–4.

53. Choudhary M, Haimes E, Herbert M et al. Demographic, medical and treatment characteristics associated with couples' decisions to donate fresh spare embryos for research. Hum Reprod 2004; 19: 2091–6.

Index

Page numbers in *italics* refer to tables and figures.